Psychological
Obesity

Psychological Care in Severe Obesity

A Practical and Integrated Approach

Edited by

Stephanie E. Cassin
Associate Professor of Psychology and Director of Clinical Training, Ryerson University, Toronto

Raed Hawa
Psychiatrist, Toronto Western Hospital Bariatric Surgery Program and Associate Professor of Psychiatry,
University of Toronto

Sanjeev Sockalingam
Psychiatrist and Psychosocial Director, Toronto Western Hospital Bariatric Surgery Program and Associate Professor
of Psychiatry, University of Toronto

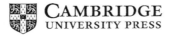
CAMBRIDGE
UNIVERSITY PRESS

CAMBRIDGE
UNIVERSITY PRESS

University Printing House, Cambridge CB2 8BS, United Kingdom

One Liberty Plaza, 20th Floor, New York, NY 10006, USA

477 Williamstown Road, Port Melbourne, VIC 3207, Australia

314–321, 3rd Floor, Plot 3, Splendor Forum, Jasola District Centre, New Delhi – 110025, India

79 Anson Road, #06–04/06, Singapore 079906

Cambridge University Press is part of the University of Cambridge.

It furthers the University's mission by disseminating knowledge in the pursuit of education, learning, and research at the highest international levels of excellence.

www.cambridge.org
Information on this title: www.cambridge.org/9781108404044
DOI: 10.1017/9781108241687

© Cambridge University Press 2018

First published 2018

Printed in the United Kingdom by Clays, St Ives plc

A catalogue record for this publication is available from the British Library.

Library of Congress Cataloging-in-Publication Data
Names: Cassin, Stephanie, editor. | Hawa, Raed, editor. | Sockalingam, Sanjeev, editor.
Title: Psychological care in severe obesity : a practical and integrated approach / edited by Stephanie Cassin, Raed Hawa, Sanjeev Sockalingam.
Description: Cambridge, United Kingdom ; New York, NY : Cambridge University Press, 2018. | Includes bibliographical references and index.
Identifiers: LCCN 2018003698 | ISBN 9781108404044 (paperback : alk. paper)
Subjects: | MESH: Obesity, Morbid – psychology | Obesity, Morbid – therapy | Obesity Management | Psychotherapy – methods
Classification: LCC RC552.O25 | NLM WD 210 | DDC 616.3/980651–dc23
LC record available at https://lccn.loc.gov/2018003698

ISBN 978-1-108-40404-4 Paperback

....

Every effort has been made in preparing this book to provide accurate and up-to-date information that is in accord with accepted standards and practice at the time of publication. Although case histories are drawn from actual cases, every effort has been made to disguise the identities of the individuals involved. Nevertheless, the authors, editors, and publishers can make no warranties that the information contained herein is totally free from error, not least because clinical standards are constantly changing through research and regulation. The authors, editors, and publishers therefore disclaim all liability for direct or consequential damages resulting from the use of material contained in this book. Readers are strongly advised to pay careful attention to information provided by the manufacturer of any drugs or equipment that they plan to use.

To my daughter, Anaiya, who I love even more than psychology.

—Stephanie E. Cassin

To Joanne, Keira, and Tayla, for their unwavering support and inspiration. My creativity could not be possible without the joy you bring me each day.

—Sanjeev Sockalingam

To Roula, for being there.

—Raed Hawa

Contents

Contributors

Molly E. Atwood
Department of Psychology, Ryerson
University, Toronto, ON, Canada

Annie Basterfield
Toronto Western Hospital
Bariatric Surgery Program,
University Health Network, Toronto,
ON, Canada

Kerri Bojman
Department of Psychology, Memorial
University of Newfoundland, St. John's,
NL, Canada

Paula M. Brochu
Department of Clinical and School
Psychology, Nova Southeastern University,
Fort Lauderdale, FL, USA

Jacqueline C. Carter
Department of Psychology, Memorial
University of Newfoundland, St. John's,
NL, Canada

Stephanie E. Cassin
Department of Psychology, Ryerson
University, the Centre for Mental
Health, University Health Network,
and the Department of Psychiatry,
University of Toronto, Toronto, ON,
Canada

Lauren David
Department of Psychology,
Ryerson University, Toronto, ON,
Canada

Chau Du
Toronto Western Hospital Bariatric
Surgery Program, University Health
Network, Toronto, ON, Canada

Erin Dunn
Department of Psychology, Simon
Fraser University, Vancouver, BC,
Canada

Alexis Fertig
University of Pittsburgh School of
Medicine, Pittsburgh, PA, USA

Aliza Friedman
Department of Psychology, Ryerson
University, Toronto, ON, Canada

Josie Geller
St. Paul's Hospital Eating Disorders
Program and the Department of Psychiatry,
University of British Columbia,
Vancouver, BC, Canada

Lorraine Gougeon
Toronto Western Hospital Bariatric
Surgery Program, University Health
Network, Toronto, ON, Canada

Raed Hawa
Toronto Western Hospital Bariatric
Surgery Program, University Health
Network, and the Department of
Psychiatry, University of Toronto, Toronto,
ON, Canada

Roger Ho
Department of Psychological Medicine,
Yong Loo Lin School of Medicine,
National University of Singapore,
Singapore

Jon Hunter
Department of Psychiatry, Mount Sinai
Hospital, and the Department of
Psychiatry, University of Toronto, Toronto,
ON, Canada

Megumi Iyar
St. Paul's Hospital Eating Disorders Program and the Department of Educational and Counselling Psychology and Special Education, University of British Columbia, Vancouver, BC, Canada

Allison C. Kelly
Department of Psychology, University of Waterloo, Waterloo, ON, Canada

Jean Kristeller
Centre for Mindful Eating, Indiana State University, Terre Haute, IN, USA

Alvona Loh
Department of Psychological Medicine, Yong Loo Lin School of Medicine, National University of Singapore, Singapore

Wynne Lundblad
University of Pittsburgh School of Medicine, Pittsburgh, PA, USA

Danielle MacDonald
Toronto General Hospital Eating Disorders Program, University Health Network, Toronto, ON, Canada

Robert Maunder
Department of Psychiatry, Mount Sinai Hospital, and the Department of Psychiatry, University of Toronto, Toronto, ON, Canada

Adrienne Mehak
Department of Psychology, Ryerson University, Toronto, ON, Canada

Rebecca L. Pearl
Perelman School of Medicine, University of Pennsylvania, Philadelphia, PA, USA

Sarah Royal
Toronto Western Hospital Bariatric Surgery Program, Toronto General Hospital Eating Disorders Program, University Health Network, Toronto, ON, Canada

Laurie A. Simontacchi
Department of Clinical and School Psychology, Nova Southeastern University, Fort Lauderdale, FL, USA

Sanjeev Sockalingam
Toronto Western Hospital Bariatric Surgery Program, the Centre for Mental Health, University Health Network, and the Department of Psychiatry, University of Toronto, Toronto, ON, Canada

Stephanie Sogg
Weight Center, Massachusetts General Hospital, and the Department of Psychiatry, Harvard Medical School, Boston, MA, USA

Marlene Taube-Schiff
Department of Psychiatry, Sunnybrook Health Sciences Centre, and the Department of Psychiatry, University of Toronto, Toronto, ON, Canada

Anna Wallwork
Toronto Western Hospital Bariatric Surgery Program, University Health Network, Toronto, ON, Canada

Susan Wnuk
Toronto Western Hospital Bariatric Surgery Program, University Health Network, and the Department of Psychiatry, University of Toronto, Toronto, ON, Canada

Richard Yanofsky
Toronto Western Hospital Bariatric Surgery Program, University Health Network, and the Department of Psychiatry, University of Toronto, Toronto, ON, Canada

Melvyn Zhang
Biomedical Institute for Global Health Research and Technology (BIGHEART), National University of Singapore, Singapore

Preface

This edited book serves as a practical and comprehensive guide to psychological care in severe obesity. Obesity is a complex disease of multifaceted environmental, genetic, and physiological etiologies. Some of the complications of obesity include cardiovascular disease, non-insulin-dependent diabetes mellitus, obstructive sleep apnea, reflux, and cancer. Given the excess mortality, substantial morbidity, and economic toll associated with obesity, it is a disease that warrants an integrated and long-term approach to care.

Beyond the use of antiobesity medications and bariatric surgery, it is imperative to consider the broad spectrum of psychological treatments within the continuum of treatments for severe obesity and its comorbidities. In this book we focus on evidence-based and emerging psychosocial interventions in the treatment of severe obesity, including motivational interviewing, cognitive-behavioral therapy, mindfulness- and compassion-focused interventions, technology-enabled psychological interventions, family-based interventions, and support groups. The book goes beyond a synthesis of the evidence base and provides practical approaches to apply these psychological therapies within the context of obesity management. The contents of these chapters also address the many psychosocial comorbidities of obesity, including disordered eating and mood, anxiety, and substance use disorders.

The reality is that empirical literature examining psychosocial interventions specifically for individuals with severe obesity is still in its infancy. Many of the time-limited psychosocial interventions that have been examined to date result in only modest and short-term weight loss. A more comprehensive and long-term treatment approach is warranted in the management of severe obesity, which may necessitate numerous medical and psychosocial interventions in sequence or combination for sustained improvement over time. Currently, no clinical guidelines exist to determine which type(s) of psychosocial interventions should be offered to particular patients with severe obesity, how those interventions should be integrated or sequenced, how long each intervention should continue, and when each intervention should be offered in the course of obesity care. The chapters in this book are intended to serve as a practical guide to help healthcare professionals make decisions regarding the types of psychosocial treatments that may be beneficial for particular issues warranting intervention and to illustrate how those treatments may be applied in clinical practice through the use of case vignettes and clinical dialogues.

A book of this magnitude would not be possible without the help of many people. We thank our contributors, who devoted extensive time and energy to each of their chapters, as well as Samantha Leung for her editorial assistance. We also thank the editorial team at Cambridge University Press, including Catherine Barnes, Nigel Graves, Sarah Marsh, David Mackenzie, Charlotte Brisley, and Allan Alphonse, for transforming our idea into a tangible product. Finally, we thank our patients, who provided us with inspiration each day to produce a resource that we hope will improve mental healthcare for all individuals being treated for severe obesity.

Psychosocial Issues in Severe Obesity

Sanjeev Sockalingam and Raed Hawa

Case Vignette

Nada is a 39-year-old married woman who works as a cashier. She is a mother of a 14-year-old daughter. Her husband, Sam, works as a truck driver. Nada has struggled with her weight over the years. Today she sees her primary care physician asking to be on a medication to help with her weight.

Nada was "chubby" as a kid. She started gaining weight around the time of her parents' divorce. At school she was bullied for being "lazy." She experimented with marijuana and started smoking at age 14. She was able to finish high school and worked as a cashier to support herself. She tried a number of yoyo diets and weight loss shakes with initial success in losing some weight followed by regaining the weight back and more. She gained more weight after her marriage at age 24. As she was planning to get pregnant, she quit smoking and gained more weight. Her pregnancy was complicated with gestational diabetes.

She describes her life as "hectic" and states that she is "on the go" all the time. Her husband spends days away from home due to long-haul driving. She has to juggle a job and a family. Her daughter is having some academic difficulties due to reported hyperactivity. She complains of general fatigue and periods of weepiness that she attributes to stress, preoccupation with her weight, and feeling "undesirable." She denies symptoms of cold or heat intolerance, nervousness, or irritability. She says that she has some difficulty sleeping and reports waking up feeling "unrested."

She also complains of occasional hip stiffness after walking for prolonged periods. The hip pain limits her ability to exercise. She is on metformin for type 2 diabetes. She is frustrated with her diabetes because her sugar levels are not under control. She has seen a dietitian but has been having difficulty following the nutrition education because "I am busy all the time."

When Nada's eating behavior was explored, she endorsed loss of control over eating, especially at night after she comes home from work and her daughter goes to bed. She feels bored, and she finds eating to be a "way out of stress." She eats large amounts while watching TV. She initially feels good but later feels "disgusted" with herself. She misses breakfast and eats "junk food" at the convenience store where she works.

On examination, her weight is 250 pounds and her height is 5 feet, 6 inches. Her body mass index (BMI) is 40 kg/m^2. Her affect is tearful, and she reports her mood as "frustrated" because of her weight struggles. She endorses sleep difficulties and low energy. She has missed work at times because of the fatigue and the hip pain. She also reports periods of irritability toward her daughter. Her thoughts are organized, and she feels demoralized and helpless to control her weight. She is not suicidal.

Introduction

This chapter provides an overview of the obesity epidemic and identifies common psychological issues facing patients with severe obesity. Prevalence rates, clinical presentations, and risk factors for a range of psychiatric disorders seen in severe obesity are discussed, including mood disorders, anxiety disorders, and eating disorders. Within the chapter, developmental factors predisposing individuals to obesity will be summarized. The chapter concludes with a summary of the role of psychosocial interventions in obesity care, specifically situating these interventions within the range of medical and surgical interventions in obesity care. The importance of psychosocial/behavioral health professionals in the management of psychological factors arising in obesity care are highlighted.

Obesity-Related Medical Comorbidities and Medical Treatments for Severe Obesity

Obesity, classified as a BMI of 30 kg/m^2 or greater, has reached epidemic proportions, with obesity rates nearly doubling since 1980 [1]. Data from the World Health Organization (WHO) suggest that in 2014 more than 600 million individuals had obesity worldwide [1], which compares with 78 million individuals with obesity in the United States [2]. Obesity is associated with a multitude of medical comorbidities, including hypertension, dyslipidemia, type 2 diabetes mellitus, coronary heart disease, sleep apnea, osteoarthritis, and some cancers. Moreover, obesity is associated with a significant increase in all-cause mortality even after considering metabolic status [3,4]. As a result, obesity is a well-recognized multiorgan disease with clear associations with a range of comorbidities including psychiatric illness.

Given the burden of severe obesity, several treatment options have been studied to determine their effectiveness in this patient population. Several medications have received indications for treating obesity and may offer benefit in the range of 3 to 9 percent weight loss (compared with placebo) beyond lifestyle counseling alone [5] (see Table 1.1).

At present, the most durable treatment for severe obesity is bariatric, or weight loss, surgery. A meta-analysis by Gloy and colleagues reported that bariatric surgery resulted in greater weight loss, remission of type 2 diabetes, and remission of metabolic syndrome compared with nonsurgical treatments [6]. Bariatric surgery includes a range of procedures that have evolved over time with advancements in surgical techniques and equipment. Bariatric surgery works through one of two mechanisms, namely, *malabsorption* and *restriction*. Weight loss from malabsorption is achieved through bypassing the first part of the small intestine, where calories are absorbed. Restriction from bariatric surgery procedures limits food intake and calories through a smaller gastric pouch. While the exact mechanisms of bariatric surgery procedures are complex and still to be determined, current nomenclature classifies the laparoscopic gastric banding (LAGB) and laparoscopic sleeve gastrectomy (LSG) as restrictive procedures and the laparoscopic Roux-en-Y gastric bypass (LRYGB) and duodenal switch as both restrictive and malabsorptive procedures. The two most common surgical procedures offered in North America are the LSG and the LRYGB. In the STAMPEDE study, bariatric surgery with intense medical management was more effective than intense medical management alone in sustained weight loss and remission of type 2 diabetes [7]. Table 1.2 lists the types of surgical treatments for severe obesity and their descriptions.

Table 1.1 Long-Term Pharmacologic Treatments for Obesity

Obesity pharmacotherapy[a]	Mechanism of action
Orlistat (Xenical)	Lipase inhibitor causing excretion of triglycerides in stool
Lorcaserin (Belviq)	Highly selective 5-HT2 C-serotonergic receptor agonist causing appetite suppression
Phentermine/ topiramate-ER (Qysmia)	Noradrenergic and GABA-receptor activator, kainate/AMPA glutamate receptor inhibitor (note: unclear mechanism of action for weight loss)
Naltrexone-SR/ bupropion-SR (Contrave)	Pro-opiomelanocortin (POMC) neurons stimulated by bupropion and naltrexone blocking autoinhibitory effects related to weight loss
Liraglutide (Saxenda)	Glucagon-like peptide receptor agonist increasing satiety and reduces food intake

[a] Listed agents have been approved by the US Food and Drug Administration (FDA) as treatments for obesity.

Table 1.2 Summary of Common Bariatric Surgery Procedures

Bariatric surgery type	Restrictive/ malabsorptive[a]	Description
Laparoscopic Roux-en-Y gastric bypass	R + M	Creation of a 20- to 30-ml gastric pouch from proximal lesser curve of stomach. A Roux-en-Y anastomosis is created from the biliopancreatic limb, alimentary limb, and remainder of the small intestine (common channel).
Laparoscopic sleeve gastrectomy	R	The majority of the greater curve of the stomach is removed to create a smaller gastric reservoir.
Laparoscopic gastric banding	R	An adjustable silicone band is placed around the cardia of stomach below the gastroesophageal junction.
Biliopancreatic diversion ± duodenal switch	R + M	This is a less common procedure, a combination of a distal gastrectomy and long Roux-en-Y reconstruction. A duodenal switch is a variant of this procedure in which the pylorus is preserved.

[a] R = restrictive; M = malabsorptive.

Obesity-Related Psychiatric Comorbidities

Relationship between Obesity and Psychiatric Illness

A bidirectional relationship exists between obesity and psychiatric illness. Obesity results in higher rates of psychiatric disorders, and certain psychiatric disorders increase the risk of obesity independent of iatrogenic factors, such as psychotropic medications. Prevalence rates of current and lifetime psychiatric disorders vary across studies depending on the assessment setting and the method of assessment, specifically self-report versus clinician-administered diagnostic tools. Lifetime rates of psychiatric disorders in patients with severe obesity approximate 70 percent in studies where the assessment was conducted by clinicians who were independent of obesity treatment programs [8]. The most common psychiatric disorders in samples of bariatric surgery candidates are mood disorders (23 percent), binge eating disorder (17 percent), and anxiety disorders (12 percent) [9].

The high rates of psychiatric comorbidity are further supported by studies showing a positive correlation between BMI and level of psychopathology, with increases in BMI resulting in higher psychopathology in individuals with obesity [10]. This relationship is further summarized in obesity staging, which has included psychological comorbidities as part of the severity classification system for obesity. For example, the Edmonton Obesity Staging System includes "obesity-related psychological symptoms" as part of its staging system to quantify obesity severity in addition to BMI [11]. In stage 2 severity in this system, moderate psychological symptoms include depression and anxiety disorders. Thus psychiatric factors are a core component of obesity care and should be assessed in order to generate comprehensive treatment plans to support patients seeking treatment for obesity.

Pathoetiology of Psychiatric Comorbidity in Severe Obesity

A myriad of pathoetiologic factors have been proposed to explain the bidirectional relationship between psychiatric disorders and obesity. Factors can be divided into biological factors, iatrogenic factors, and environmental factors. Biological factors consist of shared abnormalities in neurometabolism and neuroinflammation between obesity and psychiatric disorders, specifically using mood disorders as the paradigm. Iatrogenic factors primarily consist of medications that are often used in psychiatric treatment that can increase the risk of metabolic syndrome, specifically atypical antipsychotic medications and some antidepressants. Lastly, environmental factors consist of early-childhood adversity, which is known to increase the risk of psychiatric illness and also obesity in the long term. Each of these factors will be further discussed in this section.

Biological Factors. As mentioned earlier, aberrant neurometabolism and neuroinflammation responses are shared between psychiatric illness and obesity. These shared features are best described in mood disorder populations [12]. One potential mechanism is the hypothalamic-pituitary-adrenal (HPA) axis, which is dysfunctional in both obesity and mood disorders. Studies suggest that abdominal adiposity has been associated with abnormal HPA axis activation, including both higher and lower cortisol levels in response to stress [13–16]. Conversely, individuals exposed to chronic stress, which resulted in elevated cortisol levels, were found to have increased visceral adipose tissue [17]. In addition to obesity, both depression and bipolar disorder have been associated with abnormalities in the HPA axis. Individuals with bipolar disorder have increased cortisol secretion in euthymic, manic, and depressive states and have blunted reactivity to stress [18]. Several studies have reliably demonstrated an association between remitted and symptomatic depression with an increase in cortisol levels [19,20]. It is possible that these overlapping findings related to HPA axis abnormalities explain the relationship between mood disorders and obesity.

Obesity is also associated with immune-inflammatory dysregulation. Data from a meta-analysis have shown elevated levels of pro-inflammatory markers, such as tumor necrosis factor-alpha (TNF-α) and interleukin-6 (IL-6), in the serum of patients with bipolar or major depressive disorder [21,22]. Moreover, obesity is also associated with pro-inflammatory states, such as increased levels of C-reactive protein [23]. Therefore, pro-inflammation may be a shared pathway leading to comorbidity between obesity and psychiatric illness that warrants further study.

Adipokines in the context of obesity have been associated with mood disorders and psychopathology. Previous studies have suggested that leptin resistance in the context of abdominal obesity was a risk factor for depression in an elderly patient sample [24]. Further, a longitudinal study of patients with early-stage bipolar disorder showed an inverse relationship between adiponectin and leptin levels and depressive symptoms [25]. In this study, higher adiponectin and leptin levels were also associated with higher BMI gain. Despite these findings, the relationship between adipokines and mood symptoms has been limited by confounding variables. The heterogeneity in the association between depression and adiponectin across studies may be explained by gender differences and differences in depression severity [26]. Further, the heterogeneity in the findings between leptin and depression may be explained by differences in BMI between groups with depression and healthy control individuals in these studies [26]. Thus the role of adipokines in this relationship between psychopathology and obesity warrants further study to elucidate the nature of this relationship across patient populations.

In addition, several studies have identified an increased association between attention deficit hyperactivity disorder (ADHD) and obesity. Identification of familial risk factors from the Swedish National Registry showed an increased risk of ADHD in siblings of index males with obesity [27]. ADHD has also been observed at higher rates among patients with eating disorders, including binge eating disorder (BED) [28].

Lastly, the construct of food addiction has emerged as a possible risk factor for obesity and has been linked to hedonic drive and eating psychopathology in obesity. Strong evidence initially emerged from animal models demonstrating that rats given intermittent access to sugar ignore their usual chow over time and begin to binge on sugar solution after repeated exposures to sugar [29]. Subsequently, rats displayed signs of withdrawal when sugar was removed from their diet or naloxone was administered to block the opioid receptor effects of sugar. Further, neuroimaging studies in humans have shown deficits in dopaminergic pathways and frontal-striatal systems that are also seen in individuals who use cocaine [30]. Additional risks for overeating in obesity include genetic attenuation of dopamine transmission as a result of reduced dopamine D_2 receptor (DDR) availability, which is observed in patients addicted to substances of abuse. The Taq1A polymorphism for the A1 allele has been proposed as a genetic variant resulting in decreased DDR [31]. However, a meta-analysis has refuted the association between the Taq1A polymorphism and obesity, thus suggesting that parallels for these genetic associations cannot be made for food addiction [32]. In summary, these vulnerabilities and activation of reward pathways by highly processed foods may predispose some individuals to develop eating patterns reflective of food addiction symptomatology; however, further exploration is required to identify clear mechanisms and risk factors.

Iatrogenic Factors. Treatment of psychiatric comorbidity in patients with severe obesity may warrant the use of psychotropic medications. These medications may predispose individuals to develop metabolic side effects including weight gain and diabetes. Antipsychotic medications, such as olanzapine, clozapine, and quetiapine, carry increased metabolic risks in the long term [33,34]. Similarly, antidepressant medications, specifically mirtazapine, paroxetine, and tricyclic antidepressants, can also result in increased weight in patients with depression and anxiety [34]. Further, patients with autoimmune disorders and chronic obstructive pulmonary disease (COPD) may require treatment with steroid medications, such as prednisone, which can increase the risk of weight gain and metabolic syndrome. Therefore, pharmacotherapy for obesity-related physical and mental health comorbidities is a potential factor contributing to the co-occurrence of obesity and psychiatric illness.

Environmental Factors. Early-childhood adversity has been associated with the development of comorbid obesity and psychological distress. In the seminal Adverse Childhood Experiences study involving 13,177 patients from a large health organization in California, a history of childhood abuse was more strongly associated with a BMI of 40 kg/m^2 or greater than a BMI of 30 kg/m^2 or greater as an adult [35]. Moreover, individuals with a history of sexual abuse have higher rates of severe obesity compared with control individuals [36]. Data from a large meta-analysis consisting of 23 cohort studies involving 112,708 participants demonstrated that all types of childhood abuse were associated with adult obesity: physical (odds ratio [OR] = 1.28), emotional (OR = 1.36), sexual (OR = 1.31), and general abuse (OR = 1.45) [37]. Weight discrimination and bullying in early childhood also have been associated with a range of psychological sequelae in children and youth with obesity, including maladaptive eating behaviors, anxiety, depression, and suicidal ideation [38]. In addition, patients' early-childhood parental figures and attachment relationships may shape their perception of the world, including their relationship with healthcare providers caring for them during their obesity care (see Chapter 4). An insecure attachment (relationship) style can also contribute to disordered eating, difficulties engaging with obesity care teams, and attenuated weight loss outcomes [39]. This evidence provides compelling support that childhood adversity and attachment relationships further contribute to the development of comorbid psychiatric illness and obesity.

Specific Psychiatric Disorders in Severe Obesity

Mood Disorders

Substantial research has identified a bidirectional relationship between obesity and depression, which has been established early in life. A meta-analysis of studies examining depression rates in children and adolescents who are obese and not obese found a positive association between childhood and adolescent obesity and depression (OR = 1.34), as well as higher depressive symptoms in the patient groups with obesity [40]. A meta-analysis involving longitudinal studies showed that individuals with depression had a 58 percent increased risk of developing obesity, and individuals with obesity had a 55 percent increased risk of developing depression [41].

Among bariatric surgery candidates, rates of depression based on clinician-administered assessment approximate 19 percent, with some large multisite studies reporting rates as high as 39 percent [9,42]. Following bariatric surgery, depression tends to improve in the first year postoperatively; however, long-term data suggest that depressive symptoms can gradually increase over time [9,43]. It should be noted that depressive symptoms remain better than before surgery for most patients, although there are several reports of increased self-harm and suicide in comparison with the general population after bariatric surgery, which may be related to worsening depression [44,45]. Some studies suggest that early postoperative depression is associated with worse long-term weight loss outcomes after bariatric surgery; however, further research is needed to replicate these early findings [9,46]. Based on the current evidence, preoperative assessment and stability of depressive symptoms should be a focus of psychosocial assessment and early intervention. This should be followed by continuous monitoring and early introduction of psychological interventions after bariatric surgery to support patients' behavior changes and psychological well-being.

Several factors have been reported to increase the association between depression and obesity. Lower socioeconomic status has been associated with an increased risk of comorbid depressive disorder and obesity [47]. Additional clinical factors increasing the risk of comorbid depression and obesity include more severe obesity, binge eating and other dysregulated eating behaviors, increased physical health issues [47], body image issues such as prominent shape and weight concerns and body image dissatisfaction [47], the presence of weight-related stigma [48,49], and interpersonal stressors and decreased social activity [50,51]. Although psychological factors such as self-esteem, hostility, and maladaptive schemas also influenced the relationship between obesity and depression, gender differences emerged regarding the impact of specific psychological factors [47]. The relationship between obesity and depression was stronger for men with low interpersonal effectiveness, poor conflict resolution, and loneliness [52]. In comparison, the relationship between obesity and depression was stronger for women with greater anger, sadness, and excitement. Based on these variables, patients identified as being at high risk should be educated on potential risks. Moreover, patients who are at an increased risk of having comorbid depression and obesity may benefit from psychological interventions aimed at improving modifiable variables, such interpersonal effectiveness and self-esteem, for example.

In addition to depression, obesity has also been associated with bipolar disorder and known to influence mood outcomes in this population. A study of 644 patients with bipolar 1 and 2 disorder from the United States and Europe identified obesity and severe obesity in 21 and 5 percent of the sample, respectively [53]. Data from the National Comorbidity Survey Replication involving 9,125 respondents noted that obesity was significantly associated with a lifetime diagnosis of bipolar disorder (OR = 1.47) and had an even stronger association with a diagnosis of bipolar disorder within the last 12 months (OR = 1.61) [54]. These studies reinforce the strong link between bipolar disorder and severe obesity.

Obesity has also been associated with a worse course of illness and increased risk of mood relapse in patients with bipolar disorder. In a study comparing treatment naive female patients with bipolar disorder with control individuals without bipolar disorder, patients with bipolar disorder had higher abdominal adiposity compared with control individuals [55]. Moreover, patients with bipolar disorder who are obese have higher rates of mood recurrence compared with nonobese patients with bipolar disorder [56]. In addition, higher BMI has been associated with longer duration of illness and chronic course in bipolar disorder [57]. The impact of obesity on bipolar illness outcomes is further reinforced by neuroimaging data from patients recovered from their first manic episode, which showed a relationship between elevated BMI and gray and white matter reductions in the frontal, temporal, and subcortical limbic areas, which are all implicated in the pathophysiology of bipolar disorder. In addition to illness-related effects on obesity, it should be noted that many of the mood-stabilizing medications, such as atypical antipsychotics, lithium, and valproate, are associated with increased weight gain in the long term [58]. Therefore, treatment of obesity should be a priority in patients with bipolar disorder given the impact on mood disorder outcomes.

Bariatric surgery outcomes have been explored for patients with bipolar disorder given the high prevalence of obesity, potential benefit on mood symptoms, and limited treatments for severe obesity in this patient population. Research has been limited by small sample sizes and short-term follow-up. A matched cohort study comparing 13 patients with bipolar disorder who underwent bariatric surgery with patients with bipolar disorder who had not undergone bariatric surgery over a 2.17-year mean follow-up period showed no effect of bariatric surgery on psychiatric hospitalization rates or outpatient psychiatric utilization [59]. A retrospective study comparing patients with bipolar disorder, other psychiatric conditions, and no psychiatric illness showed no difference in weight loss outcomes one year after surgery [60]. Moreover, a prospective cohort study showed no difference in weight loss outcomes and physical quality of life one year after surgery between patients with complex psychiatric illness (including bipolar disorder), other psychiatric illness, and no psychiatric illness; however, mental quality of life was reduced in the group with more complex psychiatric illness [61]. Despite these findings suggesting that bariatric surgery does not result in worse psychiatric stability or reduced weight loss, patients with bipolar spectrum disorders are still less likely to be deemed "ready" or eligible for bariatric surgery compared with other patient groups [62]. Therefore, greater focus on psychosocial factors and treatments is needed to better support patients through this process and to anticipate potential challenges with bipolar disorder treatments and follow-up bariatric surgery care.

Anxiety Disorders

In addition to depression, anxiety is a common comorbidity in patients with obesity. Estimated prevalence rates of anxiety disorders are approximately 12 percent, although lifetime rates are as high as 31 percent [9,42]. The most common anxiety disorders in this population are specific phobias and social anxiety disorder, with lifetime rates of the latter approximating 6 percent. The *Diagnostic and Statistical Manual of Mental Disorders*, fifth edition (DSM-5) modified the criteria for social anxiety disorder to allow for the diagnosis of social anxiety even if the fears were related to a medical condition such as obesity [63].

Assessment of anxiety in the context of severe obesity is an important component of care, especially given data suggesting that anxiety can drive maladaptive eating behaviors. For example, grazing eating patterns in bariatric surgery candidates were associated with anxiety disorders in addition to BED [64]. Anxiety symptoms also follow a similar course to depressive symptoms after bariatric surgery, specifically the "honeymoon" phase with reduced anxiety within the first 6 to 12 months after massive weight loss, followed by increased anxiety beyond the initial year. Ten-year data from the Swedish Obesity Study showed an initial reduction in anxiety symptoms at one year after surgery (37 percent), but this improvement was attenuated at six years (20 percent) and at ten years after surgery (23 percent) [65]. In addition, greater improvements in anxiety, depressive symptoms, and mental quality of life after bariatric surgery predicted improvement in employment functioning [66]. Data on the long-term effects of anxiety relapse have not predicted postoperative weight loss, although there are some data that anxious relationship (attachment) style is associated with poor adherence to postoperative prescribed vitamin supplementation after LRYGB [67].

Eating Disorders

Given the high prevalence of eating disorders in patients with severe obesity, a growing body of literature has summarized the rates of eating psychopathology in patients with severe obesity and during the course of severe obesity care. Rates of BED in patients with severe obesity are estimated to be 13 to 17 percent; however, subthreshold symptoms are more prevalent [9,42]. Prevalence rates for BED have ranged from 2 to 49 percent across studies including a broad range of assessment measures that extend beyond structured psychiatric assessment and interviews [68]. When using the DSM-IV-TR diagnostic category of "eating disorder not otherwise specified" (EDNOS), approximately 27 percent of bariatric surgery candidates meet criteria for EDNOS, which captures these subthreshold eating disorder symptoms [42]. The prevalence of night eating syndrome (NES), characterized by a shift in the circadian pattern of eating that results in nocturnal hyperphagia and increased frequency of nocturnal ingestions, ranges from 2 to 20 percent across studies due to varying measures and definitions of night eating [69]. Rates of emotional eating and grazing eating patterns have ranged from 38 to 59 percent and 20 to 60 percent, respectively, among bariatric surgery candidates [70].

Both BED and NES have been associated with obesity. Studies have demonstrated higher rates of obesity in patients with BED. In the WHO World Mental Health Survey study, the percentage of patients with a lifetime diagnosis of BED who had a BMI of 35 kg/m^2 or greater was 62 percent, compared with 25 percent in patients without a diagnosis of an eating disorder [71]. Additional studies have also supported a positive association between NES and obesity [72]. Moreover, a study of correlates of NES in bariatric surgery candidates showed that NES was positively correlated with BMI and BED, which highlights that these two distinct diagnostic entities may co-occur in patient populations with severe obesity [73]. Studies suggest that the rates of comorbid BED and NES range from 7 to 25 percent [74,75]. Nonetheless, based on data comparing normal-weight individuals and those with obesity, the risk of obesity related to NES and BED appears to increase with age [76].

Although both BED and NES have been associated with severe obesity, the direction of this relationship remains unclear. Regardless, it is clear that features of BED and NES contribute to weight gain and obesity in some patients. Loss of control over eating is a core feature of BED and can persist after bariatric surgery despite restrictive procedures. Persistence of loss of control over eating after surgery can lead to problematic eating, attenuated weight loss, weight regain, and poorer quality of life [77]. Bariatric candidates with loss of control over eating have significantly higher levels of night eating, depressive symptoms, and eating disorder psychopathology with lower mental quality of life [78].

Research examining the impact of bariatric surgery on eating psychopathology has yielded mixed results. According to an observational study analyzing data from 36 patients with preoperative BED, bariatric surgery resulted in a reduction in BED symptoms in the first year after surgery [79]. This study contrasts with other studies that have shown an initial reduction in symptoms within the first 6 to 12 months after surgery with a gradual increase in BED symptoms over time. For example, one study showed an initial reduction in binge eating episodes at six months after RYGB (61.2 percent preoperatively to 30.7 percent), followed by an increase from 6 to 12 months after surgery (36.4 percent) and a further increase at 24 months after surgery (39.4 percent) [77]. In a recent review examining changes in eating psychopathology from before to after surgery, the authors concluded that several "fair-rated" studies showed significant reemergence of BED symptomatology after an initial reduction during the first 6 to 12 months after surgery [80]. Although several systematic reviews suggest that BED and NES before surgery are not robust predictors of weight loss after surgery [8,9], some studies suggest that preoperative eating psychopathology, such as loss of control over eating, may increase the risk of similar eating psychopathology after bariatric surgery [77]. Further research is needed to examine changes in BED and NES symptoms in the long term and across additional weight loss surgery populations, specifically LSG patients.

Despite these inconclusive findings, it is clear that a proportion of patients undergoing bariatric surgery will continue to have a spectrum of disordered eating. In fact, trends in severe obesity parallel evidence from previous reviews in uncomplicated obesity demonstrating improvement in eating psychopathology with weight loss. A systematic review of 134 studies in uncomplicated obesity reported an improvement in eating psychopathology, specifically cognitive restraint, control over eating, and binge eating [81]. With respect to severe obesity, approximately 25 percent of bariatric surgery patients endorsed subjective binges up to two years after surgery; however, only 3.4 percent fulfilled criteria for BED [82]. In a Longitudinal Assessment of Bariatric Surgery (LABS) Research Consortium three-year follow-up study, eating psychopathology, specifically global disordered eating, loss of control over eating, and regular evening hyperphagia, decreased in the initial year after surgery, but cravings and subjective eating binges were unchanged [83]. These improvements in global disordered eating, loss of control over eating, and evening hyperphagia continued at three years after surgery. Ten-year follow-up studies examining psychological factors related to eating after bariatric surgery have shown persistent improvements in disinhibited eating and hunger and to a lesser degree in cognitive restraint of eating [84]. Overall, the evidence to date suggests that most patients who undergo bariatric surgery experience improvements in eating psychopathology from before to after surgery.

Patients can develop serious eating psychopathology after surgery, however, and some of these conditions may be related to surgical complications or inadequate weight loss outcomes. Although vomiting may be a sign of disordered eating, it is not uncommon for patients to experience vomiting early postoperatively due to gastric discomfort or to complications such as strictures. In a sample of postoperative bariatric surgery patients, 63 percent endorsed vomiting due to gastric discomfort, whereas 12 percent attributed vomiting to shape- and weight-related concerns [82]. Rare but distressing reports of anorexia nervosa emerging after bariatric surgery have been reported, and these cases generally occur in the context of poor weight loss outcomes after surgery [85]. Moreover, patients may resume emotional eating after surgery, which can trigger nonadherence to postoperative nutrition regimens and potentially increase the risk of weight regain [86]. Postoperative psychosocial interventions have been shown to assist in reducing emotional eating in the postoperative period and will be discussed in more detail in Chapters 6, 9, 10, and 11.

Trauma and Posttraumatic Stress Disorder

As noted earlier, trauma and childhood adversity are predisposing factors for severe obesity and associated psychological distress. Studies have shown higher rates of childhood physical and sexual abuse in bariatric surgery candidates compared with a behavioral weight control group [87]. Further, higher rates of physical and sexual abuse have been reported in patients with severe obesity (class III obesity) compared with patients with class I and class II obesity [88]. In a study of 230 bariatric surgery candidates, childhood maltreatment was assessed using the Childhood Trauma Questionnaire (short form), and approximately 66 percent of the sample endorsed a history of childhood maltreatment [89]. Patients who had endorsed childhood maltreatment had a higher number of psychiatric disorders. This finding is not surprising given that childhood trauma may result in long-standing emotion dysregulation, and distress could evolve into posttraumatic stress disorder (PTSD). Childhood sexual abuse has also been associated with higher psychiatric hospitalization rates in patients who underwent bariatric surgery, specifically RYGB, although these data were limited to care received at a single center and did not capture broader hospitalizations occurring outside this site [90]. Careful inquiry about a history of trauma and consideration about potential supports across the continuum of care are important to supporting improvement in obesity-related comorbidities and quality of life during treatment for severe obesity.

Current and lifetime rates of PTSD, according to the LABS-3 study, were 3 and 11 percent, respectively, in patients with severe obesity [42]. Given the links between affective dysregulation and disordered eating, active PTSD symptoms may exacerbate affective states and increase eating psychopathology during treatment for severe obesity. Similar to childhood abuse, a current diagnosis of PTSD during the preoperative bariatric surgery assessment phase was a significant predictor of patients not completing the full assessment [91]. After weight loss surgery, a retrospective study of veterans with and without PTSD showed no significant difference in percent excess weight loss at one-year follow-up [92]. Nonetheless, obesity may be considered protective for some patients with a history of sexual abuse, and weight loss resulting in increased social attention and interaction may be perceived as distressing for some patients. As a result, PTSD symptoms should be monitored while patients are losing weight to identify signs of relapse and determine whether psychological interventions are warranted.

Role of Psychological Treatments in Severe Obesity

Although pharmacological treatments and bariatric surgery have a role in obesity treatment, the high rates of psychiatric comorbidity reinforce the need to include psychological therapies within the continuum of treatments for severe obesity. Psychological treatments may include motivational interviewing (see Section 2), cognitive-behavioral therapy (see Section 3), mindfulness-based and compassion-focused therapies (see Section 4), and additional therapies (see Section 5), which can be critical throughout the treatment continuum for severe obesity to support patient engagement, treat comorbid psychiatric conditions, enhance weight loss and psychosocial functioning, and prevent weight regain and relapse of medical and psychiatric comorbidities after initial improvements from comprehensive, multimodal severe obesity treatments. Figure 1.1 outlines the potential role of psychological treatments throughout the spectrum of severe obesity interventions.

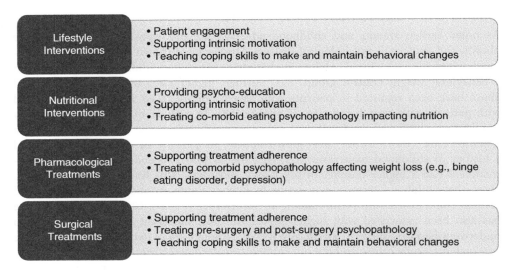

Lifestyle Interventions	• Patient engagement • Supporting intrinsic motivation • Teaching coping skills to make and maintain behavioral changes
Nutritional Interventions	• Providing psycho-education • Supporting intrinsic motivation • Treating co-morbid eating psychopathology impacting nutrition
Pharmacological Treatments	• Supporting treatment adherence • Treating comorbid psychopathology affecting weight loss (e.g., binge eating disorder, depression)
Surgical Treatments	• Supporting treatment adherence • Treating pre-surgery and post-surgery psychopathology • Teaching coping skills to make and maintain behavioral changes

Figure 1.1 Role of psychological treatments across the continuum of severe obesity interventions.

Throughout the subsequent sections of this book, psychological approaches to severe obesity management will be described and illustrated using Case Vignettes, and the empirical evidence for each approach will be reviewed.

Case Vignette Revisited

Establishing a caring and a supportive relationship with Nada is an essential step toward helping her achieve her goals. Although pharmacologic treatments should be discussed as part of Nada's obesity treatment, it is also important to engage Nada and support her motivation to lose weight and adopt healthy eating habits. Psychoeducation (about the relationship between genetics and weight, obesity and mood, as well as stress and eating) and nutrition counseling (related to her eating habits and diabetes control, regular eating and mindful eating) are important. Psychological treatments such as cognitive-behavioral therapy (addressing her cognitions of being lazy and undesirable) and mindfulness-based interventions (nonjudgmental awareness of being in the moment) can be critical throughout the treatment continuum for severe obesity. Treating Nada's comorbidities of depression, sleep disturbance, and BED (through psychopharmacology or psychological intervention) is also an essential component of the treatment.

Summary

In summary, obesity is a multisystem disease, and psychiatric illness is a significant comorbidity. There is increasing literature on the potential shared pathways and causes for obesity and psychiatric illness ranging from biological to environmental factors. Therefore, it is imperative that clinicians managing obesity consider common comorbidities such as mood disorders, anxiety disorders, and eating disorders (e.g., binge eating) in their assessment and treatment plans. Across the treatment continuum for severe obesity that extends from lifestyle and nutrition interventions to pharmacologic treatments and bariatric surgery, psychological factors can limit the effectiveness and maintenance of benefit of interventions. The remainder of this book focuses on psychological treatments to support weight loss and enhance psychosocial functioning in individuals with severe obesity, with an emphasis on practical strategies that can be incorporated into clinical practice.

Key Points

- Obesity is a multiorgan disease with a wide range of medical comorbidities (hypertension, diabetes, hyperlipidemia, and sleep apnea) and psychiatric comorbidities (mood, anxiety, and eating disorders).
- Biological (abnormal neurometabolism and neuroinflammation), iatrogenic (use of certain antipsychotics and antidepressants), and environmental (early-childhood adversity and trauma) factors should be explored when examining the relationship between obesity and psychiatric illness.
- Beyond the use of antiobesity medications and bariatric surgery, it is imperative to include psychological therapies focused on supporting motivation and developing coping skills to initiate and maintain health-related changes within the continuum of treatments for severe obesity.

References

1. World Health Organization (WHO). Obesity and overweight: fact sheet, 2016. Available at www.who.int/mediacentre/fact sheets/fs311/en/.

2. C. L. Ogden, M. D. Carroll, B. K. Kit, et al. Prevalence of obesity in the United States, 2009–2010. *NCHS Data Brief* 2012; **82**: 1–8.

3. C. K. Kramer, B. Zinman, and R. Retnakaran. Are metabolically healthy overweight and obesity benign conditions? A systematic review and meta-analysis. *Ann Intern Med* 2013; **159**: 758–69.

4. A. Berrington de Gonzalez, P. Hartge, J. R. Cerhan, et al. Body-mass index and mortality among 1.46 million white adults. *N Engl J Med* 2010; **363**: 2211–19.

5. D. Patel. Pharmacotherapy for the management of obesity. *Metabolism* 2015; **64**: 1376–85.

6. V. L. Gloy, M. Briel, D. L. Bhatt, et al. Bariatric surgery versus non-surgical treatment for obesity: a systematic review and meta-analysis of randomised controlled trials. *BMJ* 2013; **347**: f5934.

7. P. R. Schauer, D. L. Bhatt, J. P. Kirwan, et al. Bariatric surgery versus intensive medical therapy for diabetes: 5-year outcomes. *N Engl J Med* 2017; **376**: 641–51.

8. S. Sockalingam, R. Hawa, S. Wnuk, et al. Weight loss following Roux-en-Y gastric bypass surgery: A systematic review of psychosocial predictors. *Curr Psych Rev* 2011; **7**: 226–33.

9. A. J. Dawes, M. Maggard-Gibbons, A. R. Maher, et al. Mental health conditions among patients seeking and undergoing bariatric surgery: A meta-analysis. *JAMA* 2016; **315**: 150–63.

10. P. Zaninotto, M. Pierce, E. Breeze, et al. BMI and waist circumference as predictors of well-being in older adults: Findings from the English Longitudinal Study of Ageing. *Obesity (Silver Spring)* 2010; **18**: 1981–7.

11. A. M. Sharma and R. F. Kushner. A proposed clinical staging system for obesity. *Int J Obes* 2009; **33**: 289–95.

12. R. S. McIntyre, M. Alsuwaidan, B. I. Goldstein, et al. The Canadian Network for Mood and Anxiety Treatments (CANMAT) task force recommendations for the management of

patients with mood disorders and comorbid metabolic disorders. *Ann Clin Psychiatry* 2012; **24**: 69–81.

13. R. Pasquali, V. Vicennati, M. Cacciari, et al. The hypothalamic-pituitary-adrenal axis activity in obesity and the metabolic syndrome. *Ann NY Acad Sci* 2006; **1083**: 111–28.

14. L. R. Mujica-Parodi, R. Renelique, and M. K. Taylor. Higher body fat percentage is associated with increased cortisol reactivity and impaired cognitive resilience in response to acute emotional stress. *Int J Obes* 2009; **33**: 157–65.

15. A. Jones, M. R. McMillan, R. W. Jones, et al. Adiposity is associated with blunted cardiovascular, neuroendocrine and cognitive responses to acute mental stress. *PLoS One* 2012; **7**: e39143.

16. B. Kubera, C. Hubold, S. Zug, et al. The brain's supply and demand in obesity. *Front Neuroenerget* 2012; **4**: 4.

17. E. S. Brown, F. P. Varghese, and B. S. McEwen. Association of depression with medical illness: Does cortisol play a role? *Biol Psychiatry* 2004; **55**: 1–9.

18. C. Daban, E. Vieta, P. Mackin, et al. Hypothalamic-pituitary-adrenal axis and bipolar disorder. *Psychiatr Clin North Am* 2005; **28**: 469–80.

19. S. A. Vreeburg, W. J. Hoogendijk, J. van Pelt, et al. Major depressive disorder and hypothalamic-pituitary-adrenal axis activity: Results from a large cohort study. *Arch Gen Psychiatry* 2009; **66**: 617–26.

20. C. Stetler and G. E. Miller. Depression and hypothalamic-pituitary-adrenal activation: A quantitative summary of four decades of research. *Psychosom Med* 2011; **73**: 114–26.

21. M. B. Howren, D. M. Lamkin, and J. Suls. Associations of depression with C-reactive protein, IL-1, and IL-6: A meta-analysis. *Psychosom Med* 2009; **71**: 171–86.

22. K. Munkholm, M. Vinberg, and L. Vedel Kessing. Cytokines in bipolar disorder: A systematic review and meta-analysis. *J Affect Disord* 2013; **144**: 16–27.

23. J. Choi, L. Joseph, and L. Pilote. Obesity and C-reactive protein in various

populations: A systematic review and meta-analysis. *Obes Rev* 2013; **14**: 232–44.

24. Y. Milaneschi, E. M. Simonsick, N. Vogelzangs, et al. Leptin, abdominal obesity, and onset of depression in older men and women. *J Clin Psychiatry* 2012; **73**: 1205–11.

25. D. J. Bond, A. C. Andreazza, J. Hughes, et al. A longitudinal study of the relationships between mood symptoms, body mass index, and serum adipokines in bipolar disorder. *J Clin Psychiatry* 2017; **78**: 441–8.

26. A. F. Carvalho, D. Q. Rocha, R. S. McIntyre, et al. Adipokines as emerging depression biomarkers: A systematic review and meta-analysis. *J Psychiatr Res* 2014; **59**: 28–37.

27. Q. Chen, R. Kuja-Halkola, A. Sjolander, et al. Shared familial risk factors between attention-deficit/hyperactivity disorder and overweight/obesity: A population-based familial coaggregation study in Sweden. *J Child Psychol Psychiatry* 2017; **58**: 711–18.

28. B. P. Nazar, C. Bernardes, G. Peachey, et al. The risk of eating disorders comorbid with attention-deficit/hyperactivity disorder: A systematic review and meta-analysis. *Int J Eat Disord* 2016; **49**: 1045–57.

29. N. M. Avena, P. Rada, and B. G. Hoebel. Evidence for sugar addiction: behavioral and neurochemical effects of intermittent, excessive sugar intake. *Neurosci Biobehav Rev* 2008; **32**: 20–39.

30. N. Pannacciulli, A. Del Parigi, K. Chen, et al. Brain abnormalities in human obesity: A voxel-based morphometric study. *Neuroimage* 2006; **31**: 1419–25.

31. E. Stice, S. Spoor, C. Bohon, et al. Relation between obesity and blunted striatal response to food is moderated by TaqIA A1 allele. *Science* 2008; **322**: 449–52.

32. D. Benton and H. A. Young. A meta-analysis of the relationship between brain dopamine receptors and obesity: A matter of changes in behavior rather than food addiction? *Int J Obes* 2016; **40**(Suppl. 1): S12–21.

33. C. Tek, S. Kucukgoncu, S. Guloksuz, et al. Antipsychotic-induced weight gain in

first-episode psychosis patients: A meta-analysis of differential effects of antipsychotic medications. *Early Interv Psychiatry* 2016; **10**: 193–202.

34. R. Dent, A. Blackmore, J. Peterson, et al. Changes in body weight and psychotropic drugs: A systematic synthesis of the literature. *PLoS One* 2012; **7**: e36889.

35. D. F. Williamson, T. J. Thompson, R. F. Anda, et al. Body weight and obesity in adults and self-reported abuse in childhood. *Int J Obes Relat Metab Disord* 2002; **26**: 1075–82.

36. V.J. Felitti. Long-term medical consequences of incest, rape, and molestation. *South Med J* 1991; **84**: 328–31.

37. E. Hemmingsson, K. Johansson, and S. Reynisdottir. Effects of childhood abuse on adult obesity: A systematic review and meta-analysis. *Obes Rev* 2014; **15**: 882–93.

38. R. M. Puhl and K. M. King. Weight discrimination and bullying. *Best Pract Res Clin Endocrinol Metab* 2013; **27**: 117–27.

39. S. Kiesewetter, A. Kopsel, K. Mai, et al. Attachment style contributes to the outcome of a multimodal lifestyle intervention. *Biopsychosoc Med* 2012; **6**: 3.

40. Y. H. Quek, W. W. S. Tam, M. W. B. Zhang, et al. Exploring the association between childhood and adolescent obesity and depression: A meta-analysis. *Obes Rev* 2017; **18**: 742–54.

41. F. S. Luppino, L. M. de Wit, P. F. Bouvy, et al. Overweight, obesity, and depression: A systematic review and meta-analysis of longitudinal studies. *Arch Gen Psychiatry* 2010; **67**: 220–9.

42. J. E. Mitchell, F. Selzer, M. A. Kalarchian, et al. Psychopathology before surgery in the Longitudinal Assessment of Bariatric Surgery-3 (LABS-3) psychosocial study. *Surg Obes Relat Dis* 2012; **8**: 533–41.

43. J. E. Mitchell, W. C. King, J. Y. Chen, et al. Course of depressive symptoms and treatment in the Longitudinal Assessment of Bariatric Surgery (LABS-2) study. *Obesity (Silver Spring)* 2014; **22**: 1799–806.

44. J. A. Bhatti, A. B. Nathens, D. Thiruchelvam, et al. Self-harm emergencies after bariatric surgery: A population-based cohort study. *JAMA Surgery* 2016; **151**: 226–32.

45. C. Peterhansel, D. Petroff, G. Klinitzke, et al. Risk of completed suicide after bariatric surgery: A systematic review. *Obes Rev* 2013; **14**: 369–82.

46. A. Hindle, X. de la Piedad Garcia, and L. Brennan. Early post-operative psychosocial and weight predictors of later outcome in bariatric surgery: A systematic literature review. *Obes Rev* 2017; **18**: 317–34.

47. K. Preiss, L. Brennan, and D. Clarke. A systematic review of variables associated with the relationship between obesity and depression. *Obes Rev* 2013; **14**: 906–18.

48. K. E. Friedman, J. A. Ashmore, and K. L. Applegate. Recent experiences of weight-based stigmatization in a weight loss surgery population: psychological and behavioral correlates. *Obesity (Silver Spring)* 2008; **16**(Suppl. 2): S69–74.

49. E. Y. Chen, L. E. Bocchieri-Ricciardi, D. Munoz, et al. Depressed mood in class III obesity predicted by weight-related stigma. *Obes Surg* 2007; **17**: 669–71.

50. L. M. de Wit, M. Fokkema, A. van Straten, et al. Depressive and anxiety disorders and the association with obesity, physical, and social activities. *Depress Anxiety* 2010; **27**: 1057–65.

51. A. F. Jorm, A. E. Korten, H. Christensen, et al. Association of obesity with anxiety, depression and emotional well-being: A community survey. *Aust NZ J Public Health* 2003; **27**: 434–40.

52. G. J. Musante, P. R. Costanzo, and K. E. Friedman. The comorbidity of depression and eating dysregulation processes in a diet-seeking obese population: A matter of gender specificity. *Int J Eat Disord* 1998; **23**: 65–75.

53. S. L. McElroy, M. A. Frye, T. Suppes, et al. Correlates of overweight and obesity in 644 patients with bipolar disorder. *J Clin Psychiatry* 2002; **63**: 207–13.

54. G. E. Simon, M. Von Korff, K. Saunders, et al. Association between obesity and psychiatric disorders in the US adult population. *Arch Gen Psychiatry* 2006; **63**: 824–30.

55. S. B. Fleet-Michaliszyn, I. Soreca, A. D. Otto, et al. A prospective observational study of obesity, body composition, and insulin resistance in 18 women with bipolar disorder and 17 matched control subjects. *J Clin Psychiatry* 2008; **69**: 1892–900.

56. A. Fagiolini, D. J. Kupfer, P. R. Houck, et al. Obesity as a correlate of outcome in patients with bipolar I disorder. *Am J Psychiatry* 2003; **160**: 112–7.

57. C. Calkin, C. van de Velde, M. Ruzickova, et al. Can body mass index help predict outcome in patients with bipolar disorder? *Bipolar Disord* 2009; **11**: 650–6.

58. C. Torrent, B. Amann, J. Sanchez-Moreno, et al. Weight gain in bipolar disorder: Pharmacological treatment as a contributing factor. *Acta Psychiatr Scand* 2008; **118**: 4–18.

59. A. T. Ahmed, E. M. Warton, C. A. Schaefer, et al. The effect of bariatric surgery on psychiatric course among patients with bipolar disorder. *Bipolar Disord* 2013; **15**: 753–63.

60. W. C. Steinmann, K. Suttmoeller, R. Chitima-Matsiga, et al. Bariatric surgery: 1-year weight loss outcomes in patients with bipolar and other psychiatric disorders. *Obes Surg* 2011; **21**: 1323–9.

61. L. Thomson, K. A. Sheehan, C. Meaney, et al. Prospective study of psychiatric illness as a predictor of weight loss and health related quality of life one year after bariatric surgery. *J Psychosom Res* 2016; **86**: 7–12.

62. K. E. Friedman, K. Applegate, D. Portenier, et al. Bariatric surgery in patients with bipolar spectrum disorders: Selection factors, postoperative visit attendance, and weight outcomes. *Surg Obes Relat Dis* 2017; **13**: 643–51.

63. K. L. Dalrymple, E. Walsh, L. Rosenstein, et al. Modification of the medical exclusion criterion in DSM-5 social anxiety disorder: Comorbid obesity as an example. *J Affect Disord* 2017; **210**: 230–6.

64. K. P. Goodpaster, R. J. Marek, M. E. Lavery, et al. Graze eating among bariatric surgery candidates: Prevalence and psychosocial correlates. *Surg Obes Relat Dis* 2016; **12**: 1091–7.

65. J. Karlsson, C. Taft, A. Ryden, et al. Ten-year trends in health-related quality of life after surgical and conventional treatment for severe obesity: The SOS intervention study. *Int J Obes* 2007; **31**: 1248–61.

66. S. Sockalingam, S. Wnuk, K. Kantarovich, et al. Employment outcomes one year after bariatric surgery: The role of patient and psychosocial factors. *Obes Surg* 2015; **25**: 514–22.

67. S. Sunil, V. A. Santiago, L. Gougeon, et al. Predictors of vitamin adherence after bariatric surgery. *Obes Surg* 2017; **27**: 416–23.

68. K. Parker and L. Brennan. Measurement of disordered eating in bariatric surgery candidates: A systematic review of the literature. *Obes Res Clin Pract* 2015; **9**: 12–25.

69. M. de Zwaan, M. Marschollek, and K. C. Allison. The night eating syndrome (NES) in bariatric surgery patients. *Eur Eat Disord Rev* 2015; **23**: 426–34.

70. M. Opolski, A. Chur-Hansen, and G. Wittert. The eating-related behaviours, disorders and expectations of candidates for bariatric surgery. *Clin Obes* 2015; **5**: 165–97.

71. R. C. Kessler, P. A. Berglund, W. T. Chiu, et al. The prevalence and correlates of binge eating disorder in the World Health Organization World Mental Health Surveys. *Biol Psychiatry* 2013; **73**: 904–14.

72. A. R. Gallant, J. Lundgren, and V. Drapeau. The night-eating syndrome and obesity. *Obes Rev* 2012; **13**: 528–36.

73. S. L. Colles, J. B. Dixon, and P. E. O'Brien. Night eating syndrome and nocturnal snacking: Association with obesity, binge eating and psychological distress. *Int J Obes* 2007; **31**: 1722–30.

74. K. C. Allison, J. D. Lundgren, J. P. O'Reardon, et al. Proposed diagnostic criteria for night eating syndrome. *Int J Eat Disord* 2010; **43**: 241–7.

75. L. A. Berner and K. C. Allison. Behavioral management of night eating disorders. *Psychol Res Behav Manag* 2013; **6**: 1–8.

76. A. B. Goldschmidt, D. Le Grange, P. Powers, et al. Eating disorder symptomatology in normal-weight vs. obese individuals with binge eating disorder. *Obesity (Silver Spring)* 2011; **19**: 1515–18.

77. M. A. White, M. A. Kalarchian, R. M. Masheb, et al. Loss of control over eating predicts outcomes in bariatric surgery patients: A prospective, 24-month follow-up study. *J Clin Psychiatry* 2010; **71**: 175–84.

78. S. Royal, S. Wnuk, K. Warwick, et al. Night eating and loss of control over eating in bariatric surgery candidates. *J Clin Psychol Med Settings* 2015; **22**: 14–19.

79. T.A. Wadden, L. F. Faulconbridge, L. R. Jones-Corneille, et al. Binge eating disorder and the outcome of bariatric surgery at one year: A prospective, observational study. *Obesity (Silver Spring)* 2011; **19**: 1220–8.

80. M. Opozda, A. Chur-Hansen, and G. Wittert. Changes in problematic and disordered eating after gastric bypass, adjustable gastric banding and vertical sleeve gastrectomy: A systematic review of pre-post studies. *Obes Rev* 2016; **17**: 770–92.

81. T. Peckmezian and P. Hay. A systematic review and narrative synthesis of interventions for uncomplicated obesity: Weight loss, well-being and impact on eating disorders. *J Eat Disord* 2017; **5**: 15.

82. M. de Zwaan, A. Hilbert, L. Swan-Kremeier, et al. Comprehensive interview assessment of eating behavior 18–35 months after gastric bypass surgery for morbid obesity. *Surg Obes Relat Dis* 2010; **6**: 79–85.

83. M. J. Devlin, W. C. King, M. A. Kalarchian, et al. Eating pathology and experience and weight loss in a prospective study of bariatric surgery patients: 3-year follow-up. *Int J Eat Disord* 2016; **49**: 1058–67.

84. H. Konttinen, M. Peltonen, L. Sjostrom, et al. Psychological aspects of eating behavior as predictors of 10-y weight changes after surgical and conventional treatment of severe obesity: Results from the Swedish Obese Subjects intervention study. *Am J Clin Nutr* 2015; **101**: 16–24.

85. E. Conceicao, M. Orcutt, J. Mitchell, et al. Eating disorders after bariatric surgery: A case series. *Int J Eat Disord* 2013; **46**: 274–9.

86. S. Sockalingam, S. E. Cassin, S. Wnuk, et al. A pilot study on telephone cognitive behavioral therapy for patients six-months post-bariatric surgery. *Obes Surg* 2017; **27**: 670–5.

87. T. A. Wadden, M. L. Butryn, D. B. Sarwer, et al. Comparison of psychosocial status in treatment-seeking women with class III vs. class I–II obesity. *Surg Obes Relat Dis* 2006; **2**: 138–45.

88. T. A. Wadden, M. L. Butryn, D. B. Sarwer, et al. Comparison of psychosocial status in treatment-seeking women with class III vs. class I–II obesity. *Obesity (Silver Spring)* 2006; **14**(Suppl. 2): 90S–98.

89. J. E. Wildes, M. A. Kalarchian, M. D. Marcus, et al. Childhood maltreatment and psychiatric morbidity in bariatric surgery candidates. *Obes Surg* 2008; **18**: 306–13.

90. M. M. Clark, B. K. Hanna, J. L. Mai, et al. Sexual abuse survivors and psychiatric hospitalization after bariatric surgery. *Obes Surg* 2007; **17**: 465–9.

91. S. Sockalingam, S. Cassin, S. A. Crawford, et al. Psychiatric predictors of surgery non-completion following suitability assessment for bariatric surgery. *Obes Surg* 2013; **23**: 205–11.

92. D. G. Ikossi, J. R. Maldonado, T. Hernandez-Boussard, et al. Post-traumatic stress disorder (PTSD) is not a contraindication to gastric bypass in veterans with morbid obesity. *Surg Endosc* 2010; **24**: 1892–7.

The Role of Psychosocial Interventions in Supporting Medical and Surgical Treatments for Severe Obesity

Stephanie Sogg, Molly E. Atwood, and Stephanie E. Cassin

Introduction

In this chapter, we discuss the rationale for using adjunctive psychosocial interventions to support medical and surgical treatments for obesity. We provide a broad overview of the psychosocial interventions addressed in subsequent sections of this book, including motivational interviewing, cognitive-behavioral therapies (CBTs), and mindfulness- and compassion-focused therapies. We then review the current state of the empirical literature on psychosocial interventions for individuals with severe obesity.

The Role of Adjunctive Psychosocial Interventions in Supporting Medical and Surgical Treatments for Severe Obesity

Severe obesity is a complex disease with a low rate of remission and high rate of relapse [1]. Contributing to the complexity of obesity and its resistance to treatment are the many psychosocial factors of relevance to the development and maintenance of this condition. Conversely, obesity itself may engender a number of psychosocial comorbidities and challenges. Accordingly, it is evident that there is a role for behavioral health providers in the multidisciplinary treatment of obesity across the spectrum of behavioral, pharmacologic, and surgical interventions. There are many ways in which behavioral health is relevant to obesity and its treatment. First, although by no means is it accurate to assume that all individuals with obesity experience some sort of psychopathology, rates of certain types of mental health issues, particularly depression and anxiety, as well as some eating disorder symptoms, are more prevalent among people with obesity than among those without obesity (see Chapter 1) [2]. In addition, the social stigma, decreased quality of life, and medical comorbidities associated with obesity may have significant psychosocial consequences (see Chapter 3) [3]. Further, certain psychosocial factors, including symptoms of psychopathology, may pose barriers to the efficacy or tolerability of various types of weight loss treatments, and psychosocial intervention may minimize these risks and challenges.

The role of the behavioral health provider in the treatment of obesity begins with the initial evaluation, with an assessment of any psychosocial factors, including, but not limited to, symptoms of psychopathology that may contribute to the patient's weight or have an impact on treatment planning and outcome. In the initial evaluation, the behavioral health clinician gathers the information necessary to contribute to the patient's overall treatment plan. Though there are some patients for whom few or no psychosocial contributors or concerns are identified, there are many important factors to consider that may represent targets for behavioral health intervention.

Eating Pathology

A thorough behavioral health assessment should include various forms of eating pathology, such as binge eating disorder (BED), night eating syndrome (NES), sleep-related eating disorder (SRED), eating as a means of coping with negative emotions, or engaging in unhealthy compensatory behaviors for the purposes of controlling weight (e.g., self-induced vomiting, excessive exercise, laxative abuse). Some of these eating patterns may be improved with specific psychotherapeutic approaches described in subsequent chapters in this book (e.g., motivational interviewing [see Chapters 5 and 6], cognitive-behavioral therapy [see Chapters 8 and 9], mindfulness-based interventions, and compassion-focused interventions [see Chapters 10 and 11]), and for some, there is evidence that psychopharmacologic treatments can also be effective [4].

Even in the absence of clinically significant eating disorders, other behavioral patterns may present concerns or pose barriers to weight loss treatment, such as lack of consistent physical activity, unregulated and unstructured or chaotic eating schedules, meal skipping or grazing, and/or a tendency to obtain many of one's meals outside the home secondary to a demanding schedule or a deficit in necessary planning or cooking skills. These types of behavioral issues are often quite amenable to behavioral health interventions such as psychoeducation, stimulus control, and/or behavioral problem solving (see Chapters 8 and 9). In some cases, other factors confer additional vulnerability to these types of behavioral patterns. For instance, chaotic or impulsive eating patterns may be related to impairments in executive functioning, including attention deficit disorder, which is highly comorbid with obesity [5]. Individuals with executive functioning impairments may benefit from interventions designed to mitigate or compensate for these deficits. Notably, stress can contribute to or exacerbate eating pathology [6] and can create a significant barrier to improving unhealthy or chaotic eating habits. The efficacy of weight loss treatment programs may be improved with the addition of stress-management interventions.

Psychosocial Factors

Non-eating-related psychosocial factors can also contribute to weight gain or impede the outcome of weight loss treatment; therefore, assessment for such symptoms is an important part of an interdisciplinary approach to weight loss. For instance, mood and anxiety symptoms may contribute to obesity directly or indirectly through their effects on eating, motivation, or ability to make use of weight loss treatment strategies. In addition, many of the medications used to treat these symptoms have weight-promoting properties, so it may be beneficial to consider the use of less weight-promoting alternatives when feasible. Individuals with mood or anxiety disorders may use eating as a strategy to cope with or regulate these symptoms and can benefit from developing alternative coping strategies (see Chapter 16). In addition, some individuals with a trauma history describe consciously or unconsciously maintaining a higher weight as a means of protection [7]; these patients may find themselves feeling more vulnerable when anticipating or achieving significant weight loss. Assessing for such a history and discussing the potential ramifications of weight loss with the patient before and during weight loss treatment may minimize this risk or help to address it if it does occur.

Conversely, anxiety and depression symptoms may arise as the result of the discouragement, decreased self-worth, and social stigma that can accompany obesity [8–10]. Weight bias and weight-related stigma are pervasive in today's culture [3], and for some individuals, particularly those who internalize weight-related stigma [11], this stigma can contribute significantly to eating pathology, depressed mood, and anxiety symptoms (see Chapter 3) [3,12].

Behavioral health providers working with patients who have obesity should assess for such symptoms and either refer or offer interventions for symptoms causing distress or impairment in functioning. At times, distress around body image can be severe and cause significant impairment. Though such impairment, when exclusively secondary to obesity, cannot strictly be diagnosed as body dysmorphic disorder (BDD) [13], the symptoms and maladaptive cognitive patterns closely resemble BDD and may respond to intervention with a treatment protocol designed for BDD. Effective CBT-oriented treatment protocols for BDD are available [14] and may be adapted for use with individuals with obesity and significant body image distress.

Motivation

Psychosocial interventions can also be helpful in the domain of motivation. Given that any weight loss approach requires significant and sustained behavioral change, which in itself can be difficult and effortful, maintaining adequate motivation over the long term is, understandably, a challenge for many patients. This phenomenon has been conceptualized as *behavioral fatigue* [15]. Specialized interventions designed to enhance and sustain motivation can be useful with patients undergoing weight loss treatment as a means either of preparing the patient to begin weight loss treatment or of helping patients to maintain efforts over the longer term. This motivational interviewing approach will be discussed further later in this chapter and illustrated in subsequent chapters in this book (see Chapters 5, 6, and 7).

Factors Relevant to Bariatric Surgery

In addition to the roles described earlier, which are broadly relevant to working with patients in medical and/or surgical obesity programs, behavioral healthcare providers can fulfill a number of important roles in the assessment and treatment of patients undergoing bariatric surgery. Bariatric surgery is currently the most effective and durable treatment for obesity, but postoperative weight trajectories are highly variable. Approximately 50 percent of patients experience some weight regain in the first two years [16], and 24 percent experience weight regain that is considerable relative to their overall weight loss by three years after surgery [17]. Moreover, weight regain is associated with recurrence of obesity-related comorbidities [18,19]. The high rates of weight regain may be attributed in part to the fact that medical and surgical treatments for severe obesity do not directly target psychosocial factors that potentially contribute to the development and maintenance of obesity.

Bariatric surgery tends to be provided within a multidisciplinary setting, and many programs include, or work in concert with, behavioral health providers. At the preoperative evaluation stage, the behavioral health clinician should assess factors relevant to the surgical treatment process, adjustment after surgery, and long-term surgical outcome. Such factors include all the domains described earlier, but with a specific focus on how they may influence the patient's readiness for surgery and psychosocial adjustment and weight loss outcome following surgery. The behavioral health clinician can use this information to develop an individualized treatment plan for the patient designed to improve the patient's readiness for surgery and/or minimize potential challenges to successful outcome. For instance, patients exhibiting pathologic or chaotic eating patterns may benefit from behavioral interventions, before and/or after surgery as needed, to lessen the risk of these patterns contributing to suboptimal weight loss outcome or poor postoperative psychosocial adjustment. The long-term postoperative behavioral regimen is complex and requires significant and sustained effort. Thus the provision of psychoeducation, as well as interventions to address motivational, problem solving, and adherence issues may be beneficial. Patients with mood or anxiety symptoms that impair their ability to engage in consistent self-care, healthy eating, physical activity, and attendance at postoperative appointments may require extra psychological preparation and/or postoperative monitoring and support to enhance long-term outcome.

New challenges may also present themselves after surgery. Increased risks for substance abuse, compulsive behaviors, and even suicide have been documented in postoperative bariatric populations [20,21], suggesting a crucial role for the behavioral health provider in long-term postoperative monitoring and the provision of appropriate referrals and/or interventions when necessary. For some bariatric patients, the preoperative psychosocial evaluation may be their first contact with a behavioral health provider. In addition to yielding information vital to treatment planning, the preoperative psychosocial assessment visit provides an opportunity to build rapport between the patient and the behavioral health provider, making it more likely that the patient will appropriately seek behavioral health support after surgery if such a need arises.

Behavioral health clinicians are the team members best suited to develop strategies for managing patients who present challenges to the treatment team or overuse limited clinical resources secondary to psychological issues such as personality pathology [22]. They can also assist in cases where there are questions regarding competency to provide informed consent. For patients with known or suspected intellectual impairment, they can make recommendations for ways to ensure that the clinic is providing the necessary education to the patient in a modality or at a level of complexity that enhances the patient's ability to comprehend and retain that information. Additionally, given their specialized experience and training in providing psychoeducational interventions, bariatric behavioral health providers can also provide valuable input in the development of patient education materials and support group content or curricula (see Chapter 13).

Overview of Adjunctive Psychosocial Interventions in Supporting Medical and Surgical Treatments for Severe Obesity

A number of adjunctive psychosocial interventions have been used in the management of severe obesity. Some of these interventions have been examined and found to be efficacious specifically in populations with severe obesity, whereas others have not yet been examined empirically in those with severe obesity but have been found to improve weight loss, eating behaviors, physical activity, treatment adherence (e.g., medication and vitamin adherence), medical conditions (e.g., diabetes, cardiac rehabilitation, hypertension, hyperlipidemia), and body image in other populations and thus may hold promise in those with severe obesity.

The transtheoretical model of change is helpful in conceptualizing how individuals change health-related behaviors [23,24] and can be an informative guiding framework in determining which psychosocial intervention may be helpful for a particular patient at a particular point in time. Change is conceptualized as a gradual process, divided into stages characterized by differing levels of readiness for change [23,24]. Individuals in the *precontemplation* stage may or may not be aware that a problem exists. For example, an individual with obesity may not be aware that his or her weight is associated with significant morbidity or mortality *or* may not feel ready to change eating behaviors or increase physical activity at the current time despite awareness of weight-related health risks. In any event, the possibility of change is not entertained. At this stage, information, rather than advice on behavioral change, is appropriate. Individuals in the *contemplation* stage are willing to examine an issue and consider the implications of change, but feelings of ambivalence may prevent them from making a commitment to take action. For example, an individual with obesity may be aware that his or her weight is contributing to medical issues and that weight loss would likely improve these medical issues, but a number of barriers may currently exist that make it difficult to improve eating behaviors and physical activity. In addition to receiving psychoeducation, individuals at this stage must resolve their ambivalence by weighing the advantages and disadvantages of change. This can lead to the *preparation* or *determination* stage, in which individuals express a desire for behavioral change but are uncertain of how to proceed. If requested by the individual, recommendations for change are appropriate during this stage. Individuals in the *action* stage have expressed a commitment to change and are actively engaged in making changes to overcome an issue. For example, an individual with obesity may follow a balanced meal plan recommended by a dietitian and start an exercise regimen. Because this may be a difficult and stressful period, encouragement, support, and coping skills are crucial. Individuals in the *maintenance* stage focus on maintaining their changes and preventing relapse. This stage is particularly important in the management of severe obesity given the low rates of remission and high rates of relapse [1]. It is important to note that these changes are seen to be circular rather than linear, in that individuals may move forward to stages of greater readiness or, at times, even backward [25]. *Relapse* is conceptualized as part of the natural behavior change process and necessitates the repetition of earlier stages of change. For example, an individual may begin to regain some weight as a result of not adhering to his or her meal plan or exercise plan and may need to return to the preparation stage to troubleshoot some of the barriers that arose and refine the action plan.

A key assumption of the transtheoretical model is that different *processes*, or activities that facilitate modification in thinking, behavior, or affect related to a problem, predominate at different stages of change [24,26]. Although some specific assumptions of the transtheoretical model have been challenged [27], the model does have treatment implications in that a mismatch between the clinician's chosen intervention and the patient's readiness for change may have unintended consequences [28]. For example, encouraging action too soon may lead to a therapeutic rupture if an individual is not yet considering change or may increase ambivalence if an individual is still contemplating whether or not to make a change. Conversely, it can be counterproductive to thoroughly examine ambivalence about change if an individual is already taking action. It is also important to note that an individual is not simply "motivated" or "unmotivated" – "ready" or "not ready" for change. Readiness for change is dynamic rather than static and specific rather than global. That is, readiness for change fluctuates over time and differs depending on the particular change in question. For example, an individual wanting to lose weight may already be taking action to modify his or her eating behaviors but not yet feel ready to increase physical activity. Accordingly, the psychosocial interventions delivered should be tailored, taking into consideration the issue(s) to be addressed and the patient's current readiness to address each of those issues.

Motivational Interviewing

The notion that the clinician's behavior can significantly influence the patient's readiness for change, implying that motivation arises from the patient-clinician interaction rather than residing solely within the patient, led to the development of motivational interviewing (MI) [29] (see Chapters 7, 8, and 9). Motivational interviewing is a therapeutic conversation about change that employs a nonjudgmental and nonconfrontational approach to enhance intrinsic motivation for, and commitment to, a specific goal [30]. A patient's readiness for change is hypothesized to stem from both the perceived importance of the change and the confidence the patient has about successfully making the change (i.e., self-efficacy) [31]. Motivational interviewing aims to increase the importance that the patient places on change by helping the patient reflect on how the problem impinges on his or her life and what his or her goals are. Rather than advocating for the need for change, the clinician emphasizes personal choice in making decisions and draws on cognitive-dissonance theory [32], making explicit the discrepancy between the patient's long-term goals and broader personal values and the restrictions imposed by his or her current behavior. The clinician then draws on self-perception theory [33], eliciting the patient's own concerns by subtly encouraging him or her to verbally present reasons for change. This process relocates the impetus for change from the clinician to within the patient himself or herself.

Ambivalence, which refers to simultaneously desiring two incompatible things, is a common experience among individuals contemplating change. When an individual feels ambivalent about a specific goal, he or she typically voices a combination of *change talk* (i.e., self-motivational statements that favor change) and *sustain talk* (i.e., statements that oppose change) within the same conversation [30]. Although sustain talk is often attributed to patient "resistance," it is a normal and understandable aspect of ambivalence [30]. If a clinician responds to sustain talk by lecturing about the importance of change, a patient who is feeling ambivalent is likely to defend the status quo. This, in turn, reduces the likelihood of behavioral change because people become more committed to their own statements or arguments [30]. Thus MI is directive and goal directed in the sense that it seeks to explore and resolve ambivalence by strategically facilitating conversations in which people talk *themselves* into change [30].

Motivational interviewing is not a technique per se but rather a style of conversation that uses a variety of therapeutic skills to bolster readiness for change [30]. It differs from many other evidence-based treatments in that it is not a protocol-driven intervention with an accompanying treatment manual. Rather, the spirit of MI is captured by four core skills subsumed under the acronym OARS [30]. *Open-ended questions* are asked frequently throughout the conversation in a curious and nonjudgmental manner to facilitate exploration and reflection. Moreover, they can be used selectively to help guide the conversation in the direction of change. Asking the patient to elaborate on the consequences of a current behavior or the potential benefits of changing that behavior, for example, can help to resolve ambivalence and promote behavioral change because people become more committed to their own statements. *Affirming statements* are used to highlight the patient's strengths and efforts in order to provide encouragement and reinforcement and to build confidence and self-efficacy. *Reflective listening* is used to check out whether the clinician's interpretation of the patient's message corresponds with the intended meaning. In addition to providing an opportunity for the patient to listen to his or her message articulated by another person, reflective listening can also guide the conversation by selectively highlighting certain aspects of what the patient has communicated, such as the consequences of a maladaptive behaviors or the benefits of changing that maladaptive behavior or statements that the patient has made expressing the need for or commitment to change a behavior. *Summarizing* is used periodically to integrate some key points that the patient has articulated regarding his or her motivation, commitment, or plan for change and feed them back to the patient. As with open-ended questions and reflective listening, the clinician can guide the conversation by selectively choosing which points to summarize. For example, a clinician may choose to summarize the patient's reasons for needing to change and statements regarding his or her intention to change as a transition into planning for change or soliciting a commitment to take action ("So, what do you think you'll do?") [30].

Motivational interviewing is intended to guide patients through four fundamental processes leading to change – engaging, focusing, evoking, and planning [30]. During *engagement*, the clinician's goal is to develop a strong therapeutic alliance, which is essential prior to proceeding with all other processes in MI. The clinician uses the core MI skills (OARS) to thoroughly understand the patient's perspective, including both sides of his or her ambivalence, without an agenda. *Focusing* is then used to guide the direction of the conversation by helping the patient to identify an issue or behavior that he or she is feeling ambivalent about changing. Next, *evoking* is used to foster the patient's intrinsic motivation for change by eliciting his or her own reasons for change and ideas regarding the specific changes to make. The clinician listens attentively for change talk and selectively reinforces it using reflective listening, affirming, and summary statements. Finally, the conversation proceeds to *planning* for change. The clinician's goal is to foster commitment to change and work with the patient to formulate a concrete action plan. The clinician asks key questions to assess the patient's readiness to transition to this final phase of developing a plan for change and then subsequently works with the patient to develop a concrete action plan with a focus on eliciting the patient's own ideas and solutions [30]. The clinician may provide information or advice if asked or given permission by the patient, but the patient is free to choose what to do with that information [30].

Motivational interviewing was not specifically developed in response to the transtheoretical model of change, but there is some conceptual overlap, and they are compatible with one another [30]. The transtheoretical model proposes that individuals progress sequentially through different stages of change from precontemplation to maintenance and that different processes of change predominate at each stage [23,24]. Motivational interviewing is used to guide the patient through four different processes of change – engaging, focusing, evoking, planning – and these processes must occur in sequence [30]. That is, engaging is a prerequisite for MI, and planning should not occur unless the therapeutic alliance has been established, a specific issue identified, and intrinsic motivation for change elicited. The time spent on each process will differ for each patient. For example, more time will need to be spent engaging with a patient who is not yet contemplating change, and the conversation may not progress beyond that stage. In contrast, another patient may have a clear idea of what he or she needs to change and already have some ideas about how to change the behavior, in which case the conversation can proceed almost directly from engaging to planning. Given that MI is not a technique per se but rather a style of conversation or a way of working with a patient, it lends itself well to being combined with other evidence-based treatments [30]. However, it has been used as a stand-alone single-session intervention and a multisession intervention to promote engagement and enhance motivation prior to commencing an action-oriented treatment (e.g., behavioral or cognitive-behavioral therapies) and to address nonadherence issues and resolve ambivalence that may arise during the course of other treatments. As mentioned, MI is not a technique or manualized treatment protocol, but many strategies are used to guide the patient through these different processes. The reader is referred to Miller and Rollnick [30] for excellent descriptions of MI strategies and illustrative dialogues.

In the management of severe obesity, MI may be helpful in raising the topic of a patient's weight if it is posing a medical concern, providing personalized feedback regarding a patient's weight or obesity-related comorbidities, and providing psychoeducation regarding weight regulation or obesity-related comorbidities in a way that minimizes the risk of eliciting shame or defensiveness. Moreover, it may be helpful in preparing patients for medical or surgical treatments for obesity, resolving ambivalence about changing certain behaviors (e.g., increasing physical activity, improving eating behaviors, decreasing disordered eating, increasing treatment adherence), enhancing self-efficacy for change, and increasing adherence with treatment plans. Section 2 of this book goes into greater depth on MI for specific issues relevant to severe obesity, including behavioral and lifestyle changes, disordered eating, and medication and vitamin adherence.

Cognitive and Behavioral Therapies

Cognitive-behavioral therapy (CBT) is a short-term (typically 20 or fewer sessions) collaborative, skills-focused treatment that aims to teach a patient to "become his or her own therapist" (see Chapters 8 and 9). It is based on the theory that cognitions, emotions, and behaviors are all interconnected [34]. That is, the way a person interprets or appraises a situation dictates his or her emotional responses, which, in turn, influence behavioral responses. According to the principles of operant conditioning, behaviors that are positively reinforcing (e.g., increase pleasurable states) or negatively reinforcing (e.g., reduce aversive states) will be repeated. These relationships are bidirectional such that the behavioral responses also have an impact on cognitions and emotions, potentially creating a destructive feedback cycle [34]. For example, in response to being weighed at a medical weight loss program, an individual with severe obesity may have the thought, "I will never lose weight no matter what I try" or "I have so much weight to lose that nothing I do will ever make much of a difference." These automatic thoughts may lead to feelings of hopelessness, pessimism, frustration, shame, and depression. These emotions may, in turn, lead to behaviors such as social withdrawal, avoidance of activities (e.g., choosing sedentary behaviors over physical activity), and disordered eating (e.g., binge eating, emotional overeating), and these maladaptive behaviors will likely be repeated because they are rewarding in the short term (e.g., relaxing sedentary activities feel more comforting or rewarding than physical activity, binge eating and emotional overeating momentarily increase pleasure and numb negative emotions). Given that cognitions, emotions, and behaviors are interconnected, the result is essentially a self-fulfilling prophecy: binge eating, emotional overeating, and sedentary behaviors may lead to further weight gain, providing evidence to support self-defeating cognitions such as "I will never lose weight" and further intensifying negative emotions [35].

The aim of CBT is essentially to disrupt this feedback cycle. Cognitive-behavioral therapy is present focused [34]. That is, it focuses on the factors that currently maintain maladaptive thoughts and behaviors rather than the factors that contributed to their initial onset. A personalized CBT conceptualization is developed in collaboration with the patient, and treatment focuses on teaching specific cognitive and behavioral coping strategies that target the factors maintaining the current maladaptive cognitions and behaviors [34] (see Figure 8.1). Each session begins by collaboratively setting an agenda for the session, which typically consists of a brief check-in, reviewing homework from the previous session, introducing a new coping skill and applying the skill in session, and collaboratively setting new homework to practice the skill and generalize learning to the patient's environment [34]. Homework completion is a predictor of treatment outcome and thus is considered an integral component of CBT [34].

According to the CBT formulation, distorted thoughts (*cognitive distortions*) are at the root of psychopathology [34] (see Chapter 8). A few select examples of cognitive distortions include all-or-nothing thinking ("I've *totally* blown my diet, so I might as well really overdo it"), overgeneralization ("I *always* gain weight"), fortune-telling errors ("I will not be able to keep the weight off"), *should* statements ("I *should* have reached my goal weight by now"), and mind reading ("Everyone is judging me"). The goal is to reduce the strength of conviction from an absolute "truth" to a belief that can be tested and challenged.

It is important to note that cognitive distortions are not entirely "distorted." In fact, they often have some evidence to support them. It is understandable why an individual with severe obesity who has experienced many occurrences of weight-based stigma and discrimination and who has a long history of yoyo dieting with an increasing weight trajectory might have the thoughts just described. Cognitive-behavioral therapy uses cognitive restructuring techniques to examine the evidence both for and against automatic thoughts and to replace maladaptive or counterproductive thoughts with more neutral or adaptive thoughts (e.g., "I've eaten some unhealthy foods, but that doesn't mean I've totally blown my diet"; "Some people are judgmental, but the people who matter to me the most are not judging me"; "Although I haven't reached my goal weight yet, I have made some improvements to my health and I'm doing my best to continue eating better and exercising more") [34].

In addition to cognitive restructuring, clinical guidelines for the management of obesity recommend that the following cognitive and behavioral components be included in interventions: goal setting, self-monitoring (e.g., recording food consumption, physical activity, and weight), planned and structured eating, physical activity, stimulus control (e.g., strategies designed to reduce the temptation to overeat or to be sedentary), problem solving, assertiveness, relapse prevention, and strategies for dealing with weight regain [36]. Treatments that focus on behavioral strategies to promote weight loss and health behaviors in the absence of cognitive strategies are typically referred to as *behavioral lifestyle interventions*.

In the management of severe obesity, CBT may be helpful in improving behaviors and cognitions implicated in the maintenance of obesity. Specifically, it may be helpful in improving eating behaviors, physical activity, and body image, which can have benefits for both physical and psychological functioning. Moreover, with its explicit focus on relapse prevention, CBT may be helpful in maintaining behavioral and cognitive changes over time, helping to address the strong tendency for weight to be regained. Section 3 of this book goes into greater depth on CBT for specific issues relevant to severe obesity, including behavioral and lifestyle changes and disordered eating.

Mindfulness- and Compassion-Focused Therapies

Mindfulness refers to paying attention on purpose to one's experiences in the present moment with an attitude of curiosity and acceptance [37] (see Chapter 10). It is about paying attention to how things currently are as opposed to how they ideally should be. Mindfulness involves observing internal events, such as thoughts, feelings, urges, and bodily sensations, as they arise in the moment without evaluating them or trying to change their content, form, or frequency [37]. All of these internal experiences are observed as passing mental events, and as such, they do not need to be feared, avoided, terminated, distracted from, or ruminated about.

Most people spend a great deal of time in autopilot mode – ruminating about the past, worrying about the future, multitasking many competing demands, or engaging in activities while simultaneously being preoccupied with other thoughts [38]. The automatic thoughts and emotions that occur while in autopilot mode can trigger impulsive and unhelpful behaviors. For example, an individual may binge eat despite not feeling physically hungry as a conscious or unconscious strategy to avoid painful emotions [39]. Mindfulness practice involves taking a step back and learning to observe and describe an experience and to participate in that experience with full awareness [40]. Moreover, it involves approaching all experiences with a nonjudgmental stance and focusing on one thing in the moment [40]. As a result, regular practice of mindfulness is helpful in reducing reactivity to passing thoughts and emotions, thereby disrupting these autopilot tendencies and allowing people to consciously choose how to respond effectively when experiencing challenging situations or painful emotions [40].

Mindfulness training can be incorporated into individual psychotherapy sessions, but mindfulness interventions are often delivered in a multisession group format and may focus on a specific protocol, such as mindfulness-based stress reduction (MBSR) [41], mindfulness-based cognitive therapy (MBCT) [42], or mindfulness-based eating awareness training (MB-EAT) [43,44]. A number of mindfulness exercises are used to teach participants to focus on internal stimuli such as their own breath, bodily sensations, thoughts, or emotions or external stimuli such as sights, sounds, smells, tastes, or sensory experiences [41]. These include exercises such as mindful breathing, body-scan meditation, gentle yoga, and bringing mindful awareness to routine activities (e.g., walking, eating). Mindfulness is a skill that can only be cultivated with frequent practice; thus participants are expected to adopt a regular mindfulness practice outside of sessions.

Mindfulness can be used to cultivate self-acceptance [43] and is in fact a prominent component of compassion-focused interventions (see Chapter 11). True self-compassion requires the combination of three equally important core elements [45]. First, self-compassion requires *self-kindness* as opposed to self-judgment. Self-kindness involves being gentle and understanding with oneself when faced with failure, inadequacy, or suffering rather than becoming defeated, critical, or judgmental, which only serves to exacerbate painful emotions. Self-kindness involves showing oneself the same compassion, understanding, or kindness as one would show a close friend or loved one. Second, self-compassion requires appreciation of our *common humanity*, an acknowledgment that failure, inadequacy, and suffering are all part of the shared human experience, as opposed to feeling that these experiences are the burden of one individual to carry alone, leading to a sense of disconnection and isolation. Third, self-compassion requires *mindfulness* of negative thoughts and feelings, simply acknowledging and observing them as they are in the moment, without either overidentifying with them, leading to increased reactivity, or denying or dismissing them, leading to invalidation. Self-compassion–focused interventions include a number of guided meditations (e.g., compassionate body scan, loving-kindness meditation) and self-compassion exercises to foster self-kindness, a sense of common humanity, and mindfulness [45].

In the management of severe obesity, mindfulness- and compassion-focused interventions may be helpful in identifying hunger and satiety, reducing emotional eating and binge eating, reducing self-criticism, reducing pain, reducing stress, reducing depressive relapse, and improving self-acceptance and body image. In contrast to CBT, which focuses on identifying *cognitive distortions* and reframing the content of negative automatic thoughts, mindfulness- and compassion-focused interventions may be particularly helpful in managing or coping with thoughts that are not necessarily "distorted." For example, weight-based stigma and discrimination are unfortunately common experiences that contribute to negative body image, and attempting to challenge such thoughts may inadvertently lead to invalidation. In such cases, compassion-focused interventions may be helpful in acknowledging painful experiences, recognizing that many people experience obesity as well as weight-based stigma and discrimination, and treating oneself with compassion. Section 4 of this book goes into greater depth on mindfulness- and compassion-focused interventions relevant to severe obesity.

Empirical Literature on Psychosocial Interventions for Severe Obesity

This section reviews the current state of the empirical literature on psychosocial interventions used to support medical and surgical treatments for severe obesity. In some cases, there is a paucity of research examining the effectiveness and/or efficacy of the interventions specifically in populations with severe obesity (body mass index [BMI] > 40 kg/m^2). In such cases, the review of the empirical literature will be expanded to include psychosocial interventions for related issues, such as weight loss, health habits (e.g., physical activity), problematic and disordered eating behaviors, and body image disturbance.

Motivational Interviewing

Motivational Interviewing for Individuals with Severe Obesity. Although MI was initially developed to treat substance-use behaviors, in recent years it has received research attention as an intervention to help modify health behaviors such as dietary intake and physical activity and to promote weight loss. Most commonly, studies have developed and delivered adaptations of MI (AMI) for the problem of interest as opposed to pure MI interventions.

Armstrong and colleagues [46] conducted a meta-analysis of 11 randomized, controlled trials (RCTs) investigating the effectiveness of MI for reducing body weight in adults who were overweight or obese (mean BMI across studies ranged from 27 to 38 kg/m^2).

Motivational interviewing resulted in significantly greater reduction in body mass than control treatments (i.e., usual care, attention-matched control individuals; weighted mean difference of −1.47 kg). In studies reporting change in BMI, MI exhibited a greater, though nonsignificant, reduction of 0.25 kg/m^2 over and above those receiving control treatments. In studies that have reported significant weight loss, MI interventions are likely to be greater than six months in length and incorporate information regarding training in and fidelity to the intervention [46,47]. Most studies have not included assessment beyond posttreatment; thus there is limited knowledge regarding weight regain over time following MI.

Additional research supports the notion that MI delivered as an added component to a behavioral weight loss (BWL) intervention can enhance treatment adherence. For example, in a widely cited study, Smith and colleagues [48] demonstrated that incorporating MI into a BWL program significantly increased appointment attendance, completion of food diaries, and recording of blood glucose levels in a sample of 22 women with type 2 diabetes mellitus compared with BWL intervention alone. In addition, those in the MI group achieved significantly better glycemic control over the course of treatment. Similar results were obtained in a follow-up study, wherein 217 women who were overweight or obese and had type 2 diabetes were randomized to a BWL intervention plus either five sessions of MI or five sessions of an attention-matched control intervention [49]. The MI group also lost significantly more weight at 6- and 18-month follow-up than the control treatment group, and adherence to the BWL program was a strong predictor of weight loss. Several additional studies have reported comparable findings [50,51].

Recent research has also investigated the effectiveness of MI in promoting healthy eating and physical activity. In a review of 24 studies, Martins and McNeil [52] concluded that MI is effective in increasing patients' self-efficacy related to dietary choices and exercise, increasing physical activity, and increasing consumption of fruits and vegetables, both when delivered alone or in conjunction with other interventions, such as a BWL program. Although the majority of studies included in this review did not recruit overweight or obese samples, it appears that MI has a positive effect on changing behaviors associated with obesity [52].

Lastly, MI has also been applied to the treatment of eating disorders, given that many individuals with eating disorders are ambivalent about engaging in treatment and making behavioral changes. A single session of MI delivered prior to self-help treatment for binge eating has been shown to increase readiness to change, as well as confidence in the ability to control binge eating behavior in individuals with binge eating disorder [53]. Cassin and colleagues [54] also found that a single-session MI intervention plus a self-help handbook increased confidence in the ability to reduce binge eating at posttreatment compared with a control group consisting of self-help only. Those in the MI group reported greater improvement in binge eating, depressive symptoms, self-esteem, and quality of life at 16-week follow-up. In addition, a greater proportion ceased binge eating in the MI group (27.8 versus 11.1 percent) and no longer met diagnostic criteria for BED (87.0 versus 57.4 percent). Consistent with these findings, one systematic review concluded that despite limited evidence overall for the use of MI to treat eating disorders, promising findings have been observed specifically for BED and binge eating behaviors [55].

In summary, consistent with other psychosocial interventions for obesity, MI has been found to result in modest changes in weight, although it is currently unclear whether these changes are maintained long term. MI has been shown to increase adherence to other obesity interventions, as well as to promote positive change in health behaviors, including diet and physical activity. Lastly, MI has shown promise in increasing confidence and readiness to change problematic and disordered eating behaviors and may be a useful adjunct to available psychological treatments for disordered eating in order to increase actual behavior change.

Motivational Interviewing for Bariatric Surgery Patients. In the only published study of MI for bariatric patients, David and colleagues [56] randomized 51 patients at least four months after surgery to receive a single-session MI intervention either immediately or after a 12-week waitlist delay while continuing to receive routine bariatric aftercare. The intervention was tailored to address difficulty adhering to postoperative dietary guidelines. Immediately following treatment, patients reported significant improvements in readiness, confidence, and self-efficacy for change. In addition, significant improvements in binge eating symptomatology and visual analogue scale ratings of adherence to postoperative dietary guidelines were reported at 12-week follow-up. The MI group demonstrated significant improvement in confidence for change, adherence to dietary guidelines, and binge eating symptomatology over the 12-week follow-up period, whereas the waitlist control group did not. However, no significant differences between groups were found at that time point, possibly due to the small sample size in the pilot study.

Cognitive and Behavioral Therapies

Cognitive-Behavioral Therapy for Individuals with Severe Obesity. Cognitive-behavior therapy (CBT) is the most thoroughly studied psychological treatment for obesity. Multiple RCTs have examined the efficacy of CBT for weight loss in individuals with obesity. Overall, CBT has been shown to be more effective in reducing weight than waitlist control (WLC) [57,58] and usual-care control groups [59]. In addition, adding CBT to a dietetic and/or exercise intervention enhances weight loss outcomes compared with either treatment delivered alone [60–62]. When CBT has been compared with BWL interventions, the latter has been shown to result in superior effects on weight loss in the short term, but CBT produces superior results in the longer term [63].

Despite these apparent positive findings for CBT, a relatively small proportion of patients achieves clinically significant weight loss (i.e., 5 to 10 percent of initial weight). In addition, there are high rates of dropout, and weight loss is typically not sustained in the longer term, even when the minimization of weight regain is an explicit target of the intervention [64]. Yet, even in the absence of clinically significant and durable weight loss, there is evidence that CBT results in lasting improvements in psychological correlates of obesity, such as depression and self-esteem [62,65,66], health-related quality of life [57], and eating pathology, such as emotional eating and dietary restraint [59,62]. Cognitive-behavioral therapy has also been used successfully to treat negative body image in women with obesity [67].

It is well established that BED is associated with obesity. Indeed, approximately 30 percent of individuals with obesity seeking weight loss treatment [68,69] and between 10 and 27 percent of bariatric surgery candidates meet criteria for a diagnosis of BED [70–72]. Compared with individuals with obesity who do not have a comorbid eating disorder, those with comorbid BED exhibit elevated psychopathology, including anxiety, depression, low self-esteem, and poorer quality of life [73,74].

Several systematic reviews have found that CBT results in significantly greater reductions in binge eating frequency than WLC, BWL, and pharmacotherapy at both short- and the longer-term (i.e., one to two years) follow-up [75–77]. Binge eating remission rates following CBT typically range between 40 and 60 percent [78]. Despite a slight erosion of therapeutic effects in the longer term, remission rates remain high at four years following completion of treatment [79]. There appears to be no added benefit to the addition of pharmacotherapy to CBT in increasing binge eating remission rates [80,81] or in sequencing BWL following CBT in patients who do not respond to treatment [76].

With regard to the psychological features of BED, one review concluded that CBT results in improvements in anxiety, depression, self-esteem, interpersonal functioning, and overall quality of life [76]. In addition, CBT appears to result in significant improvements in concerns regarding body shape and weight, even in the absence of weight loss. Moreover, studies assessing outcomes up to one year after treatment have generally reported maintenance of changes in these variables [77].

Cognitive-behavioral therapy does not appear to result in significant weight loss in individuals with BED [82–84]. However, several studies have found that patients who are abstinent from binge eating at completion of CBT demonstrate superior and sustained weight loss up to one year after treatment compared with patients who do not achieve abstinence [83–86]. More specifically, patients who continue to binge eat following treatment also continue to gain weight, whereas patients who cease binge eating exhibit modest weight loss that is typically maintained over follow-up.

In sum, the literature regarding CBT for obesity suggests that this treatment results in durable improvements in problematic and disordered eating behaviors, as well as common psychological correlates of obesity. While CBT does produce modest weight loss immediately following treatment, these effects typically dissipate by longer-term follow-up. Given the modest impact on weight loss, research has recently started to examine the impact of CBT when used as an adjunct to surgical treatments for obesity.

Cognitive-Behavioral Therapy for Bariatric Surgery Patients. Positive outcomes following bariatric surgery depend, in part, on patients making substantial long-term behavioral and lifestyle changes and coping effectively with psychological stressors [87]. For a proportion of patients who experience suboptimal weight loss outcomes, contributing factors include nonadherence to postoperative dietary and physical activity guidelines, problematic and disordered eating patterns, and psychological difficulties such as depression and anxiety [88,89]. Consequently, interest in examining the effectiveness of CBT, delivered in either the pre- or postoperative period, has increased.

A small number of uncontrolled studies have demonstrated that CBT, when delivered to preoperative bariatric patients, results in significant reductions in binge eating behavior and eating disorder psychopathology, as well as improvements in depressive and anxiety symptoms and self-esteem [90,91]. In addition, one study found that patients who exhibited a positive response to CBT (i.e., cessation of binge eating behavior and binge eating symptomatology in the nonclinical range at posttreatment) lost significantly greater excess weight at both 6 and 12 months after surgery compared with patients who did not exhibit a positive response to CBT [92].

Compared with treatment as usual (TAU), CBT delivered preoperatively results in greater improvements in BMI, disordered eating behaviors (i.e., binge eating, emotional eating, uncontrolled eating), depression, and anxiety at posttreatment [93,94]. However, in one study, at one year after surgical follow-up, CBT was no longer superior to TAU [95]. Thus any superior effects of CBT relative to TAU in the preoperative period does not necessarily mean improved outcomes in the postoperative period.

Several preliminary studies have also examined the effectiveness of CBT for improving psychological factors and weight loss outcomes delivered in the postoperative period. For example, in a small pilot study, Beaulac and Sandre [96] delivered an eight-session CBT group intervention to 17 bariatric patients who were at least six weeks after surgery and who were experiencing psychosocial difficulties (e.g., poor mood). Results indicated a significant reduction in psychological and weight-related distress and perceived life difficulties that were maintained at three-month follow-up. Additional studies have demonstrated improvements in binge eating symptomatology (i.e., cognitions, emotions, behaviors), emotional eating, grazing, loss-of-control eating, and depressive and anxiety symptoms from pre- to posttreatment [97,98].

A small body of literature suggests that CBT aimed at increasing adherence to dietary and physical activity guidelines prior to surgery does not result in beneficial effects following surgery with respect to weight loss, adherence to dietary guidelines, or physical activity levels [99,100]. In a study conducted by Kalarchian and colleagues [101], CBT delivered during the postoperative period facilitated greater excess weight loss than WLC, and this difference was maintained up to 12 months after treatment. In addition, patients with the least amount of weight regain before receiving the intervention demonstrated superior weight loss. Greater baseline levels of depressive symptoms were also associated with greater excess weight loss in the intervention group only. Together this suggests that CBT might be most beneficial for postoperative patients with depressive symptoms and when delivered before substantial weight regain occurs [101].

Overall, the extant literature on the efficacy of CBT for bariatric surgery patients is in its infancy. However, the literature continues to develop as the role of psychosocial interventions in enhancing bariatric surgery outcomes is increasingly acknowledged. Larger RCTs are warranted to examine the impact of CBT on long-term bariatric surgery outcomes, including weight loss and psychosocial functioning. Although existing research suggests that CBT is most effective when delivered postoperatively, the literature would also benefit from a direct comparison of the effectiveness of a preoperative and postoperative CBT interventions [102].

Mindfulness- and Compassion-Focused Therapies

Mindfulness- and Compassion-Focused Therapies for Individuals with Severe Obesity. Interest in the application of mindfulness-based interventions for disordered and problematic eating behaviors has grown in recent years, and there are now several reviews summarizing this literature. For example, Katterman and colleagues [103] conducted a systematic review of 14 randomized, controlled and uncontrolled clinical trials examining the effectiveness of mindfulness in reducing binge eating and emotional eating. All studies reported a significant reduction in binge eating frequency from pre- to posttreatment, with effect sizes ranging from medium ($d = 0.43$) to large ($d = 2.08$). With respect to emotional eating, results were more equivocal, with effects ranging from small and nonsignificant ($d = 0.01$) to large and significant ($d = 0.94$). In studies that did not report a significant effect for emotional eating, participants reported low levels of emotional eating at baseline, suggesting that there was little room for improvement. Few studies compared a mindfulness-based intervention with a control or active treatment comparison group: of those that did, mindfulness was found to be superior to an assessment-only control condition in reducing binge eating and statistically equivalent to CBT. A notable strength of this review was the exclusion of studies where mindfulness was only one portion of a larger treatment protocol, which increases confidence in conclusions regarding the specific effectiveness of mindfulness in reducing problematic eating behaviors.

A second systematic review extended outcomes of interest to include *external eating*, defined as eating in response to external cues such as sight, taste, and smell [104]. Four of six studies reported a significant reduction in external eating following a mindfulness-based intervention, with effect sizes ranging from medium ($d = 0.53$) to large ($d = 0.70$). In interventions that did not result in significant improvement, mindfulness skills were delivered in one session or did not include exercises targeting mindful eating. Indeed, the most effective interventions for reducing problematic and disordered eating appear to be those that place specific emphasis on mindful eating, as opposed to more general mindfulness-based stress reduction [103–105].

Of note, only approximately two-thirds of studies included in the abovementioned reviews examined mindfulness interventions in individuals who were overweight or obese. However, a recent meta-analysis of 15 studies investigating the effectiveness of mindfulness-based interventions delivered specifically to adults who were overweight or obese reported comparable results for binge eating outcomes [106]. Furthermore, the majority of studies included across reviews have measured subclinical binge eating behavior in individuals without a diagnosis of BED. Relatively few studies have examined mindfulness-based interventions for individuals with obesity and comorbid BED, although those that have reported positive results.

For instance, Kristeller and Halett [107] reported a significant decrease in binge eating frequency from pretreatment ($M = 4.02$ per week) to posttreatment ($M = 1.57$) following a six-week mindfulness intervention. In a more recent study, Kristeller, Wolver, and Sheets [44] randomized 150 individuals who were overweight or obese (mean BMI = 40 kg/m^2; range 26 to 78 kg/m^2) to a mindfulness-based eating awareness training group (MB-EAT), a psychoeducational cognitive-behavioral intervention group (CBT), or a WLC group. Sixty-eight percent of those in the MB-EAT group no longer met criteria for BED by four-month follow-up compared with 46 percent in the CBT group and 36 percent in the WLC group; the difference between the two treatment groups was nonsignificant. A mindfulness intervention that incorporated self-compassion has also been shown to reduce binge eating severity, eating psychopathology, shame, and self-criticism in individuals who were overweight or obese and had comorbid BED [108].

With respect to weight outcomes, Katterman and colleagues [103] reported small and mostly non-significant effect sizes in their review. In the few studies that did report a significant reduction in weight, weight loss was a primary focus and outcome of the mindfulness-based intervention. O'Reilly and colleagues [104] also reported small and predominantly non-significant effect sizes (d ranged from 0.12 to 0.26), although 9 of 10 studies reviewed reported either modest weight loss or weight maintenance from pre- to posttreatment: the average reduction in body mass across studies was 4.5 kg. Comparable results were reported in a recent meta-analysis of studies that included only participants who were overweight or obese [106]. More specifically, across 15 studies, average weight loss from before to after intervention was 4.2 kg (range 0.0 to 12.0 kg). Changes in weight were sustained up to six months after treatment; no studies have determined maintenance of change beyond that time point. Taken together, it appears that mindfulness-based interventions are at least effective in preventing further weight gain, if not in facilitating weight loss. There is preliminary evidence to suggest that incorporating skills to foster self-compassion may bolster the effects of mindfulness-based interventions on weight loss [109], although this finding awaits replication.

Regardless of the impact on weight outcomes, similar to CBT, mindfulness-based interventions show promise in improving general psychopathology for individuals with obesity. For example, Rogers and colleagues [106] reported significant medium effects for depressive and anxiety symptoms from before to after treatment. However, the durability of gains beyond completion of treatment is currently unknown. Mindfulness-based interventions also result in significant improvements in body image concerns [110].

In sum, the available evidence suggests that mindfulness-based interventions are an effective treatment for binge eating, emotional eating, and external eating and exert positive effects on depression and anxiety. Mindfulness also shows promise in promoting weight maintenance. In general, the most significant findings have been obtained when mindfulness skills are designed to target eating behaviors or weight loss rather than general mindfulness-based stress reduction. Future research should examine the comparative efficacy of mindfulness-based approaches with other established obesity treatments. In general, the literature would also benefit from longer-term follow-up in order to establish maintenance of treatment gains.

Mindfulness- and Compassion-Focused Therapies for Bariatric Surgery Patients. Few published studies have examined mindfulness- or compassion-focused therapies for bariatric surgery patients. In one uncontrolled study, Leahey, Crowther, and Irwin [111] found that 10 weekly sessions of a cognitive-behavioral mindfulness intervention resulted in a reduction in binge eating and depressive symptoms and an increase in eating-related self-efficacy and emotional regulation. Overall, there was a small improvement in the percentage of weight loss patients achieved from before to after treatment. Although promising, these findings should be interpreted in light of the small sample size of seven patients and lack of a control group.

A more recent RCT compared a 10-week mindfulness intervention and a standard intervention (consisting of a one-hour individualized counseling session with a registered dietician) in 18 bariatric patients who were experiencing weight regain between one and five years after surgery [112]. There was a significant decrease in emotional eating at six-month follow-up favoring the mindfulness group. However, there was no significant change in binge eating, weight, BMI, or waist circumference from pretreatment to 12-week or 6-month follow-up in either treatment group.

In sum, research examining the effectiveness of mindfulness- and compassion-based therapies in bariatric surgery patients is still very much in its infancy. Published studies have been limited by very small sample sizes, and the findings have been mixed regarding the impact on weight and certain disordered eating behaviors. Well-designed RCTs with larger sample sizes are warranted to draw conclusions regarding the impact of mindfulness- and compassion-focused therapies in bariatric surgery patients.

Summary

Adjunctive psychosocial interventions have been used to increase motivation and promote adherence to medical and surgical treatments for severe obesity and to reduce psychopathology and problematic or disordered eating behavior that may impede the efficacy or tolerability of these treatments. In nonsurgical obese populations, research to date shows that psychosocial interventions typically result in modest reductions in weight in the short term, but weight loss is not necessarily maintained in the longer term. However, psychosocial interventions have been shown to increase confidence and readiness to change and have demonstrated actual reductions in disordered eating behaviors. Motivational interviewing in particular has also been shown to increase adherence to other obesity interventions, as well as to promote positive change in health behaviors, including diet and physical activity. In addition, positive effects on psychological correlates of obesity have been demonstrated, including reductions in depression and improvements in quality of life. A comparatively smaller body of literature suggests that psychosocial interventions may produce similar positive effects in bariatric surgery patients, although RCTs with larger sample sizes and longer follow-up are needed to draw firm conclusions.

Key Points

- For some individuals with severe obesity, psychiatric disorders and problematic or disordered eating behaviors make it difficult to initiate and adhere to medical and surgical treatments for obesity.
- Psychosocial interventions can directly address the psychosocial correlates of obesity and help promote adherence to medical or surgical interventions.
- The empirical literature on the efficacy of adjunctive psychosocial interventions suggests positive effects on eating behavior and psychosocial functioning. There is also evidence for modest short-term effects on weight loss.

References

1. K. B. Smith and M. A. Smith. Obesity statistics. *Prim Care* 2016; **43**: 121–35.

2. N. M. Petry, D. Barry, R. H. Pietrzak, and J. A. Wagner. Overweight and obesity are associated with psychiatric disorders: Results from the National Epidemiologic Survey on Alcohol and Related Conditions. *Psychosom Med* 2008; **70**: 288–97.

3. R. M. Puhl and C. A. Heuer. The stigma of obesity: A review and update. *Obesity* 2009; **17**: 941–64.

4. J. P. O'Reardon, K. C. Allison, N. S. Martino, et al. A randomized, placebo-controlled trial of sertraline in the treatment of night eating syndrome. *Am J Psychiatry* 2006; **163**: 893–98.

5. A. Raziel, N. Sakran, and D. Goitein. The relationship between attention deficit hyperactivity disorders (ADHD) and obesity. *Harefuah* 2014; **153**: 541–45.

6. J. R. W. Menzies, K. P. Skibicka, S. L. Dickson, and G. Leng. Neural substrates underlying interactions between appetite stress and reward. *Obes Facts* 2012; **5**: 208–20.

7. M. W. Wiederman, R. A. Sansone, and L. A. Sansone. Obesity among sexually abused women: An adaptive function for some? *Women's Health* 1999; **29**: 89–100.

8. K. C. Fettich and E. Y. Chen. Coping with obesity stigma affects depressed mood in African-American and white candidates for bariatric surgery. *Obesity* 2012; **20**: 1118–21.

9. K. E. Friedman, J. A. Ashmore, and K. L. Applegate. Recent experiences of weight-based stigmatization in a weight loss surgery population: psychological and behavioural correlates. *Obesity* 2008; **16**: S69–74.

10. K. E. Friedman, S. K. Reichmann, P. R. Costanzo, et al. Weight stigmatization and ideological beliefs: Relation to psychological functioning in obese adults. *Obes Res* 2005; **13**: 907–16.

11. R. A. Carels, J. Burmeister, M. W. Oehlhof, et al. Internalized weight bias: ratings of the self, normal weight, and obese individuals and psychological maladjustment. *J Behav Med* 2013; **36**: 86–94.

12. R. L. Pearl and R. M. Puhl. The distinct effects of internalizing weight bias: An experimental study. *Body Image* 2016; **17**: 38–42.

13. American Psychiatric Association (APA). *Diagnostic and Statistical Manual of Mental Disorders* (5th edn). Arlington, VA: American Psychiatric Publishing, 2013.

14. S. Wilhelm, K. Phillips, and G. Steketee. *Cognitive-Behavioural Therapy for Body Dysmorphic Disorder: A Treatment Manual.* New York, NY: Guilford Press, 2012.

15. T. A. Wadden, M. L. Butryn, and K. J. Byrne. Efficacy of lifestyle modification for long-term weight control. *Obes Res* 2004; **12**(Suppl.): 151S–62S.

16. D. O. Magro, B. Geloneze, R. Delfini, et al. Long-term weight regain after gastric bypass: A 5-year prospective study. *Obes Surg* 2008; **18**: 648–51.

17. A. P. Courcoulas, N. J. Christian, and S. H. Belle. Weight change and health outcomes at three years after bariatric surgery among individuals with severe obesity. *JAMA* 2013; **310**: 2416–25.

18. M. DiGiorgi, D. J. Rosen, J. J. Choi, et al. Re-emergence of diabetes after gastric bypass in patients with mid- to long-term follow-up. *Surg Obes Relat Dis* 2010; **6**: 249–53.

19. M. Shah, V. Simha, and A. Garg. Long term impact of bariatric surgery on body weight, comorbidities and nutritional status. *J Clin Endocrinol Metab* 2006; **91**: 4223–31.

20. O. Backman, D. Stockeld, F. Rasmussen, E. Naslund, and R. Marsk. Alcohol and substance abuse, depression and suicide attempts after Roux-en-Y gastric bypass surgery. *Br J Surg* 2016; **103**: 1336–42.

21. W. C. King, J-Y. Chen, J. E. Mitchell, et al. Prevalence of alcohol use disorders before and after bariatric surgery. *JAMA* 2012; **307**: 2516–25.

22. S. Sogg and K. E. Friedman. Getting off on the right foot: The many roles of the psychosocial evaluation in the bariatric surgery practice. *Eur Eat Disord Rev* 2015; **23**: 451–6.

23. J. O. Prochaska and C. C. DiClemente. The transtheoretical approach. In J. C. Norcross and I. L. Goldfield, eds., *Handbook of Psychotherapy Integration.* New York, NY: Basic Books, 1982: 300–34.

24. J. O. Prochaska and C. C. DiClemente. Stages and processes of self-change in smoking: Toward an integrative model of change. *J Consult Clin Psychol* 1983; **51**: 390–5.

25. J. O. Prochaska. Change at differing stages. In C. R. Snyder and R. E. Ingram, eds., *Handbook of Psychological Change.* New York, NY: Wiley, 2000: 109–27.

26. S. Sutton. Can "stages of change" provide guidance in the treatment of addictions? A critical example of Prochaska and DiClemente's model. In G. Edwards and C. Dare, eds., *Psychotherapy, Psychological Treatments, and the Addictions.* Cambridge, Cambridge University Press, 1996.

27. G. T. Wilson and T. R. Schlam. The transtheoretical model and motivational interviewing in the treatment of eating and weight disorders. *Clin Psychol Rev* 2004; **24**: 361–78.

28. S. Rollnick, P. Kinnersley, and N. Stott. Methods of helping patients with behaviour change. *BMJ* 1993; **307**: 188–90.

29. W. R. Miller and S. Rollnick. *Motivational Interviewing: Preparing People to Change Addictive Behaviours.* New York, NY: Guilford Press, 1991.

30. W. R. Miller and S. Rollnick. *Motivational Interviewing: Helping People Change* (3rd edn). New York, NY: Guilford Press, 2013.

31. B. L. Burke, H. Arkowitz, and M. Menchola. The efficacy of motivational interviewing: A meta-analysis of controlled clinical trials. *J Consult Clin Psychol* 2003; **71**: 843–61.

32. L. Festinger. *A Theory of Cognitive Dissonance.* Stanford, CA: Stanford University Press, 1957.

33. D. J. Bem. Self-perception: An alternative interpretation of cognitive dissonance phenomena. *Psychol Rev* 1967; **74**: 183–200.

34. J. S. Beck. *Cognitive Behaviour Therapy: Basics and Beyond* (2nd edn). New York, NY: Guilford, 2011.

35. S. E. Cassin, S. Sockalingham, S. Wnuk, et al. Cognitive behavioural therapy for bariatric surgery patients: Preliminary evidence for feasibility, acceptability, and effectiveness. *Cog Behav Pract* 2013; **20**: 529–43.

36. National Institute for Health and Clinical Excellence. *Obesity: Guidance on the Prevention, Identification, Assessment, and Management of Overweight and Obesity in Adults and Children* (NICE Clinical Guideline 43). London: NICE, 2006.

37. J. Kabat-Zinn. *Wherever You Go, There You Are: Mindfulness Meditation in Everyday Life*. New York, NY: Hyperion, 1994.

38. M. Williams, J. Teasdale, Z. Segal, and J. Kabat-Zinn. *The Mindful Way through Depression*. New York, NY: Guilford Press, 2007.

39. T. F. Heatherton and R. F. Baumeister. Binge eating as escape from self-awareness. *Psychol Bull* 1991; **110**: 86–108.

40. M. Linehan. *Skills Training Manual for Treating Borderline Personality Disorder*. New York, NY: Guilford Press, 1993.

41. J. Kabat-Zinn. *Full Catastrophe Living: Using the Wisdom of Your Body and Mind to Face Stress, Pain, and Illness*. New York, NY: Delacorte, 1990.

42. Z. Segal, M. Williams, and J. Teasdale. *Mindfulness-Based Cognitive Therapy for Depression*. New York, NY: Guilford Press, 2002.

43. J. L. Kristeller and R. Q. Wolever. Mindfulness-based eating awareness training for treating binge eating disorder: The conceptual foundation. *Eat Disord* 2011; **19**: 49–61.

44. J. L. Kristeller, R. Q. Wolever, and V. Sheets. Mindfulness-based eating awareness training (MB-EAT) for binge eating: A randomized clinical trial. *Mindfulness* 2014; **5**: 282–97.

45. K. Neff. *Self-Compassion: The Proven Power of Being Kind to Yourself*. New York, NY: Harper Collins, 2011.

46. M. J. Armstrong, T. A. Mottershead, P. E. Ronksley, et al. Motivational interviewing to improve weight loss in overweight and/or obese patients: A systematic review and meta-analysis of randomized controlled trials. *Obes Rev* 2011; **12**: 709–23.

47. R. D. Barnes and V. Ivezaj. A systematic review of motivational interviewing for weight loss among adults in primary care. *Obes Rev* 2015; **16**: 304–18.

48. D. E. Smith, C. M. Heckmeyer, P. P. Kratt, and D. A. Mason. Motivational interviewing to improve adherence to a behavioural weight-control program for older obese women with NIDDM: A pilot study. *Diabetes Care* 1997; **20**: 52–54.

49. D. S. West, V. DiLillo, Z. Bursac, S. A. Gore, and P. G. Greene. Motivational interviewing improves weight loss in women with type 2 diabetes. *Diabetes Care* 2007; **30**: 1081–7.

50. I. D. DiMarco, D. A. Klein, V. L. Clark, and G. T. Wilson. The use of motivational interviewing techniques to enhance the efficacy of guided self-help behavioural weight loss treatment. *Eat Behav* 2009; **10**: 134–6.

51. V. DiLillo, N. J. Siegfried, and D. West. Incorporating motivational interviewing into behavioural obesity treatment. *Cogn Behav Pract* 2003; **10**: 120–30.

52. R. K. Martins and D. W. McNeil. Review of motivational interviewing in promoting health behaviours. *Clin Psychol Rev* 2009; **29**: 283–93.

53. R. A. Vella-Zarb, J. S. Mills, H. A. Westra, J. C. Carter, and L. Keating. A randomized controlled trial of motivational interviewing plus self-help versus psychoeducation plus self-help for binge eating. *Int J Eat Disord* 2015; **48**: 328–32.

54. S. E. Cassin, K. M. von Ranson, K. Heng, J. Brar, and A. E. Wojtowicz. Adapted motivational interviewing for women with

binge eating disorder: A randomized controlled trial. *Psychol Addict Behav* 2008; **22**: 417–25.

55. L. Knowles, A. Anokhina, and L. Serpell. Motivational interventions in the eating disorders: What is the evidence? *Int J Eat Disord* 2013; **46**: 97–107.

56. L. A. David, S. Sockalingham, S. Wnuk, and S. E. Cassin. A pilot randomized controlled trial examining the feasibility, acceptability, and efficacy of adapted motivational interviewing for post-operative bariatric surgery patients. *Eat Behav* 2016; **22**: 87–92.

57. G. Marchesini, S. Natale, S. Chierici, et al. Effects of cognitive-behavioural therapy on health-related quality of life in obese subjects with and without binge eating disorder. *Int J Obes* 2002; **26**: 1261–7.

58. L. Stahre and T. Hällström. A short-term cognitive group treatment program gives substantial weight reduction up to 18 months from the end of treatment: A randomized controlled trial. *Eat Weight Disord* 2005; **10**: 51–8.

59. S. Munsch, E. Biedert, and U. Keller. Evaluation of a lifestyle change programme for the treatment of obesity in general practice. *Swiss Med Wkly* 2003; **133**: 148–54.

60. K. Dennis, K. Pane, B. Adams, and Q. Bing Bing. The impact of a shipboard weight control program. *Obes Res* 1999; **7**: 60–67.

61. D. Painot, S. Jotterand, A. Kammer, M. Fossati, and A. Golay. Simultaneous nutritional cognitive-behavioural therapy in obese patients. *Patient Educ Couns* 2001; **42**: 47–52.

62. M. Q. Werrij, A. Jansen, S. Mulkens, et al. Adding cognitive therapy to dietetic treatment is associated with less relapse in obesity. *J Psychosom Res* 2009; **67**: 315–24.

63. T. Sbrocco, R. Nedegaard, J. Stone, and E. Lewis. Behavioural choice treatment promotes continuing weight loss: Preliminary results of a cognitive-behavioural decision-based treatment for obesity. *J Consult Clin Psychol* 1999; **67**: 260–6.

64. Z. Cooper, H. A. Doll, and D. M. Hawker. Testing a new cognitive behavioural treatment for obesity: A randomized controlled trial with three-year follow-up. *Behav Res Ther* 2010; **48**: 706–13.

65. H. Nauta, H. Hospers, G. Kok, and A. Jansen. A comparison between a cognitive and a behavioural treatment for obese binge eaters and obese non-binge eaters. *Behav Ther* 2000; **31**: 441–61.

66. G. Nauta, H. Hospers, and A. Jansen. One-year follow-up effects of two obesity treatment on psychological well-being and weight. *Br J Health Psychol* 2001; **6**: 271–84.

67. J. C. Rosen, P. Orosan, and J. Rieter. Cognitive behaviour therapy for negative body image in obese women. *Behav Ther* 1995; **26**: 25–42.

68. R. L. Spitzer, S. Yanovski, T. Wadden, et al. Binge eating disorder: Its further validation in a multisite study. *Int J Eat Disord* 1993; **13**: 137–53.

69. R. H. Striegel-Moore, and D. L. Franko. Epidemiology of binge eating disorder. *Int J Eat Disord* 2003; **34**: S19–29.

70. M. A. Kalarchian, M. D. Marcus, M. D., Levine, et al. Psychiatric disorders among bariatric surgery candidates: Relationship to obesity and functional health status. *Am J Psychiatry* 2007; **164**: 328–34.

71. R. J. Marek, Y. S. Ben-Porath, A. Windover, et al. Assessing psychosocial functioning of bariatric surgery candidates with the Minnesota Multiphasic Personality Inventory-2 Restructured Form (MMPI-2-RF). *Obes Surg* 2013; **23**: 1864–73.

72. J. E. Mitchell, F. Selzer, M. A. Kalarchian, et al. Psychopathology before surgery in the Longitudinal Assessment of Bariatric Surgery-3 (LABS-3) psychosocial study. *Surg Obes Relat Dis* 2012; **8**: 533–41.

73. C. F. Telch and E. Stice. Psychiatric comorbidity in women with binge eating disorder: Prevalence rates from a non–treatment seeking sample. *J Consult Clin Psychol* 1998; **66**: 768–76.

74. G. Marchesini, E. Solaroli, L. Baraldi, et al. Health–related quality of life in obesity:

The role of eating behaviour. *Diabetes Nutr Metab* 2000; **13**: 156–64.

75. K. A. Brownley, N. D. Berkman, J. A. Sedway, et al. Binge eating disorder treatment: A systematic review of randomized controlled trials. *Int J Eat Disord* 2007; **40**: 337–48.

76. M. Duchesne, J. C. Appolinario, B. P. Range, et al. Evidence of cognitive-behavioural therapy in the treatment of obese patients with binge eating disorder. *Rev psiquiatr Rio Gd Sul* 2007; **29**: 80–92.

77. J. M. Iacovino, D. M. Gredysa, M. Altman, and D. E. Wilfley. Psychological treatment for binge eating disorder. *Curr Psychiatry Rep* 2012; **14**: 432–46.

78. G. T. Wilson, C. M. Grilo, and K. M. Vitousek. Psychological treatments of eating disorders. *Am Psychol* 2007; **62**: 199–216.

79. A. Hilbert, M. E. Bishop, R. I. Stein, et al. Long-term efficacy of psychological treatment for binge eating disorder. *Br J Psychiatry* 2012; **200**: 232–7.

80. C. M. Grilo and R. M. Masheb. A randomized controlled comparison of guided self-help cognitive behavioural therapy and behavioural weight loss for binge eating disorder. *Behav Res Ther* 2005; **43**: 1509–25.

81. V. Ricca, E. Mannucci, B. Mezzani, et al. Fluoxetine and fluvoxamine combined with individual cognitive-behaviour therapy in binge eating disorder: A one-year follow-up study. *Psychother Psychosom* 2001; **70**: 298–306.

82. W. S. Agras, C. F. Telch, B. Arnow, et al. Does interpersonal therapy help patients with binge eating disorder who fail to respond to cognitive-behavioural therapy? *J Consult Clin Psychol* 1995; **63**: 356–60.

83. C. M. Grilo, R. M. Masheb, and G. T. Wilson. Efficacy of cognitive-behavioural therapy and fluoxetine for the treatment of binge eating disorder: A randomized double-blind placebo-controlled comparison. *Biol Psychiatry* 2005; **57**: 301–9.

84. D. E. Wilfley, R. R. Welch, R. I. Stein, et al. A randomized comparison of group cognitive-behavioural therapy and group interpersonal psychotherapy for the treatment of overweight individuals with binge-eating disorder. *Arch Gen Psychiatry* 2002; **59**: 713–21.

85. W. S. Agras, C. F. Telch, B. Arnow, et al. One-year follow–up of cognitive-behavioural therapy for obese individuals with binge eating disorder. *J Consult Clin Psychol* 1997; **65**: 343–7.

86. M. J. Devlin, J. A. Goldfein, E. Petkova, et al. Cognitive behavioural therapy and fluoxetine as adjuncts to group behavioural therapy for binge eating disorder. *Obes Res* 2005; **13**: 1077–88.

87. B. K. Wolnerhanssen, T. Peters, B. Kern, et al. Predictors of outcome in treatment of morbid obesity by laparoscopic adjustable gastric banding: Results of a prospective study of 380 patients. *Surg Obes Relat Dis* 2008; **4**: 500–6.

88. M. A. Kalarchian, G. T. Wilson, R. E. Brolin, and E. Bradley. Effects of bariatric surgery on binge eating and related psychopathology. *Eat Weight Disord* 1999; **4**: 1–5.

89. P. C. Sallet, J. A. Sallet, J. B. Dixon, et al. Eating behaviour as a prognostic factor for weight loss after gastric bypass. *Obes Surg* 2007; **17**: 445–51.

90. V. Abiles, S. Rodriguez-Ruis, J. Abiles, et al. Effectiveness of cognitive-behavioural therapy in morbidity obese candidates for bariatric surgery with and without binge eating disorder. *Nutricion Hospital* 2013; **28**: 1523–9.

91. K. Ashton, M. Drerup, A. Windover, et al. Brief, four-session group CBT reduces binge eating behaviours among bariatric surgery candidates. *Surg Obes Relat Dis* 2009; **5**: 257–62.

92. K. Ashton, L. Heinberg, A. Windover, et al. Positive response to binge eating intervention enhances postoperative weight loss. *Surg Obes Relat Dis* 2011; **7**: 315–20.

93. S. E. Cassin, S. Sockalingam, C. Du, et al. A pilot randomized controlled trial of

telephone-based cognitive behavioural therapy for preoperative bariatric surgery patients. *Behav Res Ther* 2016; **80:** 17–22.

94. H. Gade, J. Hjelmesæth, J. H. Rosenvinge, and O. Friborg. Effectiveness of a cognitive behavioural therapy for dysfunctional eating among patients admitted for bariatric surgery: A randomized controlled trial. *J Obes* 2014; **21:** 127–36.

95. H. Gade, O. Friborg, J. H. Rosenvinge, M. C. Smastuen, and J. Hjelmesæth. The impact of a preoperative cognitive behavioural therapy (CBT) on dysfunctional eating behaviours, affective symptoms and body weight one year after bariatric surgery: A randomized controlled trial. *Obes Surg* 2015; **25:** 2112–19.

96. J. Beaulac and D. Sandre. The impact of a CBT psychotherapy group on post-operative bariatric patients. *SpringerPlus* 2015; **4:** 764–77.

97. S. M. Himes, K. B. Grothe, M. M. Clark, et al. Stop regain: A pilot psychological intervention for bariatric patients experiencing weight regain. *Obes Surg* 2015; **25:** 922–7.

98. S. Sockalingam, S. E. Cassin, S. Wnuk, et al. A pilot study on telephone cognitive behavioural therapy for patients six-months post-bariatric surgery. *Obes Surg* 2016; **27:** 1–6.

99. M. A. Kalarchian, M. D. Marcus, A. P. Courcoulas, Y. Cheng, and M. D. Levine. Preoperative lifestyle intervention in bariatric surgery: A randomized clinical trial. *Surg Obes Relat Dis* 2015; **12:** 180–7.

100. H. O. Lier, E. Biringer, B. Stubhaug, and T. Tangen. The impact of preoperative counseling on postoperative adherence in bariatric surgery patients: A randomized controlled trial. *Patient Educ Couns* 2012; **87:** 336–42.

101. M. A. Kalarchian, M. D. Marcus, A. P. Courcoulas, et al. Optimizing long-term weight control after bariatric surgery: A pilot study. *Surg Obes Relat Dis* 2012; **8:** 710–16.

102. M. A. Kalarchian and M. D. Marcus. Psychosocial interventions pre and post bariatric surgery. *Eur Eat Disord Rev* 2015; **23:** 457–62.

103. S. N. Katterman, B. M. Kleinman, M. M. Hood, L. M. Nackers, and J. A. Corsica. Mindfulness meditation as an intervention for binge eating, emotional eating, and weight loss: A systematic review. *Eat Behav* 2014; **15:** 197–204.

104. G. A. O'Reilly, L. Cook, D. Spruijt-Metz, and D. S. Black. Mindfulness-based interventions for obesity-related eating behaviours: A literature review. *Obes Rev* 2014; **15:** 453–61.

105. M. Mantzios and J. C. Wilson. Mindfulness, eating behaviours, and obesity: A review and reflection on current findings. *Curr Obes Rep* 2015; **4:** 141–6.

106. J. M. Rogers, M. Ferrari, K. Mosely, C. P. Lang, and L. Brennan. Mindfulness-based interventions for adults who are overweight or obese: A meta-analysis of physical and psychological health outcomes. *Obes Rev* 2016; **18:** 51–67.

107. J. L. Kristeller and C. B. Hallett. An exploratory study of a meditation-based intervention for binge eating disorder. *J Health Psychol* 1999; **4:** 357–63.

108. J. Pinto-Gouveia, S. A. Carvalho, L. Palmeira, et al. Incorporating psychoeducation, mindfulness and self-compassion in a new programme for binge eating (BEfree): Exploring processes of change. *J Health Psychol* 2016; 1–14.

109. M. Mantzios and J. C. Wilson. Exploring mindfulness and mindfulness with self-compassion-centered interventions to assist weight loss: Theoretical considerations and preliminary results of a randomized pilot study. *Mindfulness* 2015; **6:** 824–35.

110. H. J. E. M. Alberts, R. Thewissen, and L. Raes. Dealing with problematic eating behaviour: The effects of a mindfulness-based intervention on

eating behaviour, food craving, dichotomous thinking and body image concern. *Appetite* 2012; **58**: 847–51.

111. T. M. Leahey, J. H. Crowther, and S. R. Irwin. A cognitive-behavioural mindfulness group therapy intervention for the treatment of binge eating in bariatric surgery patients. *Cog Behav Pract* 2008; **15**: 364–75.

112. S. A. Chacho, G. Y. Yeh, R. B. Davis, and C. C. Wee. A mindfulness-based intervention to control weight after bariatric surgery: Preliminary results from a randomized controlled pilot trial. *Compliment Ther Med* 2016; **28**: 13–21.

Weight Stigma and Related Social Factors in Psychological Care

Paula M. Brochu, Rebecca L. Pearl, and Laurie A. Simontacchi

Case Vignette

Susan is a 55-year-old white woman with a body mass index (BMI) of 41 kg/m². She takes medication daily to control her hypertension and was recently diagnosed with sleep apnea. Susan works full time as an office manager for a computer software company. She is married with two children, and she recently became a grandmother.

Susan reports that she first identified herself as "overweight" at age 10 years. She describes being teased by peers because of her weight, and she felt pressured by her mother to begin dieting at age 12 years. As a teenager, Susan engaged in unhealthy dieting practices, such as overrestricting her food intake during the day. As a result, she would often lose control of her eating in the evening and eat large portions of food until she felt uncomfortably full.

As an adult, Susan has experienced significant weight fluctuations. She attributes her weight gain to her two pregnancies and the stress of being a working mother. Susan identifies as an "emotional eater" and will often eat to cope with stress. She describes having tried more than 10 diets over the course of her lifetime and losing up to 15 pounds several times. However, she often discontinued her diets when she hit a "plateau" and would stop losing weight despite still adhering to her dietary plan. Susan feels like a failure because she has been unable to lose more weight or maintain her losses in the long term. She reports being treated differently by employers and coworkers depending on her weight. For example, she notices that she is invited to more networking events when she is at a lower weight.

Susan describes the stress she feels each time she goes to her physician for a physical examination due to fear of being judged or criticized. She vividly recalls an incident from 15 years ago in which, during a primary care visit, the nurse was unable to measure her blood pressure because the office did not have an appropriately sized cuff to fit Susan's arm. The physician then told her that if she continued to be "morbidly obese," she was not going to live long enough to see her children grow up. When Susan attempted to describe to the physician her past weight loss attempts, she felt dismissed and was told to "just eat less." Susan still remembers the immense guilt and shame she felt on leaving that visit and how she stopped to buy two cheeseburgers at a fast-food drive-through to eat in the car on her way home in order to soothe herself.

Susan is seeking help with her eating and weight management from a psychologist. She would like to lose weight in order to increase her energy and mobility so that she can be active with her new grandchild. She would also like to alleviate her sleep apnea and reduce her need for antihypertensive medication. Susan would like help regulating her eating, and she realizes that her extreme dieting practices have not been effective. She is nervous about meeting with a new healthcare provider, given her feelings of failure about her past weight loss attempts and her previously negative healthcare experiences.

Introduction

In this chapter, the role of weight stigma in psychological care is considered. First, we define weight stigma and describe the prevalence of weight discrimination in healthcare, employment, education, interpersonal relationships, and the media. Next, we outline the consequences of weight stigma on physical and psychological health, along with four mechanisms thought to link weight stigma and health outcomes (stress, behavior changes related to eating and physical activity, healthcare underutilization, and social disconnection). We conclude by providing a series of recommendations to help healthcare providers reduce weight stigma individually, professionally, and socially.

A Note about Language

Labels are one powerful way in which stigma is expressed [1]. A common term in weight stigma research is *fat*; it is used in many of the scales that measure weight prejudice [2,3]. There are several possible reasons why: it is highly descriptive, does not imply a medical label, and recognizes advocates in the size-acceptance movement who reclaim the word. In health research, however, terms that reflect BMI tend to be used. In this literature, recent efforts have been made to use person-first language (e.g., *person with obesity*) [4]. In light of research demonstrating that higher-body-weight people view the terms *fatness* and *obesity* as undesirable in healthcare interactions and terms such as *weight* as desirable [5], throughout this chapter we use the term *body weight* to refer to a person's relative fatness or leanness [6,7]. Higher-body-weight people are those who would be deemed *overweight* or *obese* by medical classification systems or by themselves or important others.

Defining Weight Stigma

Stigma is an attribute that is perceived to be socially disadvantageous [8]. Stigmatizing characteristics discredit and devalue people in the eyes of others, marking them as different and tainted. People who exceed socially constructed weight expectations are subject to particularly severe stigmatization because their weight is often perceived as aesthetically displeasing, controllable, and a sign of moral failure [9].

Weight stigma encompasses a range of weight biases including prejudice, stereotyping, and discrimination [10]. *Weight prejudice* refers to negative attitudes and unfavorable evaluations of higher-body-weight people that are openly expressed in research studies [2,3,11]. *Weight stereotypes* are beliefs about the personal attributes and traits of higher-body-weight people, who are commonly stereotyped as lazy, sloppy, gluttonous, clumsy, unintelligent, incompetent, and lacking in willpower, self-discipline, and self-control [12]. *Weight discrimination* includes any negative, unfair, or unequal behavior or treatment accorded to higher-body-weight people because of their weight and is evident in healthcare settings [13,14].

Two explanations for why higher-body-weight people are stigmatized are (1) belief in the controllability of weight and (2) disgust. People who believe that weight is largely within a person's control (e.g., people can lose weight easily if they try) report more negative attitudes toward higher-body-weight people [2,15]. Higher-body-weight people are blamed and viewed as a failure of personal responsibility without consideration for all the genetic, biological, and environmental factors that contribute to weight [16]. This perceived violation of important values, such as hard work, self-discipline, and self-control [2], and the perceived unattractiveness of heavier bodies [17] elicit feelings of disgust. People who report feeling disgust when encountering a higher-body-weight person are more likely to believe that weight is under personal control and more strongly support discriminatory weight-based policies [18]. In fact, disgust mediates the association between perceived control and negative attitudes toward higher-body-weight people [19].

It is important to note that stigmatization processes can be directed inward. Higher-body-weight people tend to internalize weight stigma, reporting negative attitudes and beliefs about their higher-body-weight counterparts and themselves [20]. Furthermore, weight stigma can affect people who do not exceed socially constructed weight expectations because weight stigmatization contributes to fear of fat at the societal level. For example, nearly 60 percent of lower-body-weight participants in a large study stated that they would give up at least one year of their lives rather than be heavy, and 19 percent stated that they would give up 10 years or more [21].

Pervasiveness of Weight Stigma

Weight stigma is widespread. Recent estimates suggest that the prevalence of weight discrimination has increased by 66 percent over recent decades [22] and, for women, is now comparable to discrimination based on race and age [23]. The prevalence of weight discrimination is greater among women and increases as BMI increases [24]. Phenomenological research suggests that weight stigma is an almost daily experience for many higher-body-weight people [25]. Weight stigma influences experiences and outcomes across a range of life domains, including healthcare, employment, education, interpersonal relationships, and in the media [13,24]. It is important to understand not only how weight stigma is experienced in healthcare settings but also how it influences other important life outcomes and experiences because this defines the broader social context in which people live, work, learn, and interact.

Healthcare

Many health professionals report negative attitudes and stereotypes about higher-body-weight patients that are reflective of societal biases [26,27]. For example, in a large study of more than 2,000 medical doctors, all reported a strong preference for lower-body-weight people over higher-body-weight people on both explicit (i.e., self-reported) and implicit (i.e., automatic) measures [28]. In a survey of first-year medical students in training programs across the United States, the majority exhibited implicit (74 percent) and explicit (67 percent) weight prejudice [29]. Many medical doctors report experiencing negative emotional reactions (e.g., disgust) to the appearance of higher-body-weight patients, maintaining beliefs that higher-body-weight patients are unattractive, noncompliant, and weak willed [30].

Other studies have revealed that medical providers often experience disinterest in treating higher-body-weight patients and are more likely to describe interactions with higher-body-weight patients as a waste of time [31]. This may be at least partially due to the belief that higher-body-weight patients are less compliant with treatment recommendations [32]. Healthcare providers spend less time interacting with and educating higher-body-weight patients, report less respect for them, and prescribe different treatment recommendations from those given to lower-body-weight patients [31,33–35]. In one examination of nearly 2,500 higher-body-weight women, over half reported weight stigma from their medical doctors on multiple occasions [36], and this perceived negative judgment can lead higher-body-weight patients to have lower trust in their healthcare providers [37].

In one of the few studies that focus on clinical and counseling psychologists, participants reported lower expectations for a patient's prognosis, effort, and functioning if that patient was of a higher body weight [38]. Participants were more likely to view higher-body-weight patients as having an eating disorder or adjustment disorder and set weight-related treatment goals even when patients did not report any weight concerns. Young and Powell found that psychologists assign more negative psychological symptoms, diagnostic judgments, and prognoses to higher-body-weight patients [39], and the researchers attributed impaired diagnosis and clinical judgment of higher-body-weight patients to obstructed empathy among therapists. Focusing on professionals specializing in eating disorders, those who report stronger weight bias are more likely to believe that higher body weight is caused by behavioral factors such as overeating and lack of willpower, express negative attitudes and frustrations about treating higher-body-weight patients, and perceive poorer treatment outcomes for higher-body-weight patients [40].

Employment

Weight discrimination in employment has been documented at every stage of the employment cycle, from hiring and promotion through wages to firing and disciplinary treatment [41]. Compared with thinner job candidates, higher-body-weight candidates with identical credentials, skills, and training are less likely to be hired and are ascribed more negative attributes, perceived as a poor fit for the position, and assigned lower starting salaries [13]. Research demonstrates that higher-body-weight candidates are evaluated less favorably than thinner candidates who are unqualified for the position [42]. Higher-body-weight people earn approximately 90 cents for every dollar earned by their lower-body-weight counterparts, and this wage penalty is especially pronounced for women [43].

Education

Weight discrimination in education is also evident at multiple levels, from nursery school to college [44]. Many school teachers report believing that higher-body-weight people are untidy, emotional, less likely to succeed, and have family problems. Negative weight attitudes are especially pronounced among physical educators, who are more likely to associate higher-body-weight people with a lack of willpower [45]. Higher-body-weight people are underrepresented at the college level; college students are thinner on average than their peers who do not attend college [13]. Higher-body-weight students, particularly women, are less likely to receive financial support from their parents while attending college compared with their thinner counterparts [46,47]. In an analysis of graduate school admissions, higher-body-weight applicants received fewer postinterview offers of admission, even though higher-body-weight applicants received as many interview invitations as thinner applicants, and their applications were strong according to GRE scores and letters of recommendation [48].

Interpersonal Relationships

Research demonstrates that the greatest weight stigmatization comes from family members and close friends – people who might otherwise be expected to be unconditional sources of social support and safety [13]. In one study, higher-body-weight women were asked if they had ever been stigmatized or discriminated against on the basis of their weight from an extensive list of interpersonal sources [36]. The top-rated source of weight stigma in this study was family members: 72 percent of participants reported being stigmatized on the basis of their weight from family members. Moreover, 60 percent reported weight stigmatization from their friends, and 47 percent reported weight stigmatization from their spouses. In another study, higher-body-weight people were found to experience more negative weight-related interactions (e.g., name calling, derogatory statements, teasing) in the home than in any other environment [49]. The quality of romantic relationships is influenced by weight stigma as well, particularly for women who are of a higher body weight. They are described as less attractive by others and are less likely to date compared with their lower-body-weight peers [50]. Higher-body-weight women report lower-quality relationships and greater dissatisfaction with their relationships [51]. Among adolescents, higher body weight is the leading reason for bullying [52].

Media

Media representations of higher-body-weight people are largely stigmatizing [13]. News reports frequently frame higher body weight as an issue of personal responsibility, promoting messages of blame and shame [53]. In addition to this content, news stories are accompanied by images of higher-body-weight people that are stigmatizing and perpetuate negative weight stereotypes [54]. Even though higher-body-weight people make up the majority of the population, they are underrepresented in television and, when shown, are depicted in stereotypical ways [55]. Television shows such as *The Biggest Loser* perpetuate weight stereotypes, serving to reinforce and even increase negative attitudes toward higher-body-weight people among their viewers [56]. Stigmatizing visual representations of higher-body-weight people incite more negative weight attitudes, including a desire for social distance [57], and elicit support for discriminatory weight-based policies, such as denying fertility treatment to higher-body-weight women [58].

Consequences of Weight Stigma

Weight stigma is associated with a range of negative physical and psychological health outcomes [14,59–61]. Weight stigma contributes to poor health behaviors and outcomes for those targeted, including disordered eating, reduced physical activity, psychological disorders, stress-related pathophysiology, reduced quality of healthcare, and healthcare underutilization [14]. In turn, these individual health consequences lead to public health consequences. The disregard of social and environmental contributors to weight by healthcare providers, public health officials, and the general public can lead to impaired health-promotion efforts, resulting in increased weight-based health disparities and broader social inequalities. This, altogether, leads to greater morbidity and mortality risk for higher-body-weight people due to weight stigmatization processes, independent of weight status [62]. Although the likelihood of weight stigmatization increases as weight increases, weight stigma has the potential to compromise the health and well-being of virtually anybody.

Health

Experiences of weight stigmatization can contribute to and exacerbate many of the physical health problems associated with higher body weight [63]. Recent research shows that weight bias internalization predicts a metabolic syndrome when controlling for BMI and depressive symptoms among higher-body-weight participants [64]. Weight stigma mediates the association between BMI and physical health, with weight stigma concerns (i.e., concern over being stigmatized because of one's weight) serving as a stronger predictor than perceived weight discrimination (i.e., previous experiences of being discriminated against based on weight in the past) [65]. Thus, even in the absence of direct experiences of weight discrimination, the anticipation of potentially being a target of weight stigmatization can be detrimental to physical health. Perceived weight discrimination is associated with an increased mortality risk of nearly 60 percent, above and beyond a number of common risk factors, including age, gender, BMI, smoking history, physical activity, subjective health, and depressive symptoms [62]. In other words, weight stigma may shorten life expectancy.

Weight stigma increases psychological distress and compromises well-being. Weight stigma is associated with depression, low self-esteem, body image dissatisfaction, and binge eating [13]. Furthermore, weight bias internalization is associated with a number of clinical correlates, including depression, anxiety, social and behavioral problems, lower quality of life, and eating, weight, and shape concerns [66]. Demonstrating the connection between mind and body, internalized weight bias is associated with poorer health-related quality of life, an association that is mediated by depression symptoms [67]. Perceived weight discrimination is associated with increased risk for mood disorders, anxiety disorders, and substance-use disorders, with nearly one-third of higher-body-weight participants who perceived weight discrimination in the past year meeting criteria for these psychological disorders [68]. In addition, weight stigma concerns mediate the association between BMI and psychological well-being (i.e., depression, self-esteem, and quality of life) [65]. Research findings converge in identifying a history of weight-based teasing as a significant risk factor for psychological disorders [69]. Experiences of environmental barriers due to weight (e.g., chairs too small) and interpersonal weight-based criticism also predict psychological problems [70].

Research implicates weight stigma in weight gain and the maintenance of higher body weights. In a large longitudinal survey of American residents, participants who experienced weight discrimination were 2.5 times more likely to be of a higher body weight four years later and, if already of a higher body weight, were three times more likely to remain that way [71]. In a longitudinal study of girls aged 10 to 19 years, girls labeled as "too fat" in childhood were more likely to be of a higher body weight nearly a decade later, independent of initial BMI [72]. Additionally, weight bias internalization predicts weight regain rather than weight loss maintenance among participants who reported that they tried to lose or maintain their weight over the past year [73].

More research is needed to understand the pathways by which weight stigma negatively affects health and well-being. Four proposed mechanisms garnering attention in the research literature are increased stress, unhealthy behavior changes relating to eating and physical activity, healthcare underutilization, and social disconnection [59,74,75]. The research evidence regarding these mechanisms is elucidated below.

Stress

Weight stigma is physiologically and psychologically stressful. Weight stigma was associated with hypercortisolism (increased morning serum cortisol) and oxidative stress (increased F_2-isoprostanes) in a sample of higher-body-weight women [76]. Perceived stress may mediate the association between weight stigma and physiological markers of stress. In experimentally manipulated exposure to weight stigma, cortisol reactivity is observed independent of BMI [77]. Perceived weight discrimination is also associated with increased levels of C-reactive protein, a marker of systemic inflammation [78], and poorer glycemic control [79]. In a laboratory experiment, higher-body-weight women who gave a speech while videotaped (weight visible) exhibited increased blood pressure compared with higher-body-weight women who gave a speech while audiotaped (weight not visible) and lower-body-weight women regardless of visibility [80].

Stress also influences emotional processes. Higher-body-weight women manipulated to feel weight stigma in the laboratory reported more stress-related emotions (e.g., nervous, overwhelmed, uncomfortable, and worried) and self-conscious emotions (e.g., guilty, disgusted with myself, ashamed) [80,81]. In particular, shame activates cortisol secretion [82], identifying it as a key ingredient linking weight stigmatization and health outcomes [75]. Taken together, obesity-related comorbidities – including cardiovascular disease, type 2 diabetes, hypertension, insulin resistance, decreased immune functioning, cancers, and ulcers – are exacerbated by stress, and weight stigma represents a prominent stressor that thus may negatively affect health [63,76,78,80].

Behavior Change

Eating. Cortisol is a mediator of stress-induced eating because it stimulates desire for high-fat and high-sugar foods and promotes storage of excess energy as adipose tissue [75]. Thus weight stigma may initiate stress-related processes that lead to increased eating of calorie-dense foods and fat deposition in the body. Furthermore, coping with stigma requires cognitive effort to regulate stress, negative emotions, intrusive thoughts, and interpersonal anxieties [59]. Weight stigma undermines self-regulation and executive functioning; for example, higher-body-weight women manipulated to feel stigmatized based on weight demonstrated greater interference on an attentional task and reported being less capable of controlling their eating [80]. This momentary impairment to executive functioning can lead to increased eating, and experimental research shows that participants consume more snack foods and have reduced dietary health intentions when they are exposed to weight stigma [83,84].

Conversely, weight stigma may motivate people to escape stigmatization by undertaking unhealthy weight loss behaviors in an attempt to lose weight to shed the stigma [59]. A history of weight-related teasing predicts disordered eating behaviors ranging from fasting, eating little food, consuming diet pills, purging, using laxatives and diuretics, skipping meals, smoking cigarettes for weight control, and binge eating [85]. Weight teasing, body image dissatisfaction, media use, and unhealthy dieting practices are identified as risk factors for the development of eating disorders [86]. Disordered eating behaviors are not effective for weight loss and lead to weight gain and poorer physical and mental health [87].

Physical Activity. Weight stigma negatively influences participation in physical activity. Weight stigma increases the desire to avoid physical activity, even when controlling for BMI and body dissatisfaction [88]. This association is particularly evident among people who internalize weight attitudes [89]. One study found that weight bias internalization predicted less physical activity, whereas weight stigma predicted greater physical activity [90]. Weight bias internalization mediated the association between weight stigma and current physical activity levels. Importantly, this study draws a distinction between experiencing weight stigma and internalizing it. Weight stigma predicts greater participation in physical activity, consistent with the notion that people might be motivated to escape stigma and attempt to compensate by contradicting stereotypes [59,91]. Weight stigma increases controlled (versus autonomous) exercise motivation, which is accompanied by a heightened drive for thinness that may increase the risk for long-term negative health consequences [92]. However, weight bias internalization predicts less participation in physical activity, consistent with the notion that people might be motivated to avoid stigmatizing situations (e.g., the gym) [59].

Healthcare Utilization

Weight stigmatizing experiences in healthcare settings may deter higher-body-weight patients from accessing care. This can lead to avoidance of age-appropriate preventative health screenings and treatment avoidance and nonadherence [14,26]. For example, higher-body-weight women who report weight stigma barriers to healthcare utilization – such as disrespectful treatment and negative attitudes from healthcare providers, embarrassment at being weighed, unsolicited advice to lose weight, and small gowns, exam tables, and equipment – are less likely to have timely pelvic examinations, Papanicolaou (Pap) tests, and mammograms to screen for cancer [33]. Presumably due to negative interactions with healthcare providers, higher-body-weight patients are more likely to switch physicians or "doctor shop" [93]. Frequently changing healthcare providers may impair continuity of care and increases the risk of emergency department visits and hospitalizations. This points to a vicious cycle in which weight stigma in healthcare settings leads to healthcare under-utilization and avoidance, further perpetuating weight-based health disparities because it removes the possibility of early detection and introduces a critical delay in receiving treatment.

Social Disconnection

Social isolation is a risk factor and social support is a protective factor for health and well-being [94]. Weight stigma can be pervasive in interpersonal relationships, undermining the maintenance and quality of close relationships and limiting the initiation and development of new ones [59]. People report fewer positive behavioral intentions to get to know and interact with a stranger if that person is of a higher body weight [95]. Higher-body-weight people tend to have less social support and more constricted social networks, increasing the risk for depression [96]. In this way, weight stigma may thwart the fundamental human need to belong and be accepted by others. Social rejection expectations mediated the effect of weight stigma on lowered self-esteem and increased stress and shame in a sample of higher-body-weight women [81].

As is clear from the research literature, weight stigma does not benefit health. There is little evidence that weight stigma leads to weight loss or health improvements [13,14,59,75]. Even if weight stigmatization were effective under a small set of circumstances, ethically and morally it would be difficult to justify such approaches because they primarily cause harm [97]. Healthcare providers must, first, do no harm and focus on facilitating healthy behavioral change while taking steps to prevent and reduce weight stigma in psychological care.

Recommendations

In a recent survey that asked higher-body-weight women to rate the importance of various proposed stigma-reduction strategies, over 90 percent rated strategies that focused on healthcare settings as "high-importance" initiatives [98]. In addition, 79 percent identified healthcare professionals as having the potential to play a major role in reducing weight stigma. Below is a series of recommendations for reducing weight stigma in psychological care based on patient surveys, experimental evidence, and expert insights.

Self-Assessment

Healthcare professionals are advised to reflect on their own beliefs and attitudes about higher-body-weight people. Completing validated assessment tools such as the Anti-fat Attitudes Questionnaire [2], Beliefs about Obese Persons and Attitudes toward Obese Persons Scales [15], and the Implicit Association Test [99] can be an effective way to engage with one's own biases. Clinicians can also educate themselves about the complexity of obesity and weight loss in order to challenge possible misconceptions they may have about the controllability of weight and its causes and consequences [100–106]. As is the case in any psychological setting, it can be helpful to practice perspective-taking and consider the patient's history – such as the Case Vignette at the start of this chapter in which Susan felt defeated by several past weight loss attempts and experienced stigma in healthcare settings – in order to build an empathic understanding of the patient's experience and establish rapport [26,107].

Office Environment

Patient comfort in a treatment setting often begins with the physical environment. Higher-body-weight patients frequently report inadequate facilities and equipment as a deterrent to seeking clinical care [33]. To promote an atmosphere of comfort and inclusion, equipment recommendations include having wide-based chairs that are armless, properly sized gowns and blood pressure cuffs (if applicable), wide examination tables bolted to the floor with a step-stool for access (if applicable), doors and hallways that can accommodate large wheelchairs and walkers, adequate space between chairs in the waiting area through which patients can move, and bathrooms with properly mounted and secured grab bars and toilets [108].

Additionally, mental health professionals can be aware of the images in their offices, including the reading materials in the waiting area. In particular, efforts can be made to avoid hanging pictures that promote negative stereotypes or having magazines promoting the thin ideal [6]. Special effort can be taken to provide images and materials that reflect body diversity, such as positive and counterstereotypical portrayals of higher-body-weight people. Images for public use are available through several resources intended to reduce weight stigma [109–111]. In the case of Susan from the Case Vignette, one might imagine the positive impact of her seeing images in the waiting room of a higher-body-weight woman playing with her grandchildren, attending a networking event with coworkers, or shopping at a food market compared with images that promote negative weight stereotypes or the thin ideal. These changes to the office environment communicate to patients of all sizes that they are welcome.

Considering that patients report embarrassment at being weighed, weight should only be measured if it is clinically indicated [108]. If measurement of weight is necessary, healthcare professionals must use sensitivity in their weighing procedures. It is crucial to have a high-capacity scale and for the scale to be in a private room or area (rather than in the hallway or waiting area) to give patients privacy. Weight should be treated as objective clinical data and recorded without comment or judgment. Asking for permission to weigh the patient can communicate respect and patient autonomy. If the patient declines, this preference should be honored and can provide an opportunity to openly discuss the patient's discomfort or concerns.

Language

As described earlier, several studies have documented patient preferences for words used to refer to body weight. Generally, patients perceive terms such as *morbidly obese, obese, fat, excess fat, large size,* and *heaviness* to be blaming, stigmatizing, and undesirable [5]. In contrast, terms such as *weight, unhealthy weight, overweight,* and *BMI* are viewed more favorably. If providers are unsure of what words to use, they can ask patients for their preferences (e.g., "I am going to use the term *BMI* when discussing your weight today. Is that okay? Is there another term you would prefer?"). In some clinical settings, and in the context of this book, the term *severe obesity* is used as a diagnostic medical term, and patients may be exposed to this language through billing, printed visit summaries, or when discussing health comorbidities. If the term *obesity* needs to be used, it is recommended to use person-first language [4]. As reflected in Susan's reaction to being labeled as "morbidly obese," language is one way in which weight stigma is expressed and can have long-lasting consequences. It is imperative that healthcare professionals demonstrate sensitivity, flexibility, and respect in the weight language they use.

Communication

If patients bring up their weight, it is important to ask about their perspectives on their body weight rather than assume that they want to lose weight or are concerned about their weight. If there are weight concerns on the part of the patient, as much as possible the focus of weight-based interventions should be on health rather than appearance [112]. Clinicians should refrain from making statements about weight loss to improve appearance because this reinforces the notion that the patient's current appearance is unacceptable due to his or her weight. Similarly, healthcare professionals can emphasize the importance of changing health behaviors rather than focusing solely on the goal of losing weight. Many healthcare professionals advocate for focus to be placed on health and health behavior rather than weight and weight loss [6,26,100]. As described in the Case Vignette at the start of this chapter, weight loss does not always directly correspond with adherence to behavioral goals. If patients and providers are only focused on weight, patients may feel discouraged and lose motivation and confidence when they do not achieve their desired weight loss in any given week or month. However, if patients and providers are both focusing on behavioral goals and health outcomes, successes can be celebrated and rewarded even when weight does not change, thus giving patients more encouragement and support to continue sticking with their goals. Overall, emphasizing the health benefits of changing eating and physical activity habits, reducing stress, and getting adequate sleep – as in the case of Susan, focusing on how increased energy will allow her to be more active with her grandchild – is recommended to avoid perpetuating thin-ideal beauty standards and potentially contributing to internalized weight bias.

To begin the conversation about weight and changing health behaviors, healthcare professionals can use established communication techniques such as motivational interviewing (MI) [27,112] (see Chapters 2, 5, 6, and 7). Motivational interviewing is a method for eliciting patients' internal motivation for change in an empathic and nonjudgmental manner [113]. Providers can explore why health behavior change is important to the patient and how ready and confident the patient feels to make these changes. The conversation can then move to increasing readiness and confidence by setting concrete, attainable goals. The nonjudgmental aspect of MI is key for preventing patients from feeling criticized by their providers when discussing the sensitive topic of weight. Setting specific goals can increase self-efficacy for patients with internalized weight bias, who may be more prone to believing negative stereotypes and, thus, less likely to follow through on behavioral goals [114].

Psychological Interventions

Limited research has tested the effects of psychological treatment approaches on reducing internalization of and distress related to weight stigma in higher-body-weight patients. However, recent pilot studies show promising results. In one study, an eight-week cognitive-behavioral therapy (CBT) group treatment program was designed to teach participants strategies to cope with experiences of weight stigma and reduce weight bias internalization [114]. Results showed that compared with a quasi–control group, participants in the treatment group had reduced weight bias internalization and weight stereotype endorsement and increased self-efficacy to control eating and weight. Two recent open-label trials of acceptance and commitment therapy (ACT) adapted to address weight- and eating-related distress showed reduced weight self-stigma and increased health behaviors following the interventions [115,116]. Larger trials are needed to replicate these findings. However, these preliminary results suggest that it may be beneficial for healthcare professionals trained in empirically supported treatments (such as CBT and ACT) to apply these approaches to addressing weight stigma. Mindfulness, self-compassion, and self-affirmation are some additional promising theoretically driven psychological interventions that may help higher-body-weight patients cope with experiences of weight stigma [6] (see Chapters 10 and 11). For example, Susan from the Case Vignette may benefit from practicing self-compassion to address her self-blame and thoughts of being a "failure" and consequently may feel more confident to make health behavior changes.

Education and Training

Overall, more research is needed to identify effective methods for changing weight-biased attitudes, and prior research testing potential interventions has yielded mixed results [117,118]. Furthermore, only a few studies have examined the effects of weight bias reduction interventions among health professionals or trainees [119–121]. Still, training activities that provide information about weight bias, emphasize the complexity of weight, and include patient contact may help to reduce weight bias among healthcare professionals.

Incorporating *weight sensitivity* training into course curricula and/or clinical practice is strongly supported among higher-body-weight people and could help to target weight-biased attitudes early and prevent instances of weight stigmatization in psychological care [98]. Two studies of medical students found that a brief educational video about weight bias in healthcare led to decreased explicit weight bias [120,121], although one of the studies did not find a change in implicit weight bias [121]. This study also found mixed results for sustained changes in explicit weight bias six weeks following the intervention [121].

Positive contact with higher-body-weight patients, or standardized patients, may also be helpful to increase empathy and comfort when discussing weight [27,122]. For example, one study provided medical students with articles about effective communication and weight stigma prior to role-playing discussions about weight with standardized patients [119]. Results showed a short-term reduction in stereotyping and a long-term increase in empathy and confidence in weight counseling. Including nonstereotypical case examples in training may also help to reduce implicit weight bias [27].

Another proposed approach for reducing weight bias is to emphasize biogenetic causes of obesity that are outside of individual control. Persky and Eccleston found that medical students who read about genetic causes of obesity (versus behavioral causes or a control topic) reported less negative weight-based stereotypes [32]. However, participants did not show differences in the anticipated treatment adherence of a virtual higher-body-weight patient. Other studies emphasizing biogenetic explanations have found no effects on weight-biased attitudes [123,124]. One study found that biogenetic explanations reduced the likelihood that students recommended dietary consultations or other weight-related interventions, likely due to the belief that weight cannot be changed if it is biologically determined [32]. This is consistent with prior findings that patients who believe that weight is biologically determined have less self-efficacy to lose weight [125]. Overall, it is likely that higher-body-weight patients are best served by accurately identifying weight-related factors that are within their control (e.g., behaviors) and outside of their control (e.g., genes). Thus mechanisms involved in weight should be explained to trainees and patients in a nuanced manner to emphasize that biology does not definitively determine an individual's weight or health while acknowledging the role of behavior and social determinants of health as well [126]. Applied to Susan in the Case Vignette, the overall message should be one of empowerment that motivates healthy behavior change yet remains realistic to minimize unrealistic weight loss expectations and self-blame.

Advocacy

Outside of the therapeutic interaction, healthcare professionals can advocate to reduce weight bias and stigma. Prior research suggests that social consensus plays a role in perpetuating weight bias [127]. The public may be deterred from making disparaging comments about higher-body-weight people if others around them do not condone this kind of behavior. Thus clinicians can speak out when they witness injustice and contribute to building a consensus that weight stigma is not acceptable.

Providers can also educate others about the complexity of obesity in order to challenge common misperceptions. For example, eating disorder symptoms among higher-body-weight patients often go unnoticed and untreated [128]. As a thought experiment, imagine if Susan in the Case Vignette presented with a restricted diet of no more than 800 calories per day for the previous six months; weighed herself multiple times per day; measured her waist, buttocks, arms, and legs weekly; and reported being terrified of gaining weight, stating that "she would rather die than get fat and ugly." Research suggests that higher-body-weight people are at increased risk for developing eating disorders compared with any other weight group [129]. Yet the *Diagnostic and Statistical Manual of Mental Disorders* [130] requires the identification of a "significantly low body weight" for a diagnosis of anorexia nervosa. Some mental health professionals advocate for avoidance of BMI as a marker for diagnosis or recovery, focusing instead on psychological and physical health outcomes and behaviors [131].

Finally, mental health professionals can advocate for legislation to reduce systematic weight discrimination. Support for legislation protecting people from weight-based discrimination, bullying, or other forms of unfair treatment has been strongly advocated by the public and mental health professionals [132,133]. Professionals who provide psychological care to higher-body-weight patients can further promote the reduction of weight bias for their patients and the broader community by voicing support for such proposed policies and instituting them within their own clinical practices.

Summary

Weight stigma is pervasive and permeates many domains of living, including the healthcare setting. Weight stigma is associated with several physical and psychological health consequences, including increased risk for mortality and mood and anxiety disorders. Four mechanisms thought to link weight stigma and health are increased stress, dysregulation of eating and physical activity, underutilization and avoidance of healthcare, and social disconnection. It is important for health professionals to consider weight stigma in psychological care and take practical steps to reduce it. Some recommendations for reducing weight stigma include engaging in self-assessment of one's own biases; modifying office environments to be accessible, and welcoming to higher-body-weight patients; being sensitive to the weight terminology used with patients and staff; engaging in empathic and nonjudgmental communication; applying psychological interventions that address weight stigma with patients when appropriate; seeking continuing education on the complexity of obesity and weight stigma; allaying misconceptions among staff, patients, and trainees about higher-body-weight people; and engaging in advocacy for higher-body-weight people more broadly. By considering weight stigma in psychological care, healthcare professionals can drastically improve the quality of life and well-being of numerous patients who are not currently getting their needs met in the healthcare system.

Key Points

- Weight stigma is pervasive and harmful to physical and psychological health and well-being.
- Weight stigma is perpetuated, often unintentionally, in psychological care.
- Healthcare professionals must consider weight stigma in psychological care and work to reduce it.

References

1. B. G. Link and J. C. Phelan. Conceptualizing stigma. *Annu Rev Sociol* 2001; **27**: 363–85.

2. C. S. Crandall. Prejudice against fat people: Ideology and self-interest. *J Pers Soc Psychol* 1994; **66**: 882–94.

3. J. D. Latner, K. S. O'Brien, L. E. Durso, et al. Weighing obesity stigma: The relative strength of different forms of bias. *Int J Obes (Lond)* 2008; **32**: 1145–52.

4. T. K. Kyle and R. M. Puhl. Putting people first in obesity. *Obesity (Silver Spring)* 2014; **22**: 1211.

5. T. A. Wadden and E. Didie. What's in a name? Patients' preferred terms for describing obesity. *Obes Res* 2003; **11**: 1140–6.

6. C. Logel, D. A. Stinson, and P. M. Brochu. Weight loss is not the answer: A well-being solution to the "obesity problem." *Soc Pers Psychol Compass* 2015; **9**: 678–95.

7. A. Meadows and S. Daníelsdóttir. What's in a word? On weight stigma and terminology. *Front Psychol* 2016; **7**: 1527.

8. B. Major and L. T. O'Brien. The social psychology of stigma. *Annu Rev Psychol* 2005; **56**: 393–421.

9. J. Crocker, B. Cornwell, and B. Major. The stigma of overweight: Affective consequences of attributional ambiguity. *J Pers Soc Psychol* 1993; **64**: 60–70.

10. K. D. Brownell, R. M. Puhl, M. B. Schwartz, et al. *Weight Bias: Nature, Consequences, and Remedies*. New York, NY: Guilford Press, 2005.

11. P. M. Brochu, B. Gawronski, and V. M. Esses. The integrative prejudice framework and different forms of weight prejudice: An analysis and expansion. *Group Process Intergroup Relat* 2011; **14**: 429–44.

12. P. M. Brochu and V. M. Esses. What's in a name? The effects of the labels "fat" versus "overweight" on weight bias. *J Appl Soc Psychol* 2011; **41**: 1981–2008.

13. R. M. Puhl and C. A. Heuer. The stigma of obesity: A review and update. *Obesity (Silver Spring)* 2009; **17**: 941–64.

14. R. M. Puhl and C. A. Heuer. Obesity stigma: Important considerations for public health. *Am J Public Health* 2010; **100**: 1019–28.

15. D. B. Allison, V. C. Basile, and H. E. Yuker. The measurement of attitudes toward and beliefs about obese persons. *Int J Eat Disord* 1991; **10**: 599–607.

16. B. Weiner, R. P. Perry, and J. Magnusson. An attributional analysis of reactions to stigmas. *J Pers Soc Psychol* 1988; **55**: 738–48.

17. B. E. Robinson, J. G. Bacon, and J. O'Reilly. Fat phobia: Measuring, understanding, and changing anti-fat attitudes. *Int J Eat Disord* 1993; **14**: 467–80.

18. P. M. Brochu and V. M. Esses. Weight prejudice and medical policy: Support for an ambiguously discriminatory policy is influenced by prejudice-colored glasses. *Anal Soc Issues Public Policy* 2009; **9**: 117–33.

19. L. R. Vartanian. Disgust and perceived control in attitudes toward obese people. *Int J Obes (Lond)* 2010; **34**: 1302–7.

20. L. E. Durso and J. D. Latner. Understanding self-directed stigma: Development of the weight bias internalization scale. *Obesity (Silver Spring)* 2008; **16**: S80–6.

21. M. B. Schwartz, L. R. Vartanian, B. A. Nosek, et al. The influence of one's own body weight on implicit and explicit anti-fat bias. *Obesity (Silver Spring)* 2006; **14**: 440–7.

22. T. Andreyeva, R. M. Puhl, and K. D. Brownell. Changes in perceived weight discrimination among Americans, 1995–1996 through 2004–2006. *Obesity (Silver Spring)* 2008; **16**: 1129–34.

23. R. M. Puhl, T. Andreyeva, and K. D. Brownell. Perceptions of weight discrimination: Prevalence and comparison to race and gender discrimination in America. *Int J Obes (Lond)* 2008; **32**: 992–1000.

24. J. Spahlholz, N. Baer, H. -H. König, et al. Obesity and discrimination: A systematic review and meta-analysis of observational studies. *Obes Res* 2016; **17**: 43–55.

25. L. R. Vartanian, R. T. Pinkus, and J. M. Smyth. The phenomenology of weight stigma in everyday life. *J Context Behav Sci* 2014; **3**: 196–202.

26. S. M. Phelan, D. J. Burgess, M. W. Yeazel, et al. Impact of weight bias and stigma on quality of care and outcomes for patients with obesity. *Obes Rev* 2015; **16**: 319–26.

27. R. M. Puhl, S. M. Phelan, J. Nadglowski, et al. Overcoming weight bias in the management of patients with diabetes and obesity. *Clin Diabetes* 2016; **34**: 44–50.

28. J. A. Sabin, M. Marini, and B. A. Nosek. Implicit and explicit anti-fat bias among a large sample of medial doctors by BMI, race/ethnicity and gender. *PLoS ONE* 2012; **7**: e48448.

29. S. M. Phelan, J. F. Dovidio, R. M. Puhl, et al. Implicit and explicit weight bias in a national sample of 4,732 medical students: The medical student CHANGES study. *Obesity (Silver Spring)* 2014; **22**: 1201–8.

30. G. D. Foster, T. A. Wadden, A. P. Makris, et al. Primary care physicians' attitudes about obesity and its treatment. *Obes Res* 2003; **11**: 1168–77.

31. M. R. Hebl and J. Xu. Weighing the care: Physicians' reactions to the size of a patient. *Int J Obes Relat Metab Disord* 2001; **25**: 1246–52.

32. S. Persky and C. P. Eccleston. Impact of genetic causal information on medical students' clinical encounters with an obese virtual patient: Health promotion and social stigma. *Ann Behav Med* 2011; **41**: 363–72.

33. N. K. Amy, A. Aalborg, P. Lyons, et al. Barriers to routine gynecological cancer screening for white and African-American obese women. *Int J Obes (Lond)* 2006; **30**: 147–55.

34. K. A. Gudzune, M. C. Beach, D. L. Roter, et al. Physicians build less rapport with obese patients. *Obesity (Silver Spring)* 2013; **21**: 2146–52.

35. S. Persky and C. P. Eccleston. Medical student bias and care recommendations for an obese versus non-obese virtual patient. *Int J Obes (Lond)* 2011; **35**: 728–35.

36. R. M. Puhl and K. D. Brownell. Confronting and coping with weight stigma: An investigation of overweight and obese individuals. *Obesity (Silver Spring)* 2006; **14**: 1802–15.

37. K. A. Gudzune, W. L. Bennett, L. A. Cooper, et al. Patients who feel judged about their weight have lower trust in their primary care providers. *Patient Educ Couns* 2014; **97**: 128–31.

38. K. Davis-Coelho, J. Waltz, and B. Davis-Coelho. Awareness and prevention of bias against fat clients in psychotherapy. *Prof Psychol Res Pr* 2000; **31**: 682–4.

39. L. M. Young and B. Powell. The effects of obesity on the clinical judgments of mental health professionals. *J Health Soc Behav* 1985; **26**: 233–46.

40. R. M. Puhl, J. D. Latner, K. M. King, et al. Weight bias among professionals treating eating disorders: Attitudes about treatment and perceived patient outcomes. *Int J Eat Disord* 2014; **47**: 65–75.

41. B. Nowrouzi, A. McDougall, B. Gohar, et al. Weight bias in the workplace: A literature review. *Occup Med Health Aff* 2015; **3**: 206.

42. M. L. Sartore and G. B. Cunningham. Weight discrimination, hiring recommendations, person-job fit, and attributions: Fitness-industry implications. *J Sport Manag* 2007; **21**: 172–93.

43. C. L. Baum II and W. F. Ford. The wage effects of obesity: A longitudinal study. *Health Econ* 2004; **13**: 885–99.

44. R. M. Puhl and J. D. Latner. Stigma, obesity, and the health of the nation's children. *Psychol Bull* 2007; **133**: 557–80.

45. K. S. O'Brien, J. A. Hunter, and M. Banks. Implicit anti-fat bias in physical educators: Physical attributes, ideology and socialization. *Int J Obes (Lond)* 2007; **31**: 308–14.

46. C. S. Crandall. Do heavy-weight students have more difficulty paying for college? *Pers Soc Psychol Bull* 1991; **17**: 606–11.

47. C. S. Crandall. Do parents discriminate against their heavyweight daughters? *Pers Soc Psychol Bull* 1995; **21**: 724–35.

48. J. M. Burmeister, A. E. Kiefner, R. A. Carels, et al. Weight bias in graduate school admissions. *Obesity (Silver Spring)* 2013; **21**: 918–20.

49. R. M. Puhl, C. A. Moss-Racusin, M. B. Schwartz, et al. Weight stigmatization and bias reduction: Perspectives of overweight and obese adults. *Health Educ Res* 2008; **23**: 347–58.

50. V. Sheets and K. Ajmere. Are romantic partners a source of college students' weight concern? *Eat Behav* 2005; **6**: 1–9.

51. A. D. Boyes and J. D. Latner. Weight stigma in existing romantic relationships. *J Sex Marital Ther* 2009; **35**: 282–93.

52. R. M. Puhl, J. Luedicke, and C. Heuer. Weight-based victimization toward overweight adolescents: Observations and reactions of peers. *J Sch Health* 2011; **81**: 696–703.

53. S. Kim and L. A. Willis. Talking about obesity: News framing of who is responsible for causing and fixing the problem. *J Health Commun* 2007; **12**: 359–76.

54. C. A. Heuer, K. J. McClure, and R. M. Puhl. Obesity stigma in online news: A visual content analysis. *J Health Commun* 2011; **16**: 976–87.

55. B. S. Greenberg, M. Eastin, L. Hofschire, et al. Portrayals of overweight and obese individuals on commercial television. *Am J Public Health* 2003; **93**: 1342–8.

56. S. E. Domoff, N. G. Hinman, A. M. Koball, et al. The effects of reality television on weight bias: An examination of *The Biggest Loser*. *Obesity (Silver Spring)* 2012; **20**: 993–8.

57. R. L. Pearl, R. M. Puhl, and K. D. Brownell. Positive media portrayals of obese persons: Impact on attitudes and image preferences. *Health Psychol* 2012; **31**: 821–9.

58. P. M. Brochu, R. L. Pearl, R. M. Puhl, et al. Do media portrayals of obesity influence support for weight-related medical policy? *Health Psychol* 2014; **33**: 197–200.

59. J. M. Hunger, B. Major, A. Blodorn, et al. Weighed down by stigma: How weight-based social identity threat contributes to weight gain and poor health. *Soc Pers Psychol Compass* 2015; **9**: 255–68.

60. S. Papadopoulos and L. Brennan. Correlates of weight stigma in adults with overweight and obesity: A systematic literature review. *Obesity (Silver Spring)* 2015; **23**: 1743–60.

61. R. Puhl and Y. Suh. Stigma and eating and weight disorders. *Curr Psychiatry Rep* 2015; **17**: 10.

62. A. R. Sutin, Y. Stephan, and A. Terracciano. Weight discrimination and risk of mortality. *Psychol Sci* 2015; **26**: 1803–11.

63. P. Muennig. The body politic: The relationship between stigma and obesity-associated disease. *BMC Public Health* 2008; **8**: 128.

64. R. L. Pearl, T. A. Wadden, C. M. Hopkins, et al. Association between weight bias internalization and metabolic syndrome among treatment-seeking individuals with obesity. *Obesity (Silver Spring)* 2017; **25**: 317–22.

65. J. M. Hunger and B. Major. Weight stigma mediates the association between BMI and self-reported health. *Health Psychol* 2015; **34**: 172–5.

66. C. A. Roberto, R. Sysko, J. Bush, et al. Clinical correlates of the weight bias internalization scale in a sample of obese adolescents seeking bariatric surgery. *Obesity (Silver Spring)* 2012; **20**: 533–9.

67. R. L. Pearl, M. A. White, and C. M. Grilo. Weight bias internalization, depression, and self-reported health among overweight binge eating disorder patients. *Obesity (Silver Spring)* 2014; **22**: E142–8.

68. M. L. Hatzenbuehler, K. M. Keyes, and D. S. Hasin. Associations between perceived weight discrimination and the prevalence of psychiatric disorders in the general population. *Obesity (Silver Spring)* 2009; **17**: 2033–9.

69. J. S. Benas and B. E. Gibb. Weight-related teasing, dysfunctional cognitions, and symptoms of depression and eating disturbances. *Cogn Ther Res* 2008; **32**: 143–60.

70. K. E. Friedman, J. A. Ashmore, and K. L. Applegate. Recent experiences of weight-based stigmatization in a weight loss surgery population: Psychological and behavioural correlates. *Obesity (Silver Spring)* 2008; **16**: S69–74.

71. A. R. Sutin and A. Terracciano. Perceived weight discrimination and obesity. *PLoS ONE* 2013; **8**: e70048.

72. J. M. Hunger and A. J. Tomiyama. Weight labeling and obesity: A longitudinal study of girls aged 10–19 years. *JAMA Pediatr* 2014; **168**: 579–80.

73. R. M. Puhl, D. M. Quinn, B. M. Weisz, et al. The role of stigma in weight loss maintenance among U.S. adults. *Ann Behav Med* 2017; **51**: 754–63.

74. A. A. Brewis. Stigma and the perpetuation of obesity. *Soc Sci Med* 2014; **118**: 152–8.

75. A. J. Tomiyama. Weight stigma is stressful: A review of evidence for the cyclic obesity/weight-based stigma model. *Appetite* 2014; **82**: 8–15.

76. A. J. Tomiyama, E. S. Epel, T. M. McClatchey, et al. Associations of weight stigma with cortisol and oxidative stress independent of obesity. *Health Psychol* 2014; **33**: 862–7.

77. N. A. Schvey, R. M. Puhl, and K. D. Brownell. The stress of stigma: Exploring the effect of weight stigma on cortisol reactivity. *Psychosom Med* 2014; **76**: 156–62.

78. A. R. Sutin, Y. Stephan, M. Luchetti, et al. Perceived weight discrimination and C-reactive protein. *Obesity (Silver Spring)* 2014; **22**: 1959–61.

79. V. K. Tsenkova, D. Carr, D. A. Schoeller, et al. Perceived weight discrimination amplifies the link between central adiposity and nondiabetic glycemic control (HbA1c). *Ann Behav Med* 2011; **41**: 243–51.

80. B. Major, D. Eliezer, and H. Rieck. The psychological weight of weight stigma. *Soc Psychol Pers Sci* 2012; **3**: 651–8.

81. A. Blodorn, B. Major, J. Hunger, et al. Unpacking the psychological weight of weight stigma: A rejection-expectation pathway. *J Exp Soc Psychol* 2016; **63**: 69–76.

82. M. E. Kemeny, T. L. Gruenewald, and S. S. Dickerson. Shame as the emotional response to threat to the social self: Implications for behaviour, physiology, and health. *Psychol Inq* 2004; **15**: 153–60.

83. P. M. Brochu and J. F. Dovidio. Would you like fries (380 calories) with that? Menu labeling mitigates the impact of weight-based stereotype threat on food choice. *Soc Psychol Pers Sci* 2014; **5**: 414–21.

84. N. A. Schvey, R. M. Puhl, and K. D. Brownell. The impact of weight stigma on caloric consumption. *Obesity (Silver Spring)* 2011; **19**: 1957–62.

85. D. Neumark-Sztainer, N. Falkner, M. Story, et al. Weight-teasing among adolescents: Correlations with weight status and disordered eating behaviours. *Int J Obes (Lond)* 2002; **26**: 123–31.

86. J. Haines and D. Neumark-Sztainer. Prevention of obesity and eating disorders: A consideration of shared risk factors. *Health Educ Res* 2006; **21**: 770–82.

87. D. Neumark-Sztainer, M. Wall, M. Story, et al. Dieting and unhealthy weight control behaviours during adolescence: Associations with 10-year changes in body mass index. *J Adolesc Health* 2012; **50**: 80–6.

88. L. R. Vartanian, and J. G. Shaprow. Effects of weight stigma on exercise motivation and behaviour: A preliminary investigation among college-aged females. *J Health Psychol* 2008; **13**: 131–8.

89. L. R. Vartanian, and S. A. Novak. Internalized societal attitudes moderate the impact of weight stigma on avoidance of exercise. *Obesity (Silver Spring)* 2011; **19**: 757–62.

90. R. L. Pearl, R. M. Puhl, and J. F. Dovidio. Differential effects of weight bias experiences and internalization on exercise among women with overweight and obesity. *J Health Psychol* 2015; **20**: 1626–32.

91. R. Puhl and K. D. Brownell. Ways of coping with obesity stigma: Review and conceptual analysis. *Eat Behav* 2003; **4**: 53–78.

92. R. L. Pearl, J. F. Dovidio, R. M. Puhl, et al. Exposure to weight-stigmatizing media:

Effects on exercise intentions, motivation, and behaviour. *J Health Commun* 2015; **20**: 1004–13.

93. K. A. Gudzune, S. N. Bleich, T. M. Richards, et al. Doctor shopping by overweight and obese patients is associated with increased healthcare utilization. *Obesity (Silver Spring)* 2013; **21**: 1328–34.

94. S. Cohen. Social relationships and health. *Am Psychol* 2004; **59**: 676–84.

95. P. M. Brochu and M. A. Morrison. Implicit and explicit prejudice toward overweight and average-weight men and women: Testing their correspondence and relation to behavioural intentions. *J Soc Psychol* 2007; **147**: 681–706.

96. L. M. de Wit, M. Fokkema, A. von Straten, et al. Depressive and anxiety disorders and the association with obesity, physical, and social activities. *Depress Anxiety* 2010; **27**: 1057–65.

97. L. R. Vartanian and J. M. Smyth. Primum non nocere: Obesity stigma and public health. *Bioeth Inq* 2013; **10**: 49–57.

98. R. Puhl, M. Himmelstein, A. Gorin, et al. Missing the target: Including perspectives of women with overweight and obesity to inform stigma-reduction strategies. *Obes Sci Pract* 2017; **3**: 25–35.

99. Project Implicit. Preliminary information, 2011. Available at https://implicit.harvard.edu/implicit/takeatest.html.

100. L. Bacon and L. Aphromor. Weight science: Evaluating the evidence for a paradigm shift. *Nutr J* 2011; **10**: 9.

101. J.-P. Chaput, Z. M. Ferraro, D. Prud'homme, et al. Widespread misconceptions about obesity. *Can Fam Physician* 2014; **60**: 973–5.

102. K. M. Flegal, B. K. Kit, H. Orpana, et al. Association of all-cause mortality with overweight and obesity using standard body mass index categories: A systematic review and meta-analysis. *JAMA* 2013; **309**: 71–82.

103. J. M. Friedman. Modern science versus the stigma of obesity. *Nat Med* 2004; **10**: 563–9.

104. T. Mann, A. J. Tomiyama, E. Westling, et al. Medicare's search for effective obesity treatments: Diets are not the answer. *Am Psychol* 2007; **62**: 220–33.

105. X. R. Salas, M. Forhan, and A. Sharma. Diffusing obesity myths. *Clin Obes* 2014; **4**: 189–96.

106. A. J. Tomiyama, B. Ahlstrom, and T. Mann. Long-term effects of dieting: Is weight loss related to health? *Soc Pers Psychol Compass* 2013; **7**: 861–77.

107. J. Gloor and R. Puhl. Empathy and perspective-taking: Examination and comparison of strategies to reduce weight stigma. *Stigma Health* 2016; **1**: 269–79.

108. Rudd Center for Food Policy and Obesity. Preventing weight bias: Helping without harming in clinical practice. Available at www.uconnruddcenter.org/resources/bias_toolkit/index.html.

109. Obesity Action Coalition. Guidelines for media portrayals of individuals affected by obesity, 2017. Available at www.obesityaction.org/weight-bias-and-stigma/media-guidelines-for-obesity.

110. Rudd Center for Food Policy and Obesity. Rudd Center media gallery: Combating weight bias in the media, 2017. Available at www.uconnruddcenter.org/media-gallery.

111. L. Gurrieri. Stocky bodies image library. Available at http://stockybodies.com.

112. W. Dietz, S. Kahan, C. Gallagher, et al. Why weight? A guide to discussing obesity and health with your patients, 2014. Available at http://whyweightguide.org.

113. J. Hettema, J. Steele, and W. Miller. Motivational interviewing. *Annu Rev Clin Psychol* 2005; **1**: 91–111.

114. R. Pearl, C. Hopkins, R. Berkowitz, et al. Group cognitive-behavioural treatment for internalized weight stigma: A pilot study. *Eat Weight Disord* (forthcoming).

115. M. Levin, S. Potts, J. Haeger, et al. Delivering acceptance and commitment therapy for weight self-stigma through guided self-help: Results from an open pilot trial. *Cogn Behav Pract* (forthcoming).

116. L. Palmeira, J. Pinto-Gouveia, and M. Cunha. Exploring the efficacy of an acceptance, mindfulness and compassionate-based group intervention for women struggling with their weight (kg-free): A randomized controlled trial. *Appetite* 2017; **112**: 107–16.

117. S. Danielsdottir, K. O'Brien, and A. Ciao. Anti-fat prejudice reduction: A review of published studies. *Obes Facts* 2010; **3**: 47–58.

118. M. Lee, R. Ata, and M. Brannick. Malleability of weight-biased attitudes and beliefs: A meta-analysis of weight bias reduction interventions. *Body Image* 2014; **11**: 251–9.

119. R. Kushner, D. Zeiss, J. Feinglass, et al. An obesity educational intervention for medical students addressing weight bias and communication skills using standardized patients. *BMC Med Educ* 2014; **14**: 53.

120. Y. Poustchi, M. S. Saks, A. K. Piasecki, et al. Brief intervention effective in reducing weight bias in medical students. *Fam Med* 2013; **45**: 345–8.

121. J. Swift, V. Tischler, S. Markham, et al. Are anti-stigma films a useful strategy for reducing weight bias among trainee healthcare professionals? Results of a pilot randomized controlled trial. *Obes Facts* 2013; **6**: 91–102.

122. S. M. Phelan, R. M. Puhl, S. E. Burke, et al. The mixed impact of medical school on medical students' implicit and explicit weight bias. *Med Educ* 2015; **49**: 983–92.

123. N. Lippa and S. Sanderson. Impact of information about obesity genomics on the stigmatization of overweight individuals: An experimental study. *Obesity (Silver Spring)* 2010; **20**: 2367–76.

124. B. A. Teachman, K. D. Gapinski, K. D. Brownell, et al. Demonstrations of implicit anti-fat bias: The impact of providing causal information and evoking empathy. *Health Psychol* 2003; **22**: 68–78.

125. R. L. Pearl and M. S. Lebowitz. Beyond personal responsibility: Effects of causal attributions for obesity on weight-related beliefs, stigma, and policy support. *Psychol Health* 2014; **29**: 1176–91.

126. A. R. Tarlov. Public policy frameworks for improving population health. *Ann NY Acad Sci* 1999; **896**: 281–93.

127. R. M. Puhl, M. B. Schwartz, and K. D. Brownell. Impact of perceived consensus on stereotypes about obese people: A new approach for reducing bias. *Health Psychol* 2005; **24**: 517–25.

128. J. Lebow, L. A. Sim, and L. N. Kransdorf. Prevalence of a history of overweight and obesity in adolescents with restrictive eating disorders. *J Adolesc Health* 2015; **56**: 19–24.

129. A. Darby, P. Hay, J. Mond, et al. Disordered eating behaviours and cognitions in young women with obesity: Relationship with psychological status. *Int J Obes* 2007; **31**: 876–82.

130. American Psychiatric Association. *Diagnostic and Statistical Manual of Mental Disorders* (5th edn). Washington, DC: APA, 2013.

131. A. Lamarre and C. Rice. Normal eating is counter-cultural: Embodied experiences of eating disorder recovery. *J Commun Appl Soc Psychol* 2016; **26**: 126–49.

132. R. Puhl, D. Neumark-Sztainer, S. Austin, et al. Setting policy priorities to address eating disorders and weight stigma: Views from the field of eating disorders and the US general public. *BMC Public Health* 2013; **14**: 524.

133. Y. Suh, R. Puhl, S. Liu, et al. Support for laws to prohibit weight discrimination in the United States: Public attitudes from 2011 to 2013. *Obesity (Silver Spring)* 2014; **22**: 1872–9.

Engaging Individuals with Severe Obesity in Care

Jon Hunter and Robert Maunder

Introduction

The rapid increase in obesity in North America has directed increased attention toward treatments for severe obesity, including bariatric surgery. It has also become clear that people with severe obesity often have substantial needs for psychosocial intervention and support [1]. However, engaging individuals in effective treatment for severe obesity is challenging for several reasons. For those who choose surgery, adherence to aftercare is important and often quite difficult [2]. For those who choose against surgery or feel unready for it, other interventions are required to provide support and to aid in decision making.

Some predictors of poor adherence to interventions for severe obesity that have been identified, such as body mass index (BMI), age, marital status, employment status, and insurance coverage [3], provide little opportunity for attuning treatment psychologically to increase engagement and the success of interventions. Furthermore, even well-designed counseling interventions may be unsuccessful in improving outcomes [4].

In this chapter, we approach the question of how best to increase patient engagement in effective treatment of severe obesity from the perspective of attachment theory, which has several advantages as a psychological framework. These include its robust theoretical and empirical basis for understanding the role of affect regulation and close relationships in shaping health outcomes [5–7] and its applicability to a wide range of specific psychological treatment modalities.

Specific Models of Intervention

The most common framework for understanding individuals' engagement in behavioral change is Prochaska's transtheoretical model, which proposes five stages of change: precontemplation, contemplation, preparation, action, and maintenance [8] (see Chapter 2). The work of increasing engagement in treatment can be understood from this perspective as focused on helping individuals to advance from one stage to the next and to be able to recover from moving backward in these stages. A Cochrane review indicated that interventions based on the transtheoretical model improved physical activity and dietary habits in individuals who were overweight or obese, but the quality of the evidence was rated as weak due to the small number and methodologic limitations of the included studies [9], so this field continues to evolve. Motivational interviewing (MI) is the specific modality most directly linked to this therapeutic goal. The chapters in Section 2 of this book describe the current state of practice and delineate future directions in applying MI to specific goals related to treating severe obesity.

Several other evidence-based models of psychotherapy have also been adopted to complement the treatment of severe obesity. Prominent among these are cognitive-behavioral therapy (CBT), applications of which are described in Section 3 of this book, and mindfulness- and compassion-focused therapies, which are described in Section 4 of this book. The focus of this chapter is on the nonspecific therapeutic factors that are common to all of these modalities of intervention.

Common Therapeutic Factors

Insights that have accumulated about the most effective ingredients of psychotherapy may be helpful in overcoming some of the challenges of working with patients with severe obesity. In trying to identify the aspects of psychotherapy that have the largest effects, researchers distinguish between specific techniques (the things that distinguish between a therapist who is faithfully providing CBT versus one who is faithfully providing MI, for example), the common factors that are shared by all therapies (such as maintaining a therapeutic alliance and developing shared goals), expectancy (placebo effects), and changes that occur for reasons that lie entirely outside of therapy. A synthesis of evidence from several studies of these factors suggests that specific techniques account for just 15 percent of change, with twice that effect due to common factors. It is humbling to acknowledge that the power of extratherapeutic factors is even greater [10].

These data emphasize the importance of developing and maintaining the skills that allow for optimal engagement with patients. Such skills include maintaining a strong alliance (including repairing inevitable ruptures in the alliance), demonstrating empathy, developing consensus on goals, showing positive regard, collecting patient feedback, managing negative emotional responses, and remaining genuine [10,11]. In this chapter we use attachment theory as a framework from which to optimize the common factors in order to boost the effects of specific modalities of treatment.

The Relevance of Attachment to Obesity and Its Treatment

Attachment theory is a developmental theory that informs us about the roles of our closest relationships throughout life. In particular, attachment theory explains the impact of relationships on affect and behavior in adults by making explicit how these processes once emerged from relationships between infants and their parents. Several studies have examined the links between insecure patterns of attachment (described later) and obesity throughout the lifespan.

Childhood

Starting with childhood, a prospective developmental study found that low maternal sensitivity at six months of age, which is an important contributor to subsequent insecure attachment, predicted girls' BMI at two years of age [12]. Another study found that a child's BMI at three years of age is linked to the child's mother's ability to regulate her own affect and her BMI prior to pregnancy [13]. Since a parent's ability to regulate intense feelings affects his or her ability to support an infant's sense of security, this evidence suggests some potential for interactions between environmental and genetic contributions to obesity from a very early age. Similarly, a study comparing mothers who were either normal weight or obese found that obese mother-infant dyads had a lower quality of mother-child attachment. Furthermore, the child's pattern of attachment contributed to the child's BMI even after controlling for both the child's BMI at birth and the parents' BMIs [14]. Insecure infant patterns of attachment have also been linked to obesity at four years of age [15].

Adolescence

Moving forward in development to adolescence, qualitative research on teenage girls with obesity describes family conflicts in which the girls take on the family role of caring for others, without acknowledging their own emotional needs [16]. This suggests an attachment pattern known as *compulsive caregiving* [17], a type of dismissing insecure attachment in which emotional vulnerability is masked by caring for others rather than acknowledging ones' own needs. The adolescent girls in this study indicated that they use food to manage distressing emotions, which suggests how strategies to suppress emotions such as loneliness and depression might be linked to obesity.

Adulthood

In adulthood, the fearful pattern of insecure attachment is associated with higher BMI and higher waist-hip ratio [18]. This association is stronger when obesity is more severe [19]. Indeed, evidence supports the idea that a history of childhood trauma may be common among adults with obesity and that insecure attachment may mediate the relationship between early adverse experiences and adult obesity [20]. One of the leading ideas about insecure attachment diminishing healthy behaviors is that it impairs affect regulation, allowing unmodulated emotions to interfere with self-care and with healthcare relationships. Indeed, in bariatric surgery patients, emotion regulation is a link that mediates the relationship between insecure attachment and emotional eating [21]. Insecure attachment is also linked to other aspects of unhealthy eating; for example, it predicts high-caloric food intake in both children and adults [22].

Individuals with insecure attachment are more concerned about body shape, more dissatisfied with their own bodies, and more interested in cosmetic surgery than those with secure attachment [23–25]. Thus attachment insecurity leads some people to feel that love and approval depend on appearance. Being dissatisfied with one's appearance and eating excessively in response to these distressing feelings can lead to a vicious cycle of negative emotions, consumption, and negative self-image. Bearing these associations in mind, it is no surprise that insecure attachment is common in eating disorders in general and binge eating in particular [26–28].

After bariatric surgery, ongoing contact with the bariatric surgery team to continue adherence to the diet regimen has benefit for weight loss maintenance. Insecure attachment predicts poor outcomes and therefore suggests an additional need for support and adaptations in care. In particular, attachment insecurity is a risk factor for poor adherence, which leads to poor weight loss results [29]. Beyond just weight loss, insecure attachment is also associated with reduced quality of life after bariatric surgery [30].

Thus patterns of insecure attachment are highly relevant in severe obesity. First, patterns of attachment are almost always useful to bear in mind in order to adapt treatment to optimize nonspecific factors in therapy [11]. Second, insecure attachment is overrepresented among those with severe obesity for the reasons reviewed earlier. We can add to this list that insecure attachment, and particularly attachment avoidance, may be linked to a precontemplative stage of change and therefore may be more common among those who feel unready to progress with treatment. The following sections of this chapter review how a clinician can recognize different patterns of insecure attachment and use that insight to adapt treatment when insecure attachment interferes with care.

Recognizing Attachment Styles

In order to incorporate an appreciation of adult attachment patterns into the clinical care of individuals with severe obesity, a clinician needs a practical and fairly simple framework for identifying different attachment patterns. We advocate the 2 × 2 categorization of attachment patterns first introduced by Bartholomew and Horowitz [31], adapted to include subsequent research and observations about attachment in healthcare settings [32] (see Figure 4.1). In this adapted model, we recognize two dimensions of attachment insecurity, attachment anxiety and attachment avoidance, and four prototypical patterns that emerge from different degrees of insecurity on these dimensions: secure (low anxiety + low avoidance), preoccupied (anxiety > avoidance), dismissing (avoidance > anxiety), and fearful/disorganized (high anxiety + high avoidance). In this section we focus on the insecure prototypes because secure attachment is typically not associated with nonadherence or difficulties in maintaining an alliance [33,34].

Attachment Anxiety

It helps to appreciate what the two dimensions of insecure attachment represent before describing the prototypes. Attachment anxiety is characterized by a tendency toward dependency and proximity seeking, which is often accompanied by feelings of low self-worth, low confidence, and a lack of self-efficacy. Other people are expected to be inconsistently available, and fears of separation and abandonment are prominent. Individuals who are high on this dimension of insecurity express distress readily, which can be

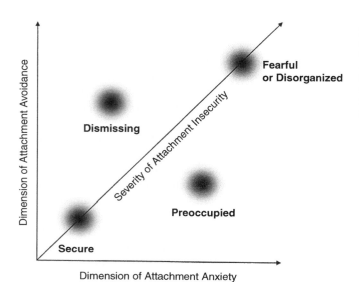

Figure 4.1 Prototypical patterns of adult attachment. (*Source:* From R. G. Maunder and J. J. Hunter, A prototype-based model of adult attachment for clinicians. *Psychodyn Psychiatry* 2012; 40: 549–73. Reprinted with permission.)

understood as a strategy to draw others toward them and thereby increase the likelihood that others will be there when they are needed [32].

Attachment Avoidance

Attachment avoidance is characterized by a preference for self-reliance and interpersonal distance. People who are high on this dimension prefer to keep any feelings of distress or vulnerability to themselves and often describe themselves as self-sufficient and not needing help or support [32]. It is helpful to conceptualize attachment avoidance as a defensive strategy – preemptively suppressing underlying feelings of insecurity in order to avoid any possibility of being shamed by another person [35].

Preoccupied Attachment

Preoccupied attachment is the result of insecurity that is based mostly on high attachment anxiety. Often the most obvious characteristic of a patient's preoccupied attachment is his or her style of communication. Preoccupied attachment often leads to a personal story that is hard to follow because the person expresses many details and intense emotions that are not organized well enough to make clear sense of them [36,37]. A listener is left with a greater appreciation of the person's sense of urgency and distress than clarity about the facts of their situation [37,38]. Many aspects of communication contribute to this dilemma, including vague words, frequent digressions, sudden changes in topics, and inattention to coherent timelines. These can all be understood as the consequences of a person telling his or her own story without keeping the needs of the listener (to make sense and stay engaged) "in mind." In fact, an inability to keep the inner worlds of others in mind (which is called *mentalization*) is an important aspect of insecure attachment of all types. In preoccupied attachment, deficits in mentalization are recognized by a story that is hard to synthesize and gives a sense of being "all evidence and no conclusion."

People with preoccupied attachment may also have difficulty reflecting on and expressing their own inner experience. They may leave it to the listener to imagine their thoughts rather than directly expressing them [39]. A person with preoccupied attachment is typically anxious about maintaining close relationships and fears abandonment, rejection, and separation [38,40,41]. As a result, expectations of others may be based on personal need (e.g., expecting rescue) or on preexisting schemas (e.g., expecting rejection) rather than on an appraisal of what the other person is actually offering or expressing [42]. A person with preoccupied attachment often feels too "clingy" or dependent for comfort [40]. In a clinical setting, preoccupied attachment may be particularly evident at the end of appointments when a patient's distress increases as he or she anticipates the looming separation.

The person with preoccupied attachment also has difficulty with agency, because he or she feels personally incapable and may compulsively turn to signal the other person to provide help. This is important because it may interfere with a preoccupied person's ability to pursue self-care effectively. Often people with this type of insecure attachment are able to identify what they *should* do while feeling quite inhibited about actually doing it [43].

Dismissing Attachment

A person who is a "textbook case" of dismissing attachment appears confident and self-reliant [40]. He or she does not ask for help, does not indicate distress, and is not inclined to pass on information that is particularly revealing [42,44]. In a conversation about intimate relationships, a person with dismissing attachment may seem not to value relationships highly and definitely indicates a preference to not depend on others [40,45]. A relationship with a spouse or romantic partner may appear cool and distant [40]. Beyond this appearance of reserve, close relationships may actually be described as aversive or "suffocating" [40,42]. Others may not be trusted because they are expected to be exploitive, unresponsive, or controlling [46].

A person with dismissing attachment may fail to communicate his or her situation effectively to a listener but does so in a way that is very different from a person with preoccupied attachment. In this case, the most striking barrier to feeling that one knows a patient well is how little information is provided or that information is provided in the form of clichés and conventional descriptions that conform to common social "scripts" but may not seem genuine [43]. The result is that an individual with dismissing attachment may seem inattentive or aloof, and his or her story lacks detail [37]. Generalizations are common but are not supplemented with examples, giving the listener the sense of a story that is "all conclusion with no evidence."

Whereas a preoccupied individual's chaotic and inconclusive style of communication may keep a listener engaged for a long time, without progressing toward a goal, the dismissing individual's communication style tends to have the effect of shutting down discussion. In each case, we interpret these results as the (possibly unconscious) goal of the interaction.

A dismissing individual typically does not seek social support when stressed [40,42]. He or she copes with stress with strategies that increase distance from emotions, such as denial and distraction [47,48].

Fearful or Disorganized Attachment

Fearful attachment combines attachment anxiety and attachment avoidance, which creates tension because these forms of insecurity pull in opposite directions. Disorganized attachment is more severe and conceptually different, marked not by a stable balance of opposing forces (as occurs with the fearful pattern) but by a disorganized fluctuation between the tendency to express distress and seek care and to shut down such expressions and avoid care [49]. In either case, the mixture of different sources and types of insecurity usually leads to markedly incoherent narratives [37]. Although these styles differ conceptually, the distinction often does not matter very much clinically because each represents a position of extreme insecurity and calls for adaptations of treatment that keep both dimensions of attachment insecurity in mind.

If attachment avoidance is understood as a strategic defense against underlying insecurity that a person feels it is best not to express or acknowledge, then fearful attachment can be understood as a partial failure of this defense, which allows attachment anxiety to break through the avoidance that is supposed to mask it [35], resulting in a sometimes contradictory combination of interpersonal anxiety and avoidant behaviors.

The key observation that identifies fearful or disorganized attachment is the tension or inconsistency between approach and avoidance. For example, these patients are the least likely to schedule routine appointments, the most likely to schedule urgent appointments, and the most likely to fail to attend [50]. The presence of suffering without help seeking may manifest as high levels of symptoms combined with low healthcare utilization [51]. Strong ambivalence in relationships may lead this person to tolerate unfair treatment in order to maintain an alliance [46,52]. This attitude may also be applied to relationships with healthcare professionals for whom a person with fearful attachment may unassertively assume that he or she has to bow to authority because "they have all the power" [46].

Fearful and disorganized attachment is often characterized by intense negative affect [38]. Emotions may be inflexibly suppressed and then erupt when stress is intolerable [35,53]. Others' unavailability may provoke anger rather than feelings of sadness and fear. When this occurs, anger may be expressed as a rejection of support that is considered to be too little, too late or insincere [54].

People with fearful attachment can be highly attuned to cues from others that predict rejection or abandonment. Sometimes this vigilant attunement creates a false impression that they are effective at mentalizing, but in truth they have difficulty understanding a wide range of intentions of others. The clue to the ineffectiveness of this hyperattentiveness is its inflexibility. Rigid expectations that others will be disappointing or harmful are not attentive to context and not easily amended by contrary evidence.

Narrative incoherence here may be similar to preoccupied attachment (excessive affect, excess words, multiple fragmented story lines, with deficits in logical organization and orientation of the listener) or dismissing attachment (suppressed affect, minimal detail, a closed, rigid, and sparse story) or may alternate emphasis between these elements.

Adapting Treatment to Patients' Attachment Styles

Of course, actual people are complicated and rarely present as "textbook cases" or prototypical examples of anything, including patterns of attachment. Nonetheless, the patterns just described often serve as a helpful guide to identifying some of the leading characteristics that interfere with establishing a strong treatment alliance. As such, they provide a clinician with a basis for adapting his or her approach in order to optimize the common factors of therapy. In each case, the goal of adapting care is to optimize a patient's opportunities to feel secure. We have described these possible adaptations in depth elsewhere and summarize them in this section [55].

Adapting to a Patient with Preoccupied Attachment

A patient with preoccupied attachment often feels inadequate to meet health challenges alone. Fear trumps other health concerns because a person who is too frightened simply cannot receive information well, appraise his or her situation accurately, or participate in problem solving. Until he or she experiences some relief, he or she cannot collaborate effectively with a healthcare provider to figure out what is wrong and what needs to be done. An effective clinician adapts his or her approach to reduce the patient's fear and to build the patient's sense of self-efficacy. These strategies can help the clinician maintain the frame of mind that optimizes the necessary changes.

Be Calm. A person with preoccupied attachment has a great deal of trouble regulating his or her own feelings of fear and distress and cannot easily use relationships as a source of calmness either. The person's anxiety feels contagious, sufficient to knock one off the course of normal clinical interactions, unless the interaction is recognized and addressed. Your own unflappable, reflective manner can model less intense reactivity for the individual and serve as a reassuring template for a more effective approach to stress and problems. Maintaining calm can be harder than it sounds because a preoccupied patient's confusing narrative style and lack of clarity about goals can be anxiety provoking.

Take Time. One of the reasons that a preoccupied patient's style can provoke anxiety or other unhelpful emotional responses is that it leads to inefficient interactions. It is easy for a busy clinician to feel that "the clock is ticking and we are getting nowhere." However, trying to speed the interaction up makes things worse, as a clinician tries to finish the patient's run-on sentences or summarize prematurely. Paradoxically, allowing the patient extra time may reduce anxiety and improve efficiency. Once this is recognized as a barrier to care, scheduling a longer appointment or even an extra one can improve the communication. Simply reducing expectations for how much can be accomplished in the time allowed can increase the effectiveness of treatment.

Take a Thoughtful History. Particularly for a preoccupied patient, feeling understood goes a long way toward increasing feelings of security, which, in turn, allows a person to focus on the challenges at hand. For a clinician, appreciating how behaviors that are counterproductive in the current circumstance were once an adaptive response to a nonoptimal environment can change the tone of the interaction and improve the therapeutic alliance. Taking a careful history can also provide opportunities to ask about and identify effective coping with stressors in the past (of which the patient may be essentially unaware because they occurred at times of high stress and so have not been experienced by him or her as good adaptations), which enhances a patient's self-confidence and self-esteem.

Use Your Observations of an Incoherent Narrative as Information. It is hard to make sense of a story that is all evidence but has no coherent conclusion. Not being able to adequately understand a patient can lead a clinician to feel inadequate or helpless. It can be very useful to realize that observations of incoherence are "diagnostic" (not in the sense of leading to a diagnosis of mental illness but rather allowing a clinician to identify the patient's attachment style). Furthermore, they provide invaluable information about how a patient is likely to communicate with others, at least at times of high stress, and how this may interfere with other relationships – a crucial observation in a clinic with many independent healthcare provider-patient relationships.

Be Predictable and Supportive. Situations in which the availability of support is uncertain or unpredictable tend to increase anxiety. You can counter this by being clear and reliable in your communications about your availability, sticking to your word and not promising more than you can follow through on (which sometimes occurs as a well-intentioned attempt to be reassuring). Similarly, being open and transparent about the reasons for questions during an interview and what can be expected in future appointments helps a preoccupied patient to feel more secure.

Remember That the Central Problem Is Fear. Discombobulating communications can confuse. Unreasonable expectations for availability can be off-putting. A person who is "too dependent" can appear to be weak. These and other manifestations of preoccupied attachment can lead a clinician to experience negative emotional reactions such as anger, helplessness, hopelessness, or rejection. Remembering that fear is the primary emotion driving all of this behavior can help a clinician to put things into a constructive context and may be a first necessary step toward repairing a rupture in what had been an otherwise positive therapeutic alliance.

Allow Your Patients to Use the Resources That Allow Them to Feel More Secure. Sometimes preoccupied patients feel more secure if they can attend an appointment with a buddy or take notes during a session or modify appointments in some other way. Where the patient's intention is regulating his or her own distress, adapting to these needs as much as possible usually helps the treatment work toward its goals.

Use the Skills of Active Listening. A skilled clinician can help an incoherent patient to tell a better-organized and more-informative story. Using skills of paraphrasing and summarizing can ensure that information is being understood accurately and help the patient to find a more succinct vocabulary. Simple questions are required more often than with other patients in order to clarify vague descriptions, make timelines explicit, and identify the important characters in anecdotes and their relationship to the patient. Sometimes we draw diagrams with the patient's input on a piece of paper or a whiteboard (e.g., a timeline, a simple flowchart to show how elements of the story relate to each other, or a family tree) in order to ensure that we have a shared understanding of a complex story.

Teach Relaxation Techniques. Once a therapeutic alliance is established, patients may benefit from learning skills to reduce anxiety, such as muscle relaxation or breathing techniques. In addition to their direct benefit, learning these skills can increase independence and self-efficacy. It is often best to wait until there are indicators of a good working alliance before introducing specific relaxation techniques, which might otherwise be misconstrued as a superficial response to a complex problem.

Break the Contingency between Expressing Distress and Getting Care. Preoccupied attachment often leads to an unfortunate cycle that is reinforced in healthcare settings. It works like this: a person with preoccupied attachment expects others to be inattentive, unavailable, or rejecting. His or her response (developing and reinforced in early development) is to send frequent and amplified signals of need (symptoms, complaints, distress) in order to keep the other person near. This sometimes leads to the desired result (reinforcing the learned reflex) but ultimately is perceived to be "too much," leading the other person to withdraw or become inattentive (reinforcing the expectation of rejection or unavailability), which restarts the cycle. It is a frustrating and sometimes painful cycle for all involved.

An alternative that can be negotiated in circumstances in which there is some ongoing therapeutic relationship is to try to break the contingency between distress and contact by providing contact that does not depend on asking for it. This means scheduled appointments (not meeting "as needed"), which are typically spaced more frequently than might otherwise be the case. According to this principle, 20 minutes every two weeks is better than 40 minutes once a month. This negotiation also includes a discussion that, as much as is safe and reasonable, issues that arise between appointments will be deferred until the next scheduled meeting. Naturally, such an arrangement only works if the appointments are reliable and predictable.

Teach Healthy Assertiveness. People with preoccupied attachment often lack a sense of agency in their lives. Teaching healthy assertiveness in situations of modest perceived conflict ("Excuse me, I think I was next in line") is a practical skill that can pay dividends both in terms of improving a sense of agency and by building confidence in the ability of therapy to support movement toward larger life goals.

Facilitate Communication and Coordination between Various Care Providers. People with preoccupied attachment often initiate relationships in which they seek care from professionals and from nonprofessionals but are less likely to terminate these relationships when they are no longer providing value. Furthermore, these caring relationships are often compromised by the fractured and incoherent nature of their communication, combined with urgent requests for help. The result can be a complex network of care providers who frequently do not have a complete picture of the patient's situation and who are not communicating with one another. It is helpful to take practical steps to opening communication and bringing some coordination to this fractured web. Negotiating that all providers will be copied on progress notes, for example, is an easily implemented step to reduce miscommunication. Similarly, within a multidisciplinary obesity clinic, for example, it is helpful to present the treatment team to the patient as working together as an integrated whole.

Adapting to a Patient with Dismissing Attachment

A person with dismissing attachment finds emotional intimacy and vulnerability to be uncomfortable. If he or she feels distress, expressing it may make him or her feel worse. There may be exceptions, but this is the usual starting point. Feeling insecure is likely to push a dismissing person to strive to appear even stronger, to dig in and distance himself or herself further from others.

Naturally, this preference for independence reduces opportunities to be supported by others. The expectation that others will disappoint, or intrude, or pressure him or her toward self-revelation also reduces collaboration. While self-reliance can be an excellent strategy when it works, it often leads to conflict when it does not work. The problems that can emerge when attachment avoidance interferes with healthcare often are the opposite of the problems that we discussed for people with preoccupied attachment. They call for different adaptations.

Respect Independence. Understanding that the suppressed emotions and interpersonal distance that are typical in dismissing attachment are a defensive strategy that developed to conceal and contain underlying insecurity may lead a clinician to want his or her patient to "open up." It is useful to remember that applying pressure in this direction is aversive and may be counterproductive. It is usually not the therapeutic goal in treating obesity to change a patient's attachment style (or defenses) but rather to adapt to them in ways that help him or her work toward health goals. While we sometimes tell a dismissing patient that he or she seems to be "too self-reliant for your own good," we do so to develop a shared under-standing of the challenges they face, not to force change. As much as possible, within the bounds of good care, we try to allow a dismissing patient to direct his or her own treatment.

Allow Your Patient to Set the Interpersonal Distance. Related to the preceding point, patients often display social cues that indicate how they wish to interact. A preoccupied patient may choose the chair nearest to the clinician; a dismissing patient, the most distant chair. Similarly a dismissing patient may prefer to be called by his or her last name and title until he or she offers permission to use his or her first name, as another example. In general, it is often helpful to respect and follow these cues, usually without identifying them out loud. Allowing a dismissing patient to set the interpersonal distance allows him or her to find the position in which the greatest sense of security is available, which facilitates the exploration and challenge that is inevitable in a therapeutic dialogue.

Clarify Cautiously. Whereas a clinician is called on to be quite active with a preoccupied patient in the service of organizing a fractured and vague narrative, a dismissing patient might find that behavior intrusive and controlling. Nonetheless, a story that communicates little because of overuse of clichéd or conventional generalizations requires some clarification. Often it is helpful to listen carefully first (following rather than leading, to avoid the unhelpful sense of conducting an interrogation) and then to inquire. As a clinician, you can point out that people experience (whatever has just been described) very differently and that you will be more helpful if you can understand just how it was in this case. Genuine curiosity, transparent statements of what seems clear and what remains to be understood, and clear links between the information that is being sought and its value in reaching the treatment goal will facilitate patient self-disclosure.

Put More Emphasis on Objective Measures of Health. People with dismissing attachment are disinclined to report that they have problems or to ask for help. As a result, their self-reports of health status on which clinicians rely to gauge their patients' needs and progress often do not provide a full or accurate picture. As much as possible, it helps to base treatment decisions on objective measures.

Use Scheduled Appointments Instead of Seeing Dismissing Patients As Needed. Interestingly, we give this same advice to preoccupied and dismissing patients, but for very different reasons. For preoccupied patients, we suggested this tactic as a step toward reducing the contingency between distress and contact. For dismissing patients, the reason is less subtle – they are loath to identify that they have needs and tend to fall out of touch if there isn't a scheduled appointment.

Negotiate and Reframe. A dialogue between equals (even if they differ in expertise) is often a framework that makes treatment more palatable for individuals with dismissing attachment. Negotiating on treatment goals and strategies is often effective and much less confrontational than other models of interactions. The idea that a patient should *comply* with what an expert and authoritative clinician prescribes is anathema. Rather, a dismissing patient may find that he or she is motivated to *adhere* to mutually agreeable changes that lead to shared goals. Reframing undesired tests or treatments as unpleasant but necessary steps toward a desired goal can also be helpful.

Use the Principles and Techniques of Motivational Interviewing. Some of the principles and techniques of MI are a very good match for dismissing individuals. "Rolling with the resistance" and arriving at goals through transparent, good-faith discussion of the pros and cons of changing or not changing can be quite acceptable to a person who does not want to be told what to do or to engage in emotional-focused conversations that make him or her feel too exposed. There is much more discussion of these approaches in Section 2 of this book.

Disconfirm Negative Expectations. Since adult attachment styles have developmental origins, it can be helpful to remember that the parenting environment that reinforces avoidant attachment consists of a consistent but aversive response to vulnerability and need. Thus your dismissing patient expects that if he or she counts on you, your response will be invalidating, belittling, or even exploitive. In the context of discussing obesity, a topic that is laden with feelings of shame, this concern is amplified. Although we do not usually aim to change a patient's attachment style, it can only help in providing a more effective alliance to consistently provide an interaction that is better than expected: understanding, respectful, curious, and supportive.

Mentalize Your Patient's Needs and Concerns. Since dismissing attachment is based upon a defensive strategy, there is often more going on than it may appear at first. Dismissing patients are not only disinclined to describe their inner worlds, but they may also lack *skills* in self-description. If the therapeutic relationship is well-enough established that a solid sense of trust can be assumed, a clinician can sometimes risk making tentative guesses about a patient's feelings, beliefs, and expectations that go beyond what has been explicitly expressed. These should usually be tentatively expressed, not as "mind reading" ("When you got angry at my question, it made me wonder if I hurt you. Sometimes feelings of hurt can trigger anger"). Extending a person's ability to reflect on his or her own inner world and what others' think and feel not only can increase opportunities for interpersonal support but also may help that person to regulate his or her own emotions.

Don't Take Anger Personally. A person with a dismissing style needs to maintain a comfortable interpersonal distance. Anger may serve this function when others are getting uncomfortably close or acting in a way that is reminiscent of a past injury. If you do something that triggers anger, it is always helpful to try to understand it (and usually helpful to try not to repeat it). Try not to act on your own sense of hurt or injustice if those feelings emerge.

Adapting to Fearful or Disorganized Attachment

It is hard to live with a pattern of attachment that is influenced by both attachment anxiety and attachment avoidance. It is also hard to try to help someone with that interpersonal pattern. Mutually contradictory strategies create a complicated mixture of approach and withdrawal or seeking and then rejecting help. Communication can be very challenging. For a patient with obesity, the demands of finding sufficient comfort to discuss one's body and adherence to prescribed regimens is often provocative, so a fearful or disorganized patient with obesity is likely to be identified as a troubled or troubling patient. It is a situation that demands patience, skill, and genuine concern to make the adaptations that can improve the situation.

Put All Your Effort into Establishing a Trusting Alliance. There is no point working on other goals until you trust one another. It is possible to waste effort for a long period of time, seeming to get nowhere, because the primary task of any therapy has been neglected. It may be a challenging task that takes some time to accomplish. A clinician needs to demonstrate reliability, make a genuine effort to be understanding and supportive, use clear and consistent communication, and work to establish shared goals in order to develop the trust on which therapeutic interventions can succeed.

Use the Skills That Work for Preoccupied and Dismissing Attachment. Since fearful and disorganized attachment involves combinations of attachment anxiety and attachment avoidance, the approaches that we have described for each of those patterns may be useful. The trick is that none of them is likely to apply consistently. A great deal of therapeutic skill and flexibility is required to identify which aspect of insecurity is currently most prominent and to respond to insecurity with suitable adaptations of technique.

Address Ruptures in the Alliance Honestly and Supportively. Even when a strong working alliance has been established, it is virtually inevitable that errors and missteps will cause hurts that interfere with that bond of trust. It is almost always constructive to identify these as they emerge, to try to understand together what has gone wrong, and then to use this collaborative enquiry as the basis for repairing the alliance and getting back to goal-directed work tasks. This can be quite challenging because it requires honesty and maturity. There is no room for the "fake apologies" that are often heard in public life, of the "sorry if you were offended, although I didn't do anything wrong" type. If you missed an appointment or failed to notify the patient of a holiday, it is best to acknowledge it straightforwardly, apologize, and not try to minimize or obfuscate the event.

Encourage Clear and Assertive Expression of Needs. The opposing pulls of attachment anxiety and attachment avoidance can lead to a variety of ways in which fearful attachment manifests. One such pattern is to live with unmet needs and unexpressed concerns, too inhibited by fear and the expectation of hostile or disappointing responses from others to give voice to these troubles. When this pattern is present, a clinician can be very helpful as a supportive coach, encouraging clear statements of needs and expectations – a special and more challenging version of the teaching of healthy assertiveness that we encourage for preoccupied attachment.

Focus on Shifting the Balance to Favor Attachment Avoidance over Attachment Anxiety. A person who is caught between attachment anxiety and attachment avoidance is usually unable to try to modify both of those drives at once. If you have to choose, it is usually easier to help a person to shift the balance toward a more prominent role for attachment avoidance. The reverse is harder because it requires giving up a defense and allowing more of the underlying distress to emerge. The readjusted balance between these opposing forces can allow a person to feel more independent control over his or her life, which can be a useful step toward other goals. Often this shift takes the form of declining to participate in interactions that are predictably hurtful (such as with relatives with whom there is a long history of repeated injurious interactions).

Attend to Overwhelming Challenges. People with fearful and disorganized attachment can easily feel overwhelmed. Sometimes the practical interventions to make challenges feel less overwhelming can pay dividends. Simple strategies such as breaking large challenges up into manageable chunks can be helpful (and are easy to miss when you feel like you are in the midst of a crisis). Interventions to reduce acute symptoms such as pain or anxiety that interfere with focusing on other tasks can also help.

Treat Mental Illness If It Is Present. All attachment styles are an aspect of normal psychology. They are understood as patterns that were learned and reinforced at a time when they were the most adaptive responses available to the interpersonal environment in which a child grew up. Nonetheless, insecure attachment, and especially disorganized attachment, is a risk factor for developing depression, anxiety disorders, and other mental illnesses. If fearful or disorganized attachment is interfering with the care of a patient with severe obesity, stay attuned to the signs that a treatable psychiatric syndrome might also be present. Often such an illness will be the most treatable part of a complex situation.

Attend to the Treatment Team. Caring for patients who are living with conflicting drives toward and away from affiliation is very challenging and can lead to strain for the clinicians who are struggling to find a workable alliance and sense that they are failing. They will need the support of the team, including a chance to vent about how problematic they find this situation, in order not to become nihilistic or blaming or even simply to withdraw.

Lastly, patients with the incoherent communication typical of fearful or disorganized individuals often do not convey clearly whether or not interventions are experienced as useful, which can, in turn, disorganize the clinician. One way to help the team or clinician relocate his or her balance with such patients is the advice to "adhere to your usual excellent standard of care." This reminder of their skill and expertise – independent of this person's confusing feedback – settles the fraught circumstance so that the person can access the best available care, and the clinician can feel more secure in his or her own behavior.

Incorporating an Attachment Perspective into a Bariatric Surgery Clinic

Sockalingam and Hawa have described an integrated multidisciplinary approach to bariatric surgery that incorporates an attachment focus into a broad psychosocial assessment [19,56]. A comprehensive assessment includes a valid self-report measure of attachment insecurity, the ECR-M16 [57,58]. Treatment team members of all disciplines are taught to appreciate the impact of attachment anxiety and attachment avoidance and use the self-report scores to identify and understand interpersonal vulnerability. Weekly team meetings in which relevant aspects of patients' care are discussed include attention to patients' attachment styles.

Team members can then tailor patients' treatment and support options to their individual needs. Patients who are challenging to engage with are understood in terms of their attachment patterns. For example, consider a patient with dismissing attachment who has difficulty feeling connected with most team members but forms a stronger alliance with a particular clinician. In this case the clinician whom the patient identifies as a "good match" may serve as his or her primary contact for longitudinal care, regardless of his or her discipline. Allowing the patient to choose his or her primary contact is an accommodation to a dismissing patient's preference for control and autonomy. The accommodation promotes a greater sense of security for the patient and a better treatment, as that clinician is backed up by the rest of the team.

Other accommodations are also possible. Patients with high attachment avoidance can be offered telephone or online psychological interventions, such as CBT, which allows them to receive treatment on their own schedule and without the experience of clinicians becoming "too close for comfort" (see Chapters 14 and 15). Some clinicians provide email access to facilitate the patient's control over communication during the postoperative phase.

Patients with preoccupied attachment receive different accommodations. These include more frequent scheduled appointments, which reduce frequent emails or phone calls when these anxiously attached patients feel overwhelmed. Attention to continuity of contact with core team members is emphasized, especially a familiar dietician, because preoccupied patients often feel unable to control eating on their own and are challenged to adhere to the postoperative diet. Dieticians who are trained in CBT techniques and are backed up by a psychologist or psychiatrist as needed will be most effective in this role.

Because relationship discontinuity triggers stress, patients with insecure attachment often benefit from a "warm handoff" when care passes from one team member to another. The familiar team member walks the patient over to the new team member and introduces them, which facilitates an easier start to the new relationship.

Finally, the importance of relationship styles to bariatric care is taught to patients in a bariatric surgery support group. Attachment theory is taught as a way to understand how people relate to one another and to provide insights into how group members' attachment styles affect their efforts to lose weight.

Summary

Engaging in treatment for obesity inevitably focuses an individual on issues intertwined with self-esteem, shame, and low self-efficacy. As a result, this work is likely to stimulate feelings of insecurity and to activate the behaviors that are characteristic of a patient's attachment style. The clinician who can recognize these patterns and adapt his or her interventions and advice to the individual will be advantaged in maintaining a therapeutic alliance and likely have greater success in his or her interventions.

As the clinic, and the relationships within it, becomes less likely to evoke fear and insecurity, or even function to increase security, the patient is freed up from his or her relationship behaviors that are intended to increase feelings of security and is better able to focus on addressing the challenges of obesity management, whether it is dietary, behavioral, medical, or surgical. Attachment theory provides an empirical basis for improving the treatment alliance and bolstering the common factors of care by individualizing treatment. A clinic for severe obesity is advantaged when its clinicians are able to identify a patient's characteristic interpersonal style and employ strategies that tailor interactions to optimize the patient's opportunities to feel secure in his or her care.

Key Points

- People with severe obesity often struggle with self-esteem, shame, and low self-efficacy. For those who choose surgical intervention, optimizing adherence to aftercare is important but difficult.
- Attending to common therapeutic factors can have a positive impact on patient engagement. These factors include maintaining a strong alliance, demonstrating empathy, developing consensus on goals, showing positive regard, collecting patient feedback, managing negative emotional responses, and remaining genuine.
- A clinic for severe obesity is advantaged when its clinicians are able to identify a patient's characteristic interpersonal style. Attachment theory provides an empirical basis for improving the treatment alliance and bolstering the common factors of care by individualizing treatment.
- Strategies consistent with an attachment framework include recognizing the type and intensity of an individual's insecurity and modifying practice to address the most pressing concerns.
- These strategies can be incorporated into the normal functioning of a bariatric service via the standardized measurement of attachment style and team meetings that tailor interventions to that style.

References

1. R. Hawa and S. Sockalingam. Introduction to severe obesity for psychiatrists. In S. Sockalingam and R. Hawa, eds., *Psychiatric Care in Severe Obesity*. Berlin: Springer, 2017: 3–4.

2. A. E. Pontiroli, A. Fossati, P. Vedani, et al. Post-surgery adherence to scheduled visits and compliance, more than personality disorders, predict outcome of bariatric restrictive surgery in morbidly obese patients. *Obes Surg* 2007; **17**: 1492–7.

3. E. Wheeler, A. Prettyman, M. J. Lenhard, et al. Adherence to outpatient program postoperative appointments after bariatric surgery. *Surg Obes Relat Dis* 2008; **4**: 515–20.

4. H. O. Lier, E. Biringer, B. Stubhaug, et al. The impact of preoperative counseling on postoperative treatment adherence in bariatric surgery patients: A randomized controlled trial. *Patient Educ Couns* 2012; **87**: 336–42.

5. J. Bowlby. *Attachment and Loss,* vol 1: *Attachment.* New York, NY: Basic Books, 1969.

6. J. J. Hunter and R. G. Maunder. Using attachment theory to understand illness behavioural. *Gen Hosp Psychiatry* 2001; **23**: 177–82.

7. R. G. Maunder and J. J. Hunter. Attachment relationships as determinants of physical health. *J Am Acad Psychoanal Dyn Psychiatry* 2008; **36**: 11–32.

8. J. O. Prochaska and C. C. Di Clemente. Transtheoretical therapy: Toward a more integrative model of change. *Psychother Theor Res Pract* 1982; **19**: 276–88.

9. N. Mastellos, L. H. Gunn, L. M. Felix, et al. Transtheoretical model stages of change for dietary and physical exercise modification in weight loss management for overweight and obese adults. *Cochrane Database Syst Rev* 2014; **2**: CD008066.

10. J. C. Norcross. *Psychotherapy That Works: Evidence-Based Responsiveness* (2nd edn). New York, NY: Oxford University Press, 2011.

11. M. Leszcz, C. Pain, J. Hunter, et al. *Acheiving Psychotherapy Effectiveness.* New York, NY: W.W. Norton, 2014.

12. B. E. Wendland, L. Atkinson, M. Steiner, et al. Low maternal sensitivity at six months of age predicts higher BMI in 48-month-old girls but not boys. *Appetite* 2014; **82**: 97–102.

13. G. de Campora, G. Larciprete, A. M. Delogu, et al. A longitudinal study on emotional dysregulation and obesity risk: From pregnancy to three years of age of the baby. *Appetite* 2016; **96**: 95–101.

14. A. Keitel-Korndorfer, S. Sierau, A. M. Klein, et al. Insatiable insecurity: maternal obesity as a risk factor for mother-child attachment and child weight. *Attach Hum Dev* 2015; **17**: 399–413.

15. S. E. Anderson and R. C. Whitaker. Attachment security and obesity in US preschool-aged children. *Arch Pediatr Adolesc Med* 2011; **165**: 235–42.

16. S. Holland, R. Dallos, and L. Olver. An exploration of young women's experiences of living with excess weight. *Clin Child Psychol Psychiatry* 2012; **17**: 538–52.

17. J. Bowlby. Making and breaking of affectional bonds: 1. Aetiology and psychopathology in the light of attachment theory. *Br. J Psychiatry* 1977; **130**: 201–10.

18. M. Hintsanen, M. Jokela, L. Pulkki-Raback, et al. Associations of youth and adulthood body-mass index and waist-hip ratio with attachment styles and dimensions. *Curr Psychol* 2010; **29**: 257–71.

19. R. G. Maunder, J. J. Hunter, and T. L. Le. Insecure attachment and trauma in obesity and bariatric surgery. In S. Sockalingam and R. Hawa, eds., *Psychiatric Care in Severe Obesity*. Berlin: Springer, 2017: 37–48.

20. A. D'Argenio, C. Mazzi, L. Pecchioli, et al. Early trauma and adult obesity: Is psychological dysfunction the mediating mechanism? *Physiol Behav* 2009; **98**: 543–6.

21. M. Taube-Schiff, J. Van Exan, R. Tanaka, et al. Attachment style and emotional eating in bariatric surgery candidates: The mediating role of difficulties in emotion regulation. *Eat Behav* 2015; **18**: 36–40.

22. A. Faber and L. Dube. Parental attachment insecurity predicts child and adult high-caloric food consumption. *J Health Psychol* 2015; **20**: 511–24.

23. G. Bosmans, L. Goossens, and C Braet. Attachment and weight and shape concerns in inpatient overweight youngsters. *Appetite* 2009; **53**: 454–6.

24. I. M. Javo and T. Sorlie. Psychosocial predictors of an interest in cosmetic surgery among young Norwegian women: A population-based study. *Plast Reconstr Surg* 2009; **124**: 2142–8.

25. B. Mayer, P. Muris, C. Meesters, et al. Brief report: Direct and indirect relations of risk factors with eating behavioural problems in late adolescent females. *J Adolesc* 2009; **32**: 741–5.

26. C. J. Patton. Fear of abandonment and binge eating: A subliminal psychodynamic activation investigation. *J Nerv Ment Dis* 1992; **180**: 484–90.

27. M. Caslini, F. Bartoli, C. Crocamo, et al. Disentangling the association between child abuse and eating disorders:

A systematic review and meta-analysis. *Psychosom Med* 2016; **78**: 79–90.

28. G. A. Tasca and L. Balfour. Attachment and eating disorders: A review of current research. *Int J Eat Disord* 2014; **47**: 710–7.

29. F. Aarts, R. Geenen, V. E. Gerdes, et al. Attachment anxiety predicts poor adherence to dietary recommendations: An indirect effect on weight change one year after gastric bypass surgery. *Obes Surg* 2015; **25**: 666–72.

30. S. Sockalingam, S. Wnuk S, R. Strimas, et al. The association between attachment avoidance and quality of life in bariatric surgery candidates. *Obes Facts* 2011; **4**: 456–60.

31. K. Bartholomew and L. M. Horowitz. Attachment styles among young adults: A test of a four-category model. *J Pers Social Psychol* 1991; **61**: 226–44.

32. R. G. Maunder and J. J Hunter. A prototype-based model of adult attachment for clinicians. *Psychodyn Psychiatry* 2012; **40**: 549–73.

33. P. Ciechanowski, J. Russo, W. Katon, et al. Influence of patient attachment style on self-care and outcomes in diabetes. *Psychosom Med* 2004; **66**: 720–8.

34. R. G. Maunder, A. Panzer, M. Viljoen, et al. Physicians' difficulty with emergency department patients is related to patients' attachment style. *Soc Sci Med* 2006; **63**: 552–62.

35. P. R. Shaver and M. Mikulincer. Attachment-related psychodynamics. *Attach Hum Dev* 2002; **4**: 133–61.

36. C. George and M. West. The development and preliminary validation of a new measure of adult attachment: The adult attachment projective. *Attach Hum Dev* 2001; **3**: 30–61.

37. E. Hesse. The adult attachment interview: Protocol, method of analysis, and empirical studies. In J. Cassidy and P. R. Shaver, eds., *Handbook of Attachment: Theory, Research and Clinical Applications* (2nd edn). New York, NY: Guilford Press, 2008: 552–98.

38. M. Mikulincer and P. R. Shaver. *Attachment in Adulthood: Structure, Dynamics, and Change.* New York, NY: Guilford Press, 2007.

39. A. Jellema. Dismissing and preoccupied insecure attachment in CAT: Some implications for CAT practice. *Clin Psychol Psychother* 2002; **9**: 225–41.

40. J. G. Allen, H. Stein, P. Fonagy, et al. Rethinking adult attachment: A study of expert consensus. *Bull Menninger Clin* 2005; **69**: 59–80.

41. M. W. Baldwin, B. Fehr, E. Keedian, et al. An exploration of the relational schemata underlying attachment styles: Self-report and lexical decision approaches. *Pers Soc Psychol Bull* 1993; **19**: 746–54.

42. W. S. Rholes, J. A. Simpson, and J. G. Stevens. Attachment orientations, social support, and conflict resolution in close relationships. In J. A. Simpson and W. S. Rholes, eds., *Attachment Theory and Close Relationships.* New York, NY: Guilford Press, 1998: 166–88.

43. C. George and M. West. The development and preliminary validation of a new measure of adult attachment: The adult attachment projective. *Attach Hum Dev* 2001; **3**: 30–61.

44. M. Main. Avoidance in the service of attachment: A working paper. In K. Immelman, G. Barlow, M. Main, and L. Petrinovitch, eds., *Behaviouralal Development: The Bielefeld Interdisciplinary Project.* New York, NY: Cambridge University Press, 1981: 651–93.

45. M. Mikulincer and O. Nachshon. Attachment styles and patterns of self-disclosure. *J Pers Soc Psychol* 1991; **61**: 321–31.

46. P. Ciechanowski and W. J. Katon. The interpersonal experience of health care through the eyes of patients with diabetes. *Soc Sci Med* 2006; **63**: 3067–79.

47. J. A. Feeney. Adult attachment, coping style and health locus of control as predictors of health behavioural. *Aust J Psychol* 1995; **47**: 171–7.

48. F. G. Lopez, A. M. Mauricio, B. Gormley, et al. Adult attachment orientations and college student distress: The mediating role of problem coping styles. *J Couns Dev* 2001; **79**: 459–64.

49. K. Lyons-Ruth and D. Jacobvitz. Attachment disorganization: genetic factors, parenting contexts, and developmental transformation from infancy to adulthood. In J. Cassidy and P. R. Shaver, eds., *Handbook of Attachment: Theory, Research, and Clinical Applications* (2nd edn). New York, NY: Guilford Press, 2008: 666–97.

50. P. Ciechanowski, J. Russo, W. Katon, et al. Where is the patient? The association of psychosocial factors and missed primary care appointments in patients with diabetes. *Gen Hosp Psychiatry* 2006; **28**: 9–17.

51. P. Ciechanowski, E. A. Walker, W. J. Katon, et al. Attachment theory: A model for health care utilization and somatization. *Psychosom Med* 2002; **64**: 660–7.

52. G. R Maio, F. D. Fincham, and E. J. Lycett. Attitudinal ambivalence toward partners and attachment style. *Pers Soc Psychol Bull* 2000; **26**: 1451–64.

53. E. Berant, M. Mikulincer, and V. Florian. The association of mother's attachment style and their psychological reactions to the diagnosis of infant's congenital heart disease. *J Soc Clin Psychol* 2001; **20**: 208–32.

54. M. L. West and A. E. Sheldon-Kellor. *Patterns of Relating: An Adult Attachment Perspective*. New York, NY: Guilford Press, 1994.

55. R. Maunder and J. Hunter. *Love, Fear, and Health: How Our Attachments to Others Shape Health and Health Care*. Toronto, University of Toronto Press, 2015.

56. S. Sockalingam and R. Hawa. Attachment style in bariatric surgery: A case study. In J. Hunter and R. Maunder, eds., *Improving Patient Treatment with Attachment Theory: A Guide for Primary Care Practitioners and Specialists*. Berlin: Springer; 2016: 145–54.

57. K. B. Pitzul, T. Jackson, S. Crawford, et al. Understanding disposition after referral for bariatric surgery: When and why patients referred do not undergo surgery. *Obes Surg* 2014; **24**: 134–40.

58. C. Lo, A. Walsh, M. Mikulincer, et al. Measuring attachment security in patients with advanced cancer: Psychometric properties of a modified and brief Experiences in Close Relationships scale. *Psychooncology* 2009; **18**: 490–9.

Motivational Interviewing for Behavioral and Lifestyle Changes in Severe Obesity

Lauren David and Stephanie E. Cassin

Case Vignette

Janice is a 44-year-old teacher who lives with her husband of 14 years and their two daughters (ages 8 and 10 years). Janice finds teaching both enjoyable and rewarding, but she has been finding it increasingly difficult to stand up for extended periods while teaching lessons due to her chronic pain condition. She also tires more easily now and often finds it difficult to maintain her energy throughout the day. By the time she returns home from work, she feels that she has little energy left to prepare meals and play with her kids. She used to pride herself on her cooking ability, but the family's busy schedule (e.g., taking their daughters to various after-school activities) leaves little time to shop for groceries and prepare homemade dinners and lunches. As a result, they order takeout food several nights a week and typically prepare quick, highly processed meals the nights they eat dinner at home.

Janice has never particularly enjoyed exercise. She had periods of being able to commit to an exercise routine as a young adult when she enrolled in a regularly scheduled exercise class when she was in school, but she found it difficult to maintain that schedule after starting full-time work and having kids. Her current exercise is typically limited to being on her feet in her classroom and playing with her kids, but her chronic pain makes it difficult to keep up with them. After the kids go to bed, Janice and her husband either watch their favorite TV series together or she relaxes while reading a book.

Janice reports struggling with her weight since adolescence and currently has a body mass index (BMI) of 42 kg/m². She has a history of yoyo dieting and weight fluctuations, but her weight has been on a steady upward trajectory since her first pregnancy at 34 years of age. In addition to experiencing chronic pain, she was also recently diagnosed with type 2 diabetes mellitus. Her husband has encouraged her to exercise more out of concern for her health, and although she agrees that it is in her best interest, she finds it difficult to push herself to exercise in the evening because it would take away from the little relaxation time she has for herself each night.

Introduction

In this chapter, we provide an overview of motivational interviewing (MI) and the rationale for using MI to promote behavioral and lifestyle changes in individuals with severe obesity. We discuss a selection of MI strategies described in Miller and Rollnick's authoritative guide on MI that may be helpful in promoting behavioral and lifestyle changes in individuals with severe obesity [1]. We return to the Case Vignette throughout the chapter using clinical dialogues to illustrate the application of select MI strategies. Finally, we review the empirical evidence regarding the effectiveness of MI in facilitating health-related lifestyle changes in patients with severe obesity.

Overview of Motivational Interviewing

Motivational interviewing (MI) is a therapeutic conversation about change that is nonconfrontational and goal directed [1]. It uses a number of different strategies to arrange conversations in such a way that patients vocalize their own motivational statements and thus talk themselves into making changes. As was mentioned in Chapter 2, ambivalence about change and low self-efficacy for change are two primary obstacles in the road to change. Motivational interviewing can be used to help patients identify and mobilize their intrinsic motivation so that they subsequently feel more ready and able to make changes.

Behavioral and lifestyle changes, such as increased physical activity, are frequently recommended to alleviate health risks in individuals with obesity. Unfortunately, many individuals face physical and psychosocial obstacles that impede the consistent implementation of healthy lifestyle choices [2]. Yet approaches in healthcare largely overlook these important determinants of health when they simply provide advice regarding necessary lifestyle changes or prescribe a "one size fits all" treatment program rather than resolve ambivalence and bolster self-efficacy on a more idiographic basis. Let's take exercise as an example. Regular and moderate physical activity is among the essential components of weight management programs as outlined by national clinical guidelines [3], and yet just over one-fifth of the population in the United States engages in the minimum recommended amount of physical activity [4]. Several studies have reported negative correlations between body weight and physical activity, as well as body weight and adherence to physical activity programs [5,6]. A follow-up empirical investigation identified an interaction between physical activity and excess body weight whereby higher excess body weight created unique challenges for engaging in exercise [7]. As a result, individuals with obesity may prefer to be active for longer periods of time instead of at higher intensities [8], prefer self-determined and unsupervised exercise [9], and exhibit a lower tolerance to high-intensity workouts [10]. Thus the findings show that the lack of autonomy in externally imposed exercise recommendations or programs could undermine patients' intrinsic motivation for engagement in physical activity [7]. In fact, the need for flexibility in physical activity recommendations is gaining empirical support, especially for individuals with obesity. For example, although the current recommendation for physical activity to prevent obesity is 45 to 60 minutes of exercise daily [3], recent research has encouraged healthcare providers to counsel individuals with obesity to gradually increase their activity level over time and to remind them that they can realize significant health benefits with just 30 minutes of daily exercise [11,12].

In the Case Vignette at the beginning of this chapter, it is apparent that there are numerous physical, psychological, and environmental obstacles inhibiting Janice's ability to initiate and maintain changes to her lifestyle. Using the core skills of MI introduced in Chapter 2 (OARS: open-ended questions, affirmations, reflections, and summaries), the clinician can intentionally guide the conversation with Janice in a manner that will facilitate her movement through the four processes of MI: *engaging* her in a therapeutic working alliance, *focusing* the direction of the session toward particular goals or issues, *evoking* her own arguments and reasons for change, and *planning* for change by making concrete steps toward her goals [1].

In this chapter, we illustrate some applications of MI strategies with patients who are having difficulty initiating or maintaining lifestyle changes, including engaging in regular physical activity, healthy eating (e.g., adequate fruit and vegetable intake, adequate water consumption, portion control, reduced saturated fat and sugar consumption), and self-care (e.g., avoidance of drugs and alcohol). The following two chapters of this book will demonstrate applications of MI for disordered eating (see Chapter 6) and medication and vitamin adherence (see Chapter 7) in individuals with severe obesity. We also review additional techniques that may be helpful for resolving stuck points that can occur within each of the four MI processes. After discussing MI processes and strategies, we will use a dialogue between Janice and her clinician to illustrate the numerous ways in which lifestyle factors associated with severe obesity can be explored and mitigated using MI.

Engaging

Engaging the patient in a working alliance is the initial stage in any therapeutic interaction and is considered to be the relational foundation of MI. The engaging process is required to establish reciprocal trust, cooperation, and respect between the clinician and patient (see Chapter 4). The time needed to engage with a patient and develop an effective working alliance can vary significantly. Engagement predicts adherence to, and benefit from, treatment regardless of the provider's approach [13]. This is consistent with findings that factors common across therapeutic orientations, such as goal consensus, alliance, empathy, expectations, and positive regard, play a significant role in treatment outcomes [14].

Numerous MI strategies aim to facilitate the development of rapport. In particular, listening to understand the patient's perspective on an issue sets the stage for engagement. Engaged listening on the part of the clinician can be conveyed to the patient through the content of his or her questions and reflections. The four core skills in MI (OARS) can be used to convey compassion and understanding to the patient. For instance, beginning the conversation with open-ended questions communicates that the clinician genuinely wants to hear about the patient's concerns, if any, and has not formed preconceived notions about them. Reflections, the act of making an educated guess about what the patient means and sharing it with him or her, communicates the clinician's genuine desire to understand the patient's perspective. Reflective listening can also serve to continuously gauge whether the clinician has accurately understood what has been communicated by eliciting corroboration from the patient. Affirmations demonstrate to the patient that the clinician is attending to his or her strengths, efforts, and resources. Finally, summarizing is helpful in assuring the patient that his or her concerns have been heard and noted as important.

Engagement can also be facilitated through nonverbal factors, including vocal tone, facial expression, and body language. For example, listening can be conveyed through undivided attention to the patient, whereby the clinician sustains eye contact and avoids taking excessive notes or engaging in other distracting behaviors. Emotional support can be communicated through the mirroring of the patient's facial expression and body language.

The establishment of a working alliance in MI, as with any other healthcare service, is key for being able to move forward with the other processes. Focusing, evoking, and planning cannot occur when the patient does not feel respected and understood, does not trust the clinician, and/or does not feel that the clinician has any agency in tailoring treatment options to his or her desires. However, when a strong working alliance has been developed and the patient feels engaged in treatment, attendance and adherence increase, which has benefits for treatment outcome.

Clinical Dialogue: Engaging

CLINICIAN: Thanks for coming in today, Janice. Your vitals look good, and it appears your medication side effects are being tolerated well. Is there anything else I can help you with?

JANICE: I just wish I had more energy. I find now that teaching my class and running around with my kids is getting to be more and more taxing for me.

CLINICIAN: That's something you mentioned briefly at your last appointment too. Can you tell me a little bit more about your concerns now? [*Open-ended question*]

JANICE: My energy and stamina seem to have decreased to the point where I'm much more burned out at the end of the day.

CLINICIAN: You're feeling much more run down than you used to. [*Reflective listening*]

JANICE: Well, it's been a gradual decline I suppose. It probably just has to do with getting older and the weight continuing to go on.

CLINICIAN: You've mentioned a few different guesses as to what may be going on, including your age and your weight. You have great insight into what may be contributing to the problem. [*Affirmation*] What else have you been considering? [*Open-ended question*]

JANICE: That's probably all it is. I should just accept it and move on to things I have control over.

CLINICIAN: It feels out of your hands, and there doesn't seem to be a way that you know of to resolve this problem. [*Reflective listening*]

JANICE: Well, I mean there are ways I've thought of, but none that I'd be able to try right now.

CLINICIAN: Would you be willing to share some of those ideas with me today? [*Open-ended question*] Regardless of whether you're ready to try them, I'm wondering if it may be beneficial for us to hear them out.

JANICE: Well, for one, I think I should be drinking more water. Also, everyone says that I should exercise more. I really don't have any time to exercise, but maybe that would make me feel more awake and increase my stamina.

CLINICIAN: You're wondering if you're drinking enough fluids and getting enough exercise, and whether those factors are affecting your energy levels. [*Reflective listening*]

JANICE: I'm definitely not drinking enough water. I'm having about four glasses, but I know the recommendation is about eight. I do what I can when it comes to exercise given my busy schedule. I mean it's not easy, but I consider running around with young kids and being on my feet all day to be enough. It's just not formal or structured and can vary depending on the day.

CLINICIAN: Your job keeps you on your feet all day, and with two young kids at home, there's quite a bit of activity there. You're also wondering whether more regular and formal exercise might help with the additional fatigue you've been feeling recently. You're finding it difficult to drink enough water each day and are also wondering whether that might be contributing to the fatigue. [*Summarizing*] Does that sum up some of the things you've been thinking about? [*Elicit patient perspective*]

Focusing

As is the case with Janice, patients with severe obesity often present with multiple physical and/or psychological comorbidities that warrant intervention. Focusing is an important process in MI that involves the patient and clinician collaboratively developing and maintaining a direction in the conversation about change once rapport has been sufficiently developed. The clinician works with the patient to decide what is most important, logical, and/or practical to focus on first and prioritizes goals accordingly. Clarifying the goals and direction provides the foundation for the two subsequent processes of MI, evoking and planning.

Many MI strategies can be helpful in sorting through different options and focusing on one or more change goals. An agenda is a valuable asset in this respect. An *agenda* is a prioritized list of items to be addressed in the consultation or in future sessions and is comprised of information from various sources, including the patient, the clinician, and the treatment setting. Typically patients come to sessions with their own goals, concerns, and ideas and thus are usually the primary source of items for the agenda. When a patient possesses little awareness of the importance of making a lifestyle change or is not yet contemplating making a particular important change, the clinician may play a larger role in developing the agenda than he or she otherwise might. The clinician brings an area of expertise to the consultation and, through the process of engagement, typically holds some ideas of behaviors that might be beneficial to address. Finally, the treatment setting where the consultation is taking place can also influence the agenda items because the agency may be designed, funded, and staffed to provide certain services or address specific issues. When it comes to lifestyle and behavioral changes pertaining to obesity, these may include a diabetes management program, a physical fitness facility, or a dietician's office. Once an agenda is established, many MI strategies can be used to focus on a starting point.

When a patient presents with multiple issues and it is unclear where to begin, one technique to try is agenda mapping [1]. Agenda mapping involves listing all potential topics of conversation to form an overview of available directions for the consultation. The patient can be asked to list any concerns he or she would like to discuss. The clinician is advised to remain open and curious to the concerns raised by the patient and to ask for permission to discuss any additional concerns that are not mentioned by the patient. Providing unsolicited advice to a patient regarding needed behavior changes can feel abrasive to the patient, particularly when discussing an individual's weight. This underscores the value of engaging the patient in a therapeutic alliance before focusing on goals. Furthermore, by asking permission, the clinician is showing respect for the patient and reinforcing the patient's autonomy while also ensuring that all potential ideas that may prove to be relevant to the patient are on the table. Motivational interviewing is not about persuading people to do something that is against their values, goals, or best interests, and decisions about any personal change ultimately remain with them. Thus it is imperative for the clinician to tolerate the uncertainty that comes with the focusing process in order to resist problem solving for the patient. Furthermore, the clinician should retain an awareness of opportunities to reinforce the patients' autonomy when it comes to decision making in the focusing process. Motivational interviewing–driven ways to accomplish this task are to remind the patient that the mapping task and other areas of concern can be revisited as needed and to continually check in with the patient during the focusing process to ensure that the direction is a collaborative one.

The focusing process may deter patients who are in the action stage and have already decided to change. If a patient has already established a clear goal, the objectives of the focusing process have already been accomplished, and the clinician can move directly to the evoking process.

Clinical Dialogue: Agenda Mapping and Focusing

CLINICIAN: You mentioned at our last two appointments that you wished you had more energy, and it sounds like that's an issue that may be worth discussing further. How do you feel about taking some time in today's appointment to explore the issue in more detail? [*Asking permission to focus*]

JANICE: That would be okay.

CLINICIAN: You noted several behaviors that may be affecting your energy levels, including fluid intake and exercise. [*Reflecting*] Are there any other ideas you're wondering about? [*Open-ended question*]

JANICE: I think that covers it.

CLINICIAN: I'm wondering if it is okay with you if we also talk about your eating in this context? Sometimes our diet plays a role in our energy levels. [*Asking permission to add to the agenda*]

JANICE: Sure, what about it?

CLINICIAN: You've already mentioned fluid intake, which is an excellent suggestion. [*Affirmation*] We also know that iron or vitamin D deficiencies can result in feelings of fatigue. What does your daily intake of those nutrients look like? [*Open-ended question*]

JANICE: I take a multivitamin daily, so I feel good about that.

CLINICIAN: It's good that you're in the regular habit of taking a multivitamin. [*Affirmation*] Have there been any changes to your eating that may play a role in you feeling more tired? [*Open-ended question*]

JANICE: Well, I have to admit that my eating has not been the best lately. By the time I come home from teaching all day, I have no energy for preparing meals. I loved cooking, but now the family schedule has gotten too crazy. Even buying groceries is difficult.

CLINICIAN: You're not cooking as much as you used to. [*Reflective listening*]

JANICE: We've gotten into a bad habit of ordering takeout food several nights a week.

CLINICIAN: Eating out has become more routine because it's more convenient given your family's schedule. [*Reflective listening*]

JANICE: I still make meals most of the time, but they tend to be quick meals. I'm using more ready-made meals. I hate doing it, but I'm not sure what else to try.

CLINICIAN: How do you see this being connected to your fatigue? [*Open-ended question*]

JANICE: I know I'm not getting the nutrients I used to. Plus, eating more processed foods has led me to put on some weight, which can't be helping things.

CLINICIAN: The way you've been eating recently has not been as nutritious, which has been directly and indirectly contributing to your energy levels being lower. [*Reflective listening*]

JANICE: That's my guess.

CLINICIAN: That's a really important hypothesis. Can we add that idea to the agenda?

JANICE: Sure.

CLINICIAN: So far, we've talked about a few different ideas when it comes to your fatigue. On our agenda, we are considering the roles of water consumption, physical activity, and nutrient-rich foods. Are we missing anything? [*Agenda mapping*]

JANICE: I don't think so.

CLINICIAN: Of those options, what do you think we should focus on first? [*Agenda mapping*]

JANICE: I'm not the expert; you tell me [*laughing*]!

CLINICIAN: Well, actually, I really believe you're the expert on what you need! I'm here to be a sounding board, but I'm really curious to know which of the ideas we listed currently feels the most important to address? [*Reinforcing autonomy*]

JANICE: Well, I have some ideas as to how to tackle the water intake. I'm feeling more stuck about the exercise and diet given my lack of time and energy.

CLINICIAN: You're certainly not alone in finding it difficult to change your exercise and eating habits. Which issue feels more urgent for you? [*Agenda mapping*]

JANICE: Both are. I do worry that even if I work on one, the other one will just continue to get worse.

CLINICIAN: Can you help me understand how the exercise and eating are linked for you? [*Open-ended question*]

JANICE: Well, when I'm not taking care of myself in one way, it tends to generalize. So, if I'm eating badly, I don't feel motivated to work out, and vice versa.

CLINICIAN: If you were to think about the behavior most linked to the fatigue, what would it be? [*Agenda mapping*]

JANICE: That's an interesting perspective. I do have a sense that the physical activity is important in that respect.

CLINICIAN: Sounds like by increasing your physical activity, it may set you up to feel more energized and also to feel more able to problem solve the difficulties you are facing with cooking healthy meals. [*Reflective listening*]

JANICE: I think so!

CLINICIAN: Would it be helpful for us to take some time to dive into physical activity a bit more and speak further about your thoughts and feelings around exercise? [*Asking permission to focus*]

Evoking: Strategies for Eliciting and Responding to Change Talk

With a sufficient working alliance developed and a clear direction established, the patient and clinician can move toward strengthening motivation for making lifestyle changes that have a positive impact on weight-related issues. While engaging and focusing are common practices across many treatment approaches, evoking is relatively unique to MI. The clinician has two central tasks during this stage: listening for change talk and responding appropriately when change talk occurs. When a person feels ambivalent, it is normal to hear both change and sustain talk mixed together, even within the same sentence [1]. For example, the person may make a self-motivational statement that favors changing an aspect of his or her lifestyle and then immediately articulate an argument for not changing. A high ratio of sustain talk in comparison with change talk predicts maintenance of the current behavior. In contrast, a high ratio of change talk in comparison with sustain talk, particularly during the latter part of the conversation, predicts behavior change. Therefore, the primary goal of the evoking process is to have the patient discuss the desire, need, or intention to change [1].

The most useful way to help a patient feel more ready to change is to facilitate the vocalization of change talk, including statements that express a desire to change (e.g., "I would like to work out"), an ability to change (e.g., "I know I can work out more if I set my mind to it"), specific reasons for change (e.g., "I want to be fit in order to be a good role model for my children"), and need for change (e.g., "I cannot continue my deskbound lifestyle") [1]. By responding to change talk using the core MI skills, the clinician can yield additional or more detailed change talk and the patient's ideas for how he or she might approach it. This includes asking open-ended questions to which the answer is change talk, selectively affirming and reflecting change talk, as well as summarizing the change talk that the patient has communicated so that he or she can hear it all at once [1]. When core MI skills are used to reinforce and emphasize change talk, it encourages more detailed discussion of change talk on the part of the patient, thus strengthening his or her commitment to change in the process.

One strategy the clinician can use to evoke change talk is the *importance ruler* [1]. This technique first acquires an assessment of the current importance of change from the patient's perspective on a scale from 1 to 10 and then allows the patient to process his or her response by elaborating on the reasons change is important. Another useful strategy is to ask the patient to *look back at the past* when things were going well for him or her or to *envision the future* after he or she has successfully made changes (e.g., "If you felt stronger physically, how do you imagine things would be different in the future?") [1]. *Querying the extremes* can be used when the clinician senses that there is very little desire for change at present [1]. This technique involves the juxtaposition of the consequences that may occur with and without changing. *Exploring values and goals* can also facilitate the process of evoking [1]. A patient's broader life goals represent an important potential source of motivation for change. When provided with the opportunity to reflect on life values, the ways in which current behaviors are incompatible with longer-term goals can be identified. These discrepancies are helpful when focusing because they can identify particular behaviors with the greatest adverse impact on important areas of the patient's life.

In addition to eliciting change talk, the clinician can use the core skills of MI to hone in on and respond to self-motivational statements. For example, the clinician may ask evocative open-ended questions for which change talk is the answer, invite the patient to elaborate on change talk (e.g., "Can you say a little bit more about the ways in which you imagine your health improving if you were able to exercise regularly?"), selectively reflect the change talk back to the patient, and summarize the patient's self-motivational statements [1]. These core skills aim to elicit more specific change talk, which increases accountability and makes change more likely to occur. Some patients may present with specific goals in mind and feel prepared to work toward them. With such individuals, the clinician can transition into the planning phase.

Clinical Dialogue: Evoking and Responding to Change Talk

CLINICIAN: You mentioned earlier that everyone says you should exercise more. I'm curious to hear your own thoughts about the ways in which exercise might benefit you personally? [*Open-ended questions to elicit change talk*]

JANICE: Well, I think it might improve my fatigue. I know working out is also good for my chronic pain. [*Change talk*]

CLINICIAN: You're aware that working out is important for managing your chronic pain. Can you tell me more about your understanding of why that is? [*Open-ended questions to elicit change talk*]

JANICE: I've done my research and have found studies showing that exercise makes the muscles stronger around the joints, which relieves tension. And it makes you feel better emotionally, which helps you mentally cope better with the pain.

CLINICIAN: There is exciting evidence in the literature showing that exercise allows for physical and emotional management of chronic pain conditions like yours. [*Reflection of change talk*]

JANICE: Yes, but I just wish I enjoyed exercising! It's so frustrating. [*Sustain talk*]

CLINICIAN: It's very frustrating to learn that something you don't enjoy doing can help with the pain. [*Straight reflection*]

JANICE: Yes, and I just feel ashamed that I'm not working out. I look at everyone else and feel embarrassed that I can't just spend 30 minutes of my day doing something for my health. [*Change talk*]

CLINICIAN: It doesn't require a lot of time to do something that you know would be helpful, and then there's added shame when you see others doing it. [*Reflective listening*] Who do you compare yourself to? [*Open-ended questions to elicit change talk*]

JANICE: Well, my husband gets off work earlier, so he gets to the gym many days. He often tells me about how great it feels. I judge myself harshly because I don't get the same activity in. I think he may think I'm lazy. Plus, there are those other moms I told you about! [*Change talk*]

CLINICIAN: There are a number of people around you working out outside of work, and you're judging yourself for not doing the same. [*Reflective listening*]

JANICE: Exactly. It really makes me feel badly about myself and about the example I set for my kids. [*Change talk*]

CLINICIAN: You're also worried about your children not seeing you engage in a healthy active lifestyle. How would you like them to see you? [*Open-ended question to elicit change talk*]

JANICE: I know that modeling these things is important. If they saw me engaging in healthy routines that involved even small amounts of exercise, then it could help them recognize its importance. [*Change talk*]

CLINICIAN: You feel that your behaviors rub off on them, and that is a reason you feel badly about not getting much exercise. [*Reflective listening*] What impact does that have on you? [*Open-ended question*]

JANICE: Well, I'm feeling frustrated that I've fallen off the wagon and sad that my weight is an issue. And also anxious for the future and whether things will get better. [*Change talk*]

CLINICIAN: You've mentioned a number of reasons why continuing on the way you have been is creating difficulties for you. What might be the three best reasons to change? [*Open ended question*]

JANICE: I would definitely say my health and my kids – both at home and at work. And if I felt that I was a good role model for my kids, then I would feel better about myself as a mother and as a teacher. [*Change talk*]

CLINICIAN: What needs to happen now for you to get started on the path to making things better for your kids and yourself? [*Open ended question*]

JANICE: This is where I struggle. I see my options but don't think I know what is best for me right now. Or if I'm even ready to change right now while things are so busy.

CLINICIAN: Maybe you're not ready to make a change right now. Perhaps the pain is too much, and you're too busy at the moment to take a step toward exercising more. [*Amplified reflection*]

JANICE: But that's what I've told myself for the past five years, that I'm not ready. Now I feel like I need to do it whether I feel 100 percent ready or not. [*Change talk*]

CLINICIAN: You feel this change is necessary, regardless of whether you feel absolutely ready. [*Amplified reflection*] On a scale from 0 to 10, where 0 means "not at all important" and 10 means "extremely important," how important would you say it is for you to incorporate more formal exercise into your routine? [*Importance ruler*]

JANICE: I would say a 9.

CLINICIAN: Wow, that's a really a high number. What puts you at a 9 and not a 5?

JANICE: My health is not very good for my age, and I really, really want to feel better. I would be able to if I could get into a routine. [*Change talk*]

CLINICIAN: You are yearning to feel better and are sensing that some more structure will help you make the change necessary to achieve that result. [*Reflective listening*]

JANICE: I would probably have more energy to run around with my kids, and that's very important to me. [*Change talk*]

CLINICIAN: The time is now! Suppose you continue on as you have been, without changing. What do you imagine is the worst thing that could happen with your relationship to your children? [*Querying the extremes*]

JANICE: They will grow up with an absent and tired mom. I know it sounds dramatic, but being able to play with them is the most important thing, especially as they grow up with more technology and screens. I need to be a presence and model a healthy, active lifestyle for them, even if I am overweight. I can't keep on like this, or else I will miss valuable time with them. [*Change talk*]

CLINICIAN: You feel strongly that you can't keep going on the way things are and that something has to change. [*Reflective listening*] What could be the best result in five years if you did make a change? [*Querying the extremes*]

JANICE: I would be setting my children up to not engage in the same behaviors that lead to me being overweight. They could grow up feeling like a healthy, active lifestyle is routine and easy for them, which is something I never had. [*Change talk*]

CLINICIAN: What are you prepared to do now to make that happen? [*Open-ended question*]

JANICE: I'm willing to exercise more. It won't be easy given my busy schedule, but I can start exercising two days a week. [*Change talk*]

CLINICIAN: You will make working out two days a week a priority, for you and your children. [*Reflective listening*]

JANICE: Modeling important values for them and being there for them is everything. [*Change talk*]

Responding to Sustain Talk

When working to evoke change talk, the clinician will almost inevitably hear sustain talk, which is a natural by-product of ambivalence. Rather than perceiving such statements as resistance, clinicians using MI are urged to conceptualize this type of language as an expected reaction to challenges, fears, or lack of readiness on the road to change. Thus an important skill within the evoking process is appropriately responding to sustain talk. Sustain talk is not to be dismissed or ignored in MI. When the patient feels that his or her reasons for not changing are unexplored, dismissed, or misunderstood, it can raise defensiveness about the possibility of making changes. A number of MI strategies can be used to selectively emphasize change talk while also exploring the other side of ambivalence (sustain talk) with compassion and openness.

Several types of reflective responses can be helpful in responding to sustain talk, including straight reflection, amplified reflection, and double-sided reflection [1]. During a *straight reflection*, the clinician paraphrases the patient's words or even repeats them verbatim. Such reflections acknowledge the patient's statement without encouraging embellishment of the idea. An *amplified reflection* goes one step further, whereby the clinician makes a bolder statement about how the patient's words could be interpreted. For example, if the patient stated, "I am not willing to start going to the gym," the clinician could amplify his or her response by reflecting, "You're never going to work out again." An overstatement of the patient's words conjures the other side of ambivalence, which is change talk. For instance, if the patient hears that the clinician thinks that he or she would *never* exercise, he or she may be inclined to challenge the extreme language of the reflected information (e.g., "I didn't say that I'm never going to exercise again; I just don't see myself going to a gym because I don't like exercising in front other people"). A *doubled-sided reflection* supports both sustain and change talk (e.g., "You're not keen on going to the gym, but you're concerned about your diabetes and might consider other forms of exercise") in order to validate both sides of the ambivalence. By strategically placing the change talk in the latter half of the reflection, greater emphasis is placed on last point the patient hears.

Another technique that can be helpful when responding to sustain talk is to strategically agree with the patient. In a strategy referred to as *agreeing with a twist* [1], the clinician sides with the patient's sustain talk. When the clinician joins the patient's team and agrees with the patient's sustain talk, it becomes difficult for the patient to argue against the clinician. One way to achieve this is emphasizing the patient's autonomy. By highlighting the patient's personal autonomy to choose whether or not to make any changes at the present time, the clinician signals to the patient that he or she is on the same side. Acknowledging the patient's autonomous choice to *not* change the status quo can exert a paradoxical effect of increasing motivation for change. Another technique is the *running head start* [1], which can help the clinician move more quickly to hearing change talk by first identifying, normalizing, and validating the motivations for not changing. The head start can be achieved by purposefully asking open-ended questions about the patient's main motivations for not changing, which then presents an opportunity to ask about the downside of the status quo and advantages of change (e.g., "Many people find it difficult to exercise regularly, and it sounds like there are a lot of reasons why working out is not in the cards for you right now. I'm curious to know about any concerns you may have about not exercising"). This strategy is only recommended when the patient seems reluctant to discuss reasons for change. In the event that the patient has vocalized change talk to explore, it can be counterproductive to revisit the reasons for maintaining the status quo.

Clinical Dialogue: Responding to Sustain Talk

CLINICIAN: You mentioned that this concern around your fitness level has emerged from comparing yourself with others. Can you tell me more about that? [*Open-ended question to elicit change talk*]

JANICE: Yes! I don't know where they get the energy! They are on the treadmill in the evenings and playing tennis on the weekend. I just need to get off my feet during my spare time. [*Sustain talk*]

CLINICIAN: You work really hard at being a teacher and a mom, and when you have time off, the last thing you want to be doing is working out. [*Amplified reflection*]

JANICE: Well, I wouldn't say it's the last thing, but it's definitely not high on my priority list. I would much rather relax by reading a book or watching television with my husband. That's what makes me feel better. [*Sustain talk*]

CLINICIAN: By not working out, you have more time for relaxing and spending time with your partner. [*Straight reflection*]

JANICE: Yes. Those activities are my favorite, especially after a long day. [*Sustain talk*]

CLINICIAN: That makes lots of sense to me. We know that certain behaviors continue because they serve a function or help us in some way. When not exercising leaves room for pleasurable activities, it's logical why increasing physical activity would be difficult.

[*Agreeing with a twist*] What are the other good things about not working out? [*Running head start*]

JANICE: As you know, my chronic pain has been very debilitating. When I bend down or walk for long periods of time, it flares up and can affect me for hours. Working out has been known to make my pain worse in the short term. [*Sustain talk*] However, I know it is good for my pain in the long run. [*Change talk*]

CLINICIAN: Working out makes the pain worse for a few hours, and yet you're aware that in the long term it is helpful in improving your pain. [*Double-sided reflection*]

JANICE: It's hard to do something to help yourself down the road when it hurts in the meantime.

CLINICIAN: Absolutely. That is a difficult position to be in – knowing short-term difficulties lead to long-term improvements. [*Double sided reflection*]

JANICE: It is! I wish there was an easier fix.

CLINICIAN: You are waiting for an alternate solution because the options you have for working out are too tough for you right now. [*Amplified reflection*]

JANICE: I don't think my current options are all too tough for me. I mean I am doing a lot already, like walking to work. It's not that big of a problem.

CLINICIAN: You've implemented a number of great steps to improve your exercise. [*Affirmation*] You're walking to work, and that's sufficient. [*Amplified reflection*]

JANICE: Well, it isn't really, but I have higher priorities right now. I have to think about my children and their wellness first. [*Sustain talk*]

CLINICIAN: Your priorities are always with your kids, and sometimes that means there's no time for what you need. [*Amplified reflection*]

JANICE: Well, I mean part of being a good mother is taking care of myself too. [*Change talk*] But not at the expense of spending too much time away from them. [*Sustain talk*]

CLINICIAN: You want to prioritize your children and yourself [*Double-sided reflection*] But it's really difficult to do everything at the same time. [*Agreeing with a twist*]

JANICE: Well, I think there's a balance I could strike. [*Change talk*]

CLINICIAN: I think you're probably right, and yet it is really up to you what balance makes sense for you and your family. [*Reinforcing autonomy*]

JANICE: It's hard to imagine anyone with kids finding the right balance.

CLINICIAN: It feels daunting to make an attempt to do it all, and yet I also heard you say that there may be a way to plan a balance. [*Summarize change talk*] Where does that leave you right now? [*Open-ended question*]

Exchanging Information

As a clinician, it can be tempting to share expertise, especially if it is perceived to be helpful for a patient. However, from a patient-centered perspective, it is easy to overestimate how much information and advice patients need to be given. For example, relatively few maladaptive habits persist simply because an individual lacks knowledge that the behavior is harmful or unhelpful. For instance, it is common knowledge that an active lifestyle has many health benefits. Providing a patient with unsolicited information that he or she is already aware of can be unhelpful and counterproductive. Motivational interviewing strategies can help clinicians structure the complex interaction of providing information that may help the patient make changes.

The guidelines for information exchange can be summarized as *elicit-provide-elicit* (EPE) [1]. First, it is important to assess the patient's prior knowledge (e.g., "Tell me what you already know about the recommendations for physical activity"). By eliciting the patient's understanding before providing information, the clinician explores the patient's previous knowledge and queries his or her interest in receiving certain pieces of information. This technique helps the clinician avoid repeating information that patients already know and positions patients to assert their own reasons for change. When a patient asks for advice pertaining to the presenting concern, the clinician may invite the patient to explain what type information he or she is searching for or interested in (e.g., "What have you been wondering about exercise that I might be able to clarify for you?"). In the event that the patient does not ask for suggestions but the clinician feels that he or she has some information to offer that may be helpful, the clinician may then ask explicit permission to provide some additional information that is aligned with the patient's needs and strengths (e.g., "Would you like to know about the current physical activity recommendations for your age?"). Asking permission to share information acknowledges the patient's autonomy to agree or disagree with the information provided, which typically increases the patient's willingness to hear what the clinician says. In the spirit of MI, the clinician aims to deliver this information with reference to other people who are experiencing a similar concern or condition to the patient, leaving it to the patient to judge how this information might apply to him or her (e.g., "Would it be alright if I told you about a few forms of exercise that some other people with chronic pain have found pretty tolerable?"). The clinician should then present the information clearly, in manageable doses, and using autonomy-supportive language (e.g., "Some other people with chronic pain have found walking, swimming, yoga, pilates, and strength training pretty tolerable. Of course, it's really up to you to experiment and see what feels manageable"). The clinician should ideally offer a variety of options so that the patient can consider a range of possibilities and choose among them. Then the clinician can inquire about the patient's understanding of the information that has been shared (e.g., "What do you make of these recommendations for physical activity?") and assess the extent to which the information that has been presented is relevant to the patient's goals. This approach acknowledges the patient's freedom to disregard the advice provided, which can exert a paradoxical effect of making it more likely that the patient will be receptive to the advice.

As illustrated in the following conversation, MI strategies can be used to elicit change talk and prompt Janice to generate her own ideas about how she can begin to get started with formal exercise.

Clinical Dialogue: Exchanging Information

JANICE: I'm still struggling to think of quick activities I can do during my busy weekdays and also longer ones I can do on the weekends that won't really activate my chronic pain. [*Sustain talk*]

CLINICIAN: Perhaps we should pick a place to start. Should we first discuss brief workouts that you can do during the weekdays or longer activities on the weekends? [*Focusing*]

JANICE: I'm not sure.

CLINICIAN: This may or may not be relevant to you deciding where to focus first. [*Reinforcing autonomy*] But I do have some information regarding the optimal length of time for exercise for individuals with chronic pain. Would you like to hear those ideas? [*Asking permission*]

JANICE: Yes!

CLINICIAN: There are published guidelines for incorporating brief exercise throughout your day, especially as a start, to work up to a full workout when pain may be an obstacle. Brief exercises may be anywhere from 5 to 10 minutes. [*Providing information*] What do you make of those guidelines? [*Eliciting patient perspective*]

JANICE: That makes sense to me. I also agree from past experience that it would be logical to see when I can start doing brief exercises during the day rather than longer workouts on weekends. Plus that would also save the weekends for me to rest and spend time with my family.

CLINICIAN: That sounds like a great place to start for many reasons. Do you have a sense of a time during the weekday you could squeeze in 5 to 10 minutes of physical activity? [*Open-ended question*]

JANICE: The lunch hour is reserved for eating and lesson preparation. But the morning and afternoon recesses would work. They are about 20 minutes each.

CLINICIAN: That would leave you enough time to get in a brief workout and get ready for when your students come back in. [*Reflective listening*]

JANICE: Exactly.

CLINICIAN: Do you have any ideas about quick exercises you may be able to do during that time period? [*Elicit previous knowledge*]

JANICE: Not really. I was hoping that whomever I saw today might have some ideas.

CLINICIAN: What have you been wondering about exercise that I might be able to clarify for you? [*Query interest*]

JANICE: I would like to hear what you suggest in terms of a few quick exercises that have worked for other people with chronic pain?

CLINICIAN: There are recommendations for strength-based, low-impact exercises that build strength in your muscles but don't take a toll on your joints. These include swimming, yoga, and the elliptical; however, those options are less popular for some people because they require access to facilities. Another option is partial weight-bearing exercises, which means you will use lighter weights even if you are capable of lifting more. Given that it requires little equipment, it tends to be a good option for people who are short on time. [*Provide information*] In addition, walking is a great form of exercise that requires no equipment. Of course, it is up to you, but those are some suggestions. [*Reinforcing autonomy*]

JANICE: I like the idea of doing a few exercises with weights but am worried it will activate my pain.

CLINICIAN: That is a valid concern. [*Affirmation*] The guidelines do suggest being cautious to avoid pushing yourself into more intense discomfort. One way to monitor this is to rate your pain on a scale from 0 (no pain at all) to 10 (most pain imaginable) before you work out. During your exercise, stop or adapt the movements if you notice your pain levels increase by more than two points from where you started. What are your thoughts about that option? [*Eliciting patient perspective*]

JANICE: I'm feeling more hopeful. I'm glad there's a way I can check if I'm making my pain worse.

CLINICIAN: It feels hopeful to have guidelines based on the research that help you implement exercises that you know will be good for you and minimize risk. [*Reflective listening*] Furthermore, stretching is important to loosen tight muscles and improve range of motion. [*Provide information*] How does that sound? [*Eliciting patient perspective*]

JANICE: I like that idea. Perhaps one recess I can do the stretches, and then maybe the other I can try the weights.

CLINICIAN: That sounds like a really great option for you in light of everything we have discussed. Given those ideas, what is the next step for you? [*Open-ended question*]

Evoking Hope and Confidence

Patients with severe obesity are typically well aware that excess weight is associated with adverse health effects but lack confidence in their ability to make impactful changes. Low self-efficacy can stem from repeated "failed" diets, intensive exercise programs, and New Year's resolutions. Overall readiness for change depends on both the perceived importance of change and confidence in one's ability to change. Particularly when it comes to lifestyle changes that are inherently long term, individuals are unlikely to commit to making a change unless they have some confidence that it is possible for them to maintain change in the long run. Motivational interviewing aims to both resolve ambivalence about change and enhance the patient's confidence for change.

The clinician can strategically use the core MI skills to bolster self-efficacy in patients who may not yet feel able to make a lifestyle change. For example, the clinician can use a line of open-end questioning that elicits *confidence talk*, which is change talk that pertains to ability (e.g., "What gives you some confidence that you can start exercising regularly?") [1]. One way to achieve this objective is to use open-ended questioning to elicit examples of changes that the patient has made in the past and explore the skills used to achieve these changes. This technique is known as *reviewing past successes* [1]. Reflecting on difficult changes that have already been made can be helpful in identifying strategies that worked well in the past and particular skills or personal qualities that may be generalized and applied in the current context. If the patient recalls occasions where change has not been successful, the clinician can reframe this situation in a way that encourages further attempts. This can be accomplished by reframing the label of "failures" as "tries" and looking for evidence that demonstrates how each "try" is a necessary step toward successful change by teaching the patient what did and did not work. The clinician may also use the *confidence ruler* to assess the patient's confidence in his or her ability to make changes [1]. Similar to the importance ruler, with the *confidence ruler*, the clinician asks the patient how confident he or she feels about making a particular change if he or she decides to, on a scale from 0 to 10, where 0 is "not at all confident" and 10 is "extremely confident." The clinician follows up this question with open-ended questions that are likely to elicit statements of confidence, such as why the patient is at that number and not a lower one. Finally, *hypothetical thinking* is a strategy that poses the notion that the patient will succeed, and the patient is asked to identify the strategies that most likely helped him or her succeed.

Increased self-efficacy is one important channel by which MI effects change. Motivational interviewing strategies can be used to strengthen self-efficacy across the focusing, evoking, and planning processes. For example, during the focusing and planning processes, a patient may feel better able to make a change when there is discussion of various options, ideas, and strategies rather than a single one that may feel too difficult. Asking patients to share their own ideas regarding change and reminding them of their personal autonomy in the decision making inherently fosters self-efficacy (e.g., "You are the expert on yourself, and ultimately it's up to you to decide what will work best for you").

Clinical Dialogue: Strengthening Self-Efficacy

CLINICIAN: I'm wondering if we could shift gears a little bit and talk about other changes you have made. I'm curious to know about other changes you have made in the past that may have proven difficult or required you to learn something new or take a risk. [*Reviewing past successes*]

JANICE: Well, going back to teacher's college was a tough choice. It required more education and money.

CLINICIAN: And what made you decide to make that change? [*Open-ended question*]

JANICE: I knew it was important for my future.

CLINICIAN: After you decided it was important for your future to return to college, how did you make that change? [*Open-ended question*]

JANICE: Well, I took my time in deciding whether this was the best plan for me and consulted friends and family. I set up a budget so that I could afford the tuition. But once I made the decision, I was motivated to make it work.

CLINICIAN: Sounds like once you committed to the idea, you were determined to follow through. [*Reflective listening*]

JANICE: That's generally how I am. I'm motivated by fear of failure. But sometimes that makes me not want to set goals in the first place.

CLINICIAN: So you're cautious about setting goals because of fear of not reaching them. And, when you do set goals, you use that to motivate you to achieve them. [*Reflective listening*] What obstacles did you face in going back to school, and how did you surmount them? [*Open-ended question*]

JANICE: The financial situation was difficult, so I really found planning ahead was the most helpful in that respect.

CLINICIAN: What type of planning was involved? [*Open-ended question*]

JANICE: Setting a budget, looking into hours for part-time work, and setting aside study time.

CLINICIAN: Sounds like a lot of preparation was needed to get you to where you are now! [*Affirmation*] What personality traits drove you to make all these changes that ultimately allowed you to return to school? [*Open-ended question*]

JANICE: Well, I'm a natural organizer, so I'm diligent with planning.

CLINICIAN: How might that apply in this scenario, where you want to find a way to incorporate exercise into a routine?

JANICE: Well, I guess I can get organized and creative about finding ways to build exercise into my day. But it still just feels like there's not enough time.

CLINICIAN: Has there been another change that you've made in the past despite feeling like there wasn't enough time? [*Open-ended question*]

JANICE: Well, returning to school full time certainly required a lot of time [*laughing*]. Also, being a working mom, I encounter this difficulty all the time!

CLINICIAN: How have you surmounted that obstacle in the past?

JANICE: I make time for things that are important. For example, when my dad became sick, I made it a priority to see him and buy his groceries. Plus, after a while, it didn't feel like such a chore.

CLINICIAN: When you prioritized helping your father, it became a natural part of your routine and even an enjoyable one at that.

JANICE: Yes. I have never really thought about it in those terms.

CLINICIAN: Can you tell me about a time when it was difficult to work out but you did anyway?

JANICE: Well, for a period of time, I did go on walks on the weekends because I knew I should be getting more exercise.

CLINICIAN: Tell me about what it took to get out for a walk on those days?

JANICE: I just told myself it was nonnegotiable. Something I had to do for myself to keep me healthy.

CLINICIAN: Sounds like, in the same way with your education, when you put something high on your list of importance, you really are able to make things happen despite obstacles.

JANICE: Definitely. But even with the walking, I didn't keep it up for more than a month or two. I have tried to increase my activity lots of times, and I've never been able to keep it going. Even with all my determination!

CLINICIAN: You hit unforeseen obstacles, which made it difficult to maintain. [*Amplified reflection*]

JANICE: That's true.

CLINICIAN: Given what you know about yourself from those attempts, how could you make this change more successful? [*Confidence talk*]

JANICE: Back then, I would get caught up in these set rules I had for myself about how much I needed to do. If I'm more flexible with my guidelines, maybe when I miss a day I will feel more able to start up again.

CLINICIAN: It's been helpful to have past experience trying things out because you are now equipped with information about the potential downside of setting rigid rules for working out. [*Reflective listening*]

JANICE: Yes, it is helpful to know so that I don't make the same mistake again.

CLINICIAN: Let's check in regarding your confidence at this very moment to increase your physical activity levels. How confident are you that you could do some form of exercise during your recess breaks if you decided to? On a scale from 0 to 10, where 0 is "not at all confident" and 10 is "extremely confident," where would you say you are? [*Confidence ruler*]

JANICE: A 6.

CLINICIAN: Past the halfway mark! What brings you to a 6 rather than, say, a 5?

JANICE: Well, I have committed to periods of exercise before. I exercised regularly in the past when I took workout classes during university.

CLINICIAN: You've been successful at working out regularly in the past. [*Reflective listening*] What would it take for you to move one notch higher – from a 6 up to a 7?

JANICE: Well, back then, the gym was located at my university, and I had periods of time between classes to fill. It became an easy part of my schedule. If I found a way to make exercise an easy part of my schedule now, then I would have more confidence that I could stick to it.

CLINICIAN: I'm hearing that your confidence in your ability to increase your physical activity would increase if you felt you could incorporate it into your routine. [*Reflective listening*] Let's suppose that you did succeed, and you're looking back on yourself five years from now. What are the strategies for incorporating exercise into your routine that would have most likely worked? [*Hypothetical thinking*]

JANICE: I suppose it is doing a bit of exercise on my weekends and some during my workdays but not trying to do too much at once or holding myself to rigid standards.

Planning

When the clinician has a good sense that the patient feels able to make changes, the clinician can explore some concrete plans that the patient is willing to try out. The final stage of MI is the planning process, which captures the progression of formulating a specific course of action. The planning stage is a crucial one because individuals equipped with a specific plan for change are more likely to carry it out. The clinician may only begin the process of planning following the development of a working alliance, the clarification of a direction and goals for change, and the elicitation of change talk.

Prior to developing an action plan, clinicians are advised to test the patient's readiness to proceed [1]. If the planning stage is premature, it can strengthen ambivalence and risk progress made. To ensure that this does not occur, the clinician can *test the waters* by asking the patient directly if it is an appropriate time to start the planning process (e.g., "Would it make sense at this point to start thinking about how you could make this change, or would that be rushing into things?") [1]. The clinician can also summarize the conversation thus far to ensure that the planning stage is not premature. *Recapitulation* is a transitional collecting summary of the change talk that serves to make salient all the change talk the patient has vocalized throughout the conversation [1]. Such a summary provides an ideal opening to then ask the patient poignant *key questions* that help evoke change talk (e.g., "So what do you think you'll do?"). The pairing of recapitulation and key questions allows the patient to hear all the arguments for change and then decide what he or she is going to do about it [1].

During the planning stage, it is critical that the other three MI processes remain active. For example, the planning process should make time for continually clarifying and specifying goals in order to confirm the main goal being addressed by the plan. *Confirming the goal* is a technique to ensure that the clinician and patient are on the same page regarding which subgoal will be pursued first [1]. The patient's reasons for change should continue to be evoked during the planning stage in order to reinforce commitment to using the strategies developed to achieve the goals. It can be helpful to collaboratively develop an itemized list of options that may be used to achieve the patient's goal and to elicit the patient's ideas about each of the various options [1]. The clinician can conclude the conversation with an open-ended question designed to strengthen commitment (e.g., "What steps are you ready to take this week?") and praise the patient's openness to making a plan. When developing a plan in MI, it is important to encourage the patient to identify small, manageable steps that he or she can realistically accomplish. It can be important to check in around resources needed to make the change (e.g., running shoes, gym membership) or social supports that may be helpful to put in place. It can be helpful to offer the patient a summary of the plan so that both the patient and the clinician are on the same page. With any plan, it is important to anticipate what obstacles may get in the way of change and to troubleshoot how the patient can respond if and when they come up [1].

Patients are most likely to commit to making changes if they develop a specific action plan and vocalize their intention to carry it out. Thus it can be helpful for the patient to complete a worksheet that summarizes some of the main discussion points, including the patient's goal, various options for achieving the goal, an action plan, potential barriers to achieving the goal, and some proposed solutions to overcome barriers.

Clinical Dialogue: Making a Plan

CLINICIAN: I get the sense we are developing some ideas as to how to approach increasing your physical activity this time around. Should we discuss these ideas further and perhaps start to put a plan together, or is that getting too ahead of things? [*Testing the waters*]

JANICE: Sure, I think I'm feeling ready for that!

CLINICIAN: We have spoken about a lot of different ideas today. We started by talking about how your lack of energy is making your job more difficult and affecting your ability to keep up with your kids at home. You've voiced worries about how your current activity level is negatively affecting your chronic pain, as well as other elements of your physical health. And, most important, you mentioned concerns about the impact on your children if you don't make exercise a priority. [*Recapitulation*] It's really in your hands what, if anything, you choose to do. So what do you think you'll do? [*Key question*]

JANICE: I'm thinking it's time for a new approach to working out.

CLINICIAN: Are you willing to think about the actual steps you might take to increase your physical activity two days per week? [*Confirm the goal*]

JANICE: I'm ready to start taking baby steps.

CLINICIAN: You're ready to commit to gradual changes. [*Reflective listening*] What ideas do you have as to how you might get started with this? [*Eliciting patient's ideas*]

JANICE: Well, we've already spoken about weight-bearing exercises during recess.

CLINICIAN: That sounds like one really great option. Can we brainstorm a few others? [*Brainstorming options*]

JANICE: Sure. Walking is always a good idea for me. I find it enjoyable on the weekends, but only when the weather is nice. I could also swim laps while my kids do their swimming lessons this fall.

CLINICIAN: These are great ideas. Would it be okay if I listed the options we have spoken about so far? [*Itemize the options*] We have brief weight-bearing activities during recess, walking on the weekends, and swimming laps. Are there any other ideas you're wondering about that we've missed?

JANICE: Well, we did talk about how when I work out more I can probably start eating better as well.

CLINICIAN: You're very insightful into how taking care of yourself through physical activity can promote taking care of yourself in other ways, such as prioritizing healthy eating. [*Affirmation*] I do recall you saying that in the past, trying to do too much too soon in the change process can make change more difficult for you. I'm not sure if this is something relevant to you now at this stage of the planning process, and, of course, feel free to disregard, but I want to check in with you to see whether it feels reasonable to include both exercise and eating in your plan at this stage?

JANICE: Ah yes, I'm getting ahead of myself. Let's stick to one thing at a time and revisit the idea of eating better the next time we meet.

CLINICIAN: Great! What might be that one change you could start with this week? Which option do you feel ready to do? [*Eliciting patient's ideas*]

JANICE: Let's start with weights during recess. It doesn't take away from my evening relaxation time and will give me a stress break during the day.

CLINICIAN: That sounds like a really good idea for all the reasons you mentioned. How much activity are you willing to do during the recess time? [*Eliciting patient's ideas*]

JANICE: Recess is 20 minutes, so I could do 10 minutes to allow for some preparation and some cool-down time.

CLINICIAN: Wonderful. What steps are you willing to take this week to get started with this change? [*Eliciting patient's ideas*]

JANICE: Well, I don't have weights. I can borrow some from a friend when I see her tomorrow. I know she won't mind.

CLINICIAN: Great. So by tomorrow you should have weights in hand. And once you have the weights, what is the next step? [*Eliciting patient's ideas*]

JANICE: Well, I'll just do a few exercises two days a week at afternoon recess. That seems reasonable enough.

CLINICIAN: It does to me as well. Do you have a sense of which exercises you'd like to try? [*Eliciting patient's ideas*]

JANICE: There are online video resources that can give me some ideas. I also have a physiotherapist that I can ask.

CLINICIAN: Great ideas! Physiotherapists are well versed on those types of options. When is your next appointment with the physiotherapist?

JANICE: The day after next. But that means I won't know what type of weight I need when I see my friend.

CLINICIAN: The timing does seem a little tricky. How do you want to handle that? [*Open-ended question, reinforcing autonomy*]

JANICE: Well, I could get the lightest she has and start with those. Or I can ask to borrow a few different weights and then see what my physiotherapist has to say.

CLINICIAN: Excellent problem solving. Speaking of which, what other obstacles might arise when making this change? [*Troubleshoot*]

JANICE: Well, it may pose a problem if I can't get the weights in time or my friend won't let me borrow them.

CLINICIAN: Any ideas as to how you could navigate that difficulty if it came up? [*Troubleshoot*]

JANICE: I think I've heard soup cans are good replacements. I have those at home.

CLINICIAN: Now you are really starting to have a concrete plan in the works. [*Affirmation*] Can we write these down on a planning for change worksheet so that we don't forget what we spoke about? [*Planning*]

JANICE: That sounds great.

CLINICIAN: I think it's wonderful that you're so open to making a plan. [*Affirmation*]

Empirical Support for the Effectiveness of Motivational Interviewing for Behavioral and Lifestyle Changes in Severe Obesity

Research on MI for behavioral and lifestyle changes has increased at a rapid rate over the past two decades. Many randomized, controlled trials (RCTs) have been conducted, and more recently, a handful of systematic reviews and meta-analyses have been conducted to synthesize the key findings across numerous studies. Although few studies have examined

MI specifically in populations with severe obesity, many have examined MI for weight management, as well as behavioral health and medical issues common among individuals with severe obesity.

A systematic review and meta-analysis of 72 RCTs examining the efficacy of MI for a variety of behavioral lifestyle issues and diseases concluded that MI outperforms traditional advice giving [15]. Motivational interviewing demonstrated a significant effect in 74 percent of RCTs. Although the studies included in the review and meta-analysis were not limited to populations with obesity, the meta-analysis indicated significant effects of MI for improving BMI, total blood cholesterol, and systolic blood pressure.

A systematic review and meta-analysis of 11 RCTs examining the efficacy of behavioral change interventions using MI in individuals who are overweight or obese concluded that MI enhances weight loss [16]. Motivational interviewing was delivered by a variety of healthcare professionals including nurses, dieticians, health promotion specialists, exercise specialists, and psychologists. It was associated with greater reduction in body mass than in a variety of control groups (e.g., standard care with a physician or dietician, standard behavioral weight loss intervention, printed educational materials). Motivational interviewing demonstrated an overall medium effect on weight loss. The authors noted that studies offering MI as an adjunct to group-based behavioral weight loss interventions demonstrated the greatest weight loss and suggested that MI likely enhances weight loss by improving adherence to behavioral weight loss interventions.

A systematic review of 24 studies examining the efficacy of MI for weight loss among adults in primary care settings reported that patients receiving MI lost at least 5 percent of initial body weight in 54 percent of studies included in the review [17]. The MI interventions were delivered by a variety of healthcare professionals, including physicians, nurses, dieticians, and exercise specialists. The control conditions typically consisted of standard dietary advice or usual care. Motivational interviewing resulted in significantly greater weight loss than the control conditions in 38 percent of studies. The authors concluded that MI has the potential to improve weight loss and weight-related variables among adults in primary care settings, but the amount of weight loss was quite modest in most studies. The authors noted that the studies in which patients achieved 5 percent weight loss were more likely to provide individual MI sessions as opposed to group MI sessions and to incorporate the use of telephone calls and technology (e.g., emails).

A review of studies examining the efficacy of MI for diet and exercise (24 studies) and diabetes management (9 studies) concluded that MI is efficacious in promoting health behaviors [18]. Studies examining MI alone and in combination with other interventions suggest that MI is effective in improving diet and exercise. Patients who received MI reported increased self-efficacy, physical activity, and fruit and vegetable consumption and reduced caloric intake and BMI. Studies examining MI alone and in combination with other interventions suggest that MI is effective in improving diabetes management. Patients who received MI reported increased self-efficacy, glucose control, physical activity, and dietary changes and reduced weight. The authors noted that many of the changes were maintained one to two years following the MI intervention but cautioned that follow-up data beyond two years were not available and are important to collect in order to determine the longer-term impact of MI interventions in promoting health behaviors.

A recent systematic review examined the potential of MI to address lifestyle factors relevant to multimorbidity in healthcare settings [19]. Lack of exercise, lack of fruit and vegetable consumption, and excess weight are all associated with increased risk of multiple co-occurring long-term conditions, and it has been suggested that MI may be effective in improving lifestyle factors implicated in multimorbidity [20]. Similar to the findings of previous reviews and meta-analyses, the systematic review concluded that MI is effective in improving diet and exercise and weight management [19]. The authors noted that the research conducted to date has primarily examined MI for specific diseases and that additional research is needed to examine whether the benefits of MI for these specific diseases also extend to multimorbidity. This recommendation is particularly relevant for the clinical management of severe obesity given that obesity significantly increases the odds of multimorbidity [21].

Collectively, the findings across review papers and meta-analyses suggest that MI is effective in improving weight loss, but the amount of weight loss from before to after the intervention is generally quite modest considering participants' initial body weight. Although MI alone is unlikely to lead to clinically significant weight loss in individuals with severe obesity, it may nonetheless be helpful in promoting a number of health behaviors that can improve quality of life and may also be a useful adjunct to medical or surgical treatments for obesity.

A recent study examined the efficacy of MI in postoperative bariatric surgery patients who were having difficulty adhering to the postoperative dietary guidelines [22]. Participants were randomly assigned to receive a single-session MI intervention either immediately (MI group) or following a 12-week delay while continuing to receive standard bariatric care (waitlist control group). Participants reported significant improvements in their readiness, confidence, and self-efficacy for change immediately following the MI intervention. The MI group reported improvements on some measures of adherence to dietary guidelines over the 12-week follow-up period, whereas the control group did not. Although preliminary, the results of this pilot study suggest that MI is feasible to deliver, acceptable to bariatric patients, and holds promise to improve confidence for change and adherence to dietary guidelines postoperatively. Additional longitudinal research is needed to examine whether increased confidence and postoperative adherence translates into greater percentage weight loss and/or improved weight maintenance over time. A recent study in nonbariatric participants with obesity who lost at least 5 percent of their initial body weight in the past year reported that MI has a promising impact on weight loss maintenance [23].

Summary

Motivational interviewing can be used to resolve ambivalence and increase self-efficacy in individuals with severe obesity who are pondering lifestyle changes. For every MI strategy that may facilitate a patient's movement toward change, there are many examples of ways in which healthcare professionals can inadvertently reinforce sustain talk, undermine self-efficacy, and increase defensiveness. Providing patients with unsolicited advice can feel helpful in the moment on the part of the clinician but has a paradoxical effect based on what we know about the strategies that help move people toward making difficult health-related changes. The empirical research on MI for lifestyle and behavior changes lends support to the notion that clinicians need to meet patients where they are at, to view patients as experts and as autonomous decision makers in their own lives, and to let go of the urge to persuade or coerce patients in favor of joining with the patient to explore the possibility of change together.

Key Points

- Motivational interviewing is helpful in resolving ambivalence about change and increasing self-efficacy for change in individuals with obesity.
- The core MI skills (OARS: open-ended questions, affirmations, reflections, summaries) are useful in helping individuals with obesity move through the processes of making lifestyle changes.
- Additional MI strategies are useful for navigating stuck points in conversations about lifestyle changes. Strategies such as agenda mapping, asking permission, reinforcing autonomy, importance and confidence rulers, recapitulation, and troubleshooting can be used throughout the processes of engaging, focusing, evoking, and planning to work with patients effectively toward their health-related goals.
- Research suggests that MI is effective in promoting a number of health behaviors that can improve quality of life and potentially weight loss in individuals with obesity.

References

1. W. R. Miller and S. Rollnick. *Motivational Interviewing*, vol. 3: *Helping People Change*. New York, NY: Guildford Press, 2012.

2. A. E. Bauman, R. S. Reis, J. F. Sallis, et al. Correlates of physical activity: Why are some people physically active and others not? *Lancet* 2012; **380**: 258–71.

3. National Institute for Health and Care Excellence. *Obesity: Identification, Assessment, and Management*. National Heart, Lung, and Blood Institute, 2014. Available at www.nice.org.uk/guidance/cg189.

4. Centers for Disease Control and Prevention. QuickStats: Percentage of US adults who met the 2008 federal physical activity guidelines for aerobic and strengthening activity by sex – National Health Interview Survey, 2000–2014. *MMWR Morbid Mortal Weekly Rep* 2016; **65**: 485. Available at http://dx.doi.org/10.15585/mmwr.mm6518a9.

5. I. Bautista-Castano, J. Molina-Cabrillana, J. A. Montoya-Alonso, et al. Variables predictive of adherence to diet and physical activity recommendations in the treatment of obesity and overweight in a group of Spanish subjects. *Int J Obes Relat Metab Disord* 2004; **28**: 697–705.

6. W. W. Tryon, J. L. Goldberg, and D. F. Morrison. Activity decreases as percentage overweight increases. *Int J Obes Relat Metab Disord* 1992; **16**: 591–5.

7. P. Ekkekakis and E. Lind. Exercise does not feel the same when you are overweight: The impact of self-selected and imposed intensity on affect and exertion. *Int J Obes* 2006; **30**: 652–60.

8. M. Fogelholm, K. Kukkonen-Harjula, A. Nenonen, et al. Effects of walking training on weight maintenance after a very-low-energy diet in premenopausal obese women. *Archi Intern Med* 2000; **160**: 2177–84.

9. M. G. Perri, A. D. Martin, E. A. Leermakers, et al. Effects of group-versus home-based exercise in the treatment of obesity. *J Consult Clin Psychol* 1997; **65**: 278–85.

10. E. Mattsson, U. E. Larsson, and S. Rossner. Is walking for exercise too exhausting for obese women? *Int J Obes Relat Metab Disord* 1997; **21**: 380–6.

11. J. O. Hill and H. R. Wyatt. Role of physical activity in preventing and treating obesity. *J Appl Psychol* 2005; **99**: 765–70.

12. J. M. Jakicic and A. D. Otto. Treatment and prevention of obesity: What is the role of exercise? *Nutr Rev* 2006: **64**: S57–61.

13. W. P. Henry, H. H. Strupp, T. E. Schacht, et al. Psychodynamic approaches. In A. E. Bergin and S. L. Garfield (eds.), *Handbook of Psychotherapy and Behaviour Change* (4th edn). New York, NY: Wiley, 1994: 467–508.

14. G. W. M. Wampold, M. Moody, F. Stich, et al. A meta-analysis of outcome studies

comparing bona fide psychotherapies: Empirically, "all must have prizes." *Psychol Bull* 1997; **3**: 203–15.

15. S. Rubak, A. Sandboek, T. Lauritzen, et al. Motivational interviewing: A systematic review and meta-analysis. *Br J Gen Pract* 2005; **55**: 305–12.

16. M. J. Armstrong, T. A. Mottershead, P. E. Ronksley, et al. Motivational interviewing to improve weight loss in overweight and/or obese patients: A systematic review and meta-analysis of randomized controlled trials. *Obes Rev* 2011; **12**: 709–23.

17. R. D. Barnes and V. Ivezaj. A systematic review of motivational interviewing for weight loss among adults in primary care. *Obes Rev* 2015; **16**: 304–18.

18. R. K. Martins and D. W. McNeil. Review of motivational interviewing in promoting health behaviours. *Clin Psychol Rev* 2009; **29**: 283–93.

19. K. J. McKenzie, D. Pierce, and J. M. Gunn. A systematic review of motivational interviewing in healthcare: The potential of motivational interviewing to address the lifestyle factors relevant to multimorbidity. *J Org Chem* 2015; **5**: 162–74.

20. M. Fortin, J. Haggerty, J. Almirall, et al. Lifestyle factors and multimorbidity: A cross sectional study. *BMC Public Health* 2014; **14**: 686.

21. C. B. Agborsangaya, E. Ngwakongnwi, M. Lahtinen, et al. Multimorbidity prevalence in the general population: The role of obesity in chronic disease clustering. *BMC Public Health* 2013; **13**: 1161.

22. L. David, S. Sockalingam, S. Wnuk, et al. A pilot randomized controlled trial examining the feasibility, acceptability, and efficacy of adapted motivational interviewing for post-operative bariatric surgery patients. *Eat Behav* 2016; **22**: 87–92.

23. S. A. Simpson, R. McNamara, C. Shaw, et al. A feasibility randomized controlled trial of a motivational interviewing-based intervention for weight loss maintenance in adults. *Health Technol Assess* 2015; **19**: 1–409.

Chapter 6

Motivational Interviewing for Disordered Eating in Severe Obesity

Josie Geller, Megumi Iyar, and Erin Dunn

Introduction

One of the greatest challenges in the treatment of severe obesity is addressing patient self-criticism and shame. Paradoxically, in an effort to promote rapid weight loss, it is common for these important maintaining features of obesogenic eating behaviors to be overlooked. In our clinical experience, addressing self-compassion and self-acceptance is key to engaging patients in treatment and supporting sustained behavior change.

This chapter outlines our approach to addressing these issues using a motivational interviewing (MI) framework [1]. It is based on an overarching *mission statement* that guides our interventions, namely, "to develop and foster a *trusting, supportive* relationship that promotes patient *self-awareness, self-acceptance*, and *responsibility for change*" [2]. A central feature of MI is establishing a collaborative partnership wherein the patient feels accepted, understood, and empowered. Motivational interviewing embodies the spirit (compassion, curiosity, warmth) and offers the method (engage, focus, evoke, plan) and the skills (reflective listening, open-ended questions, summarizing, affirming, informing with permission) to meet these core therapeutic goals.

In this chapter, we begin by providing a rationale for each component of the mission statement. We subsequently provide Case Vignettes illustrating how MI tools can be used to achieve the mission statement goal. The chapter ends with final notes on MI and its role in addressing self-criticism and shame in this population.

Trust and Support

In order to build a safe and trusting space for patients to share their feelings about change (e.g., ambivalence, fear of failure) and the challenges they face, clinicians need to convey acceptance and empathy and to role-model compassion. This stance is especially important when working with individuals with severe obesity. Given that weight bias is common in Western society (see Chapter 3), patients will naturally be attuned to the therapist's attitudes toward weight. It is essential for therapists to be aware of any unhelpful attitudes or feelings they may have about body size and be willing to overcome any barriers to showing warmth, respect, and curiosity. This stance is important to maintain, independent of the patient's weight status or success at behavior change. Therapists showing acceptance and empathy toward themselves can also inspire patients to experiment with cultivating these qualities within themselves.

Self-Awareness

Self-criticism can interfere with curiosity and attunement to one's experiences, which are needed to have the capacity to identify and address barriers to change. Having one's thinking characterized by a running dialogue of judgments about one's flaws makes it difficult to be aware of present-moment feelings or sensations. In MI, therapist empathy and curiosity give the patient permission to drop internal judgments and be more contemplative, which can lead to both parties having a deeper shared understanding of the patient's experience. For instance, self-awareness may lead to the insight that eating binges typically occur when a patient is feeling sad or lonely. This is the first step in determining the most helpful course of action.

Self-Acceptance

Self-compassion is characterized by mindfulness, the recognition that suffering and feelings of inadequacy are part of the human experience, and self-kindness, particularly in times of difficulty [3] (see Chapter 11). Self-compassion increases the likelihood of sustained motivation in the face of the inevitable challenges that accompany attempts to change eating behaviors (e.g., "I'm doing the best I can. Setbacks are part of being human"). When a patient slips into habitual problematic patterns of behavior, or when he or she is unable to meet his or her treatment goals, it is important to note that these experiences are common to all humans (e.g., "Change is hard. Everyone makes mistakes"). The MI clinician's modeling of an open-minded, nonjudgmental attitude helps the patient feel more self-accepting and break the cycle of frustration, criticism, shame, self-punishment, and hopelessness that often results (ironically) in use of the problematic behavior. Other MI strategies that can be used to facilitate self-acceptance are reviewing the pros and cons of self-criticism and exploring higher values. In our previous example, a patient who becomes aware that he or she is prone to bingeing when he or she is sad or lonely can practice simply allowing the feelings without judgment or evaluation, recognizing that feelings of loneliness are shared by most of us, and having an aspiration to be as kind as possible to himself or herself by experimenting with ways to be nurturing and supportive.

Responsibility for Change

There are a number of ways in which MI helps patients take responsibility for change in order to accomplish their goals. First, simply exploring the pros and cons of change without judgment helps the patient and therapist review previous change attempts and identify existing skills that may be helpful to capitalize on in future change attempts. This review process also gives the therapist an opportunity to call attention to the patient's ongoing commitment to change. Second, helping patients connect with their higher values can assist in resolving ambivalence, increasing motivation to change, and establishing collaborative treatment goals. Increasing awareness about patients' greatest aspirations in life, possibly by exploring what they anticipate they would want for themselves in the future, helps reinforce their commitment and responsibility to change. Insight about the function and consequences of the behaviors, as well as barriers to making changes, can also help patients become more self-compassionate. Finally, a key feature of MI is the therapist stating that he or she is not invested in convincing the patient to change; rather, the therapist's wish is to support patient autonomy so that the patient makes his or her own decision about change. This critical stance ensures that the therapist and patient remain on the same side and prevents the patient from feeling defensive or pressured.

Case Vignettes

Diana: Raising Self-Awareness

Diana is a single 25-year-old university student who recently moved away from home to pursue her master's degree in library science. Although she reports struggling with her eating since she was a child, she came to therapy because of her concern about recent weight gain. She reports feeling like her eating has been out of control, and she has been forced to purchase new clothes due to substantial weight gain. In the first few sessions, Diana identified times in which her eating was most problematic. She noted that the binges usually occur when she comes home from school and can persist into the evening until she goes to bed. Diana was asked to monitor her eating and identify problematic days. She was initially reluctant to do so, but after reassurance from her therapist that doing this exercise was exclusively for learning (and that there would be no judgment about her eating), she agreed to record her eating for one week. Diana came to today's session expressing frustration that her eating did not go well and that "for no good reason" she was unable to stick to her meal plan. She said she felt disgusted with herself and her inability to get her eating on track. She described two episodes in which she ate more than she had planned and ended up subsequently feeling a loss of control for the rest of the day.

DIANA: I am so frustrated! I feel like I have no will power and that this is a hopeless situation. I don't understand why I can't get more control over my eating.

CLINICIAN: It sounds like you had a rough week. It took a lot of courage to keep food records, and increasing awareness of some of the difficulties can make things feel tougher, at least initially. I hope you aren't being hard on yourself. When we planned to monitor your eating, our objective was to learn as much as we could about the tough times. How about we use your records now to see what was happening when things got off track?

DIANA: Okay. I guess we can try, though I think it was just me not being able to stick to the plan.

CLINICIAN: Okay, well how about we pick one of the difficult times, like on Thursday when you mentioned that you overate when you got home from work?

DIANA: Ya, that day was a disaster. I meant to have a healthy snack so I wouldn't be too full later on when I was meeting friends for dinner. But I ended up having way too much and by dinner time felt overfull and awful.

CLINICIAN: Okay, so things didn't go according to your initial plan. I'm curious, what was going on for you that day? For instance, do you remember how you were feeling about going out that night?

DIANA: I was mostly really looking forward to it! I hadn't seen a couple of my friends for a while – one of them for over a year.

CLINICIAN: Cool. I noticed you said "mostly" looking forward to it. Did you have any other feelings?

DIANA: Well ... I was exhausted. I had stayed up late every night that week crunching deadlines for school and studying for exams, and I handed in my last huge assignment that day. Part of me was so tired I wished I could just go home and relax and have a quiet night to myself.

CLINICIAN: That's understandable. I know how hard you work at school and in your part time job. It sounds like you had an intense work week and could have used some self-care and down time.

DIANA: Ya ... a night off would have been nice.

CLINICIAN: So you were tired and would have welcomed a lower-key night than you had planned . . . that can be hard. [*Diana nods in agreement*] I'm wondering what else was going on that day? I noticed from your food records that you didn't have breakfast and that you had only eaten an apple at lunch. Were you feeling hungry when you got home?

DIANA: Actually, I was starving!

CLINICIAN: Ah ... do you think that might have contributed to what happened with your eating?

DIANA: [*Nods*] Ya, I feel silly because I know I am more prone to bingeing when I am superhungry.

CLINICIAN: Yes, you mentioned that was something you were working on. Any thoughts about what might have gotten in the way of having regular meals that day?

DIANA: Well, I'm a bit shy about this . . . but anticipating the evening was actually worrying me a lot.

CLINICIAN: How so?

DIANA: Well . . . I know I look different from how I looked the last time some of my friends saw me, and I have been feeling quite self-conscious. I even considered canceling because I didn't want them to see me until I had lost some of this weight. So I was trying to cut back on my food all week, thinking maybe if I lost a couple of pounds I wouldn't feel so uncomfortable.

CLINICIAN: Ah ... so you had some worries about meeting your friends, and that led to cutting back from having regular meals, which made you more at risk physiologically to binge. I'm wondering if on top of being hungry there was a connection between worrying about bingeing?

DIANA: I'm not sure. Sometimes when I feel overwhelmed, eating is nice ... kind of like shutting the world out.

CLINICIAN: You are certainly not alone in that. Many of us find that eating can help give us a break from difficult feelings like general overwhelm, anxiety, or self-criticism. So maybe that's another possible factor contributing to your eating that day?

DIANA: Ya ... I hadn't actually made that connection before.

CLINICIAN: Thanks for being so open to recording your experiences this week and exploring factors that may have been at play. I'm thinking we have learned a lot and that you were dealing with a number of challenges that day! At the start of our conversation you said you were feeling frustrated and like there was "no good reason" for your eating going off track. I'm curious, what are your thoughts now?

DIANA: [*Nods*] Ya ... now that we have talked about it, I guess the binge wasn't quite as random as I thought.

In this example, the therapist used MI techniques to increase awareness of factors contributing to Diana's binge eating. This has the potential to accomplish two objectives: (1) reduce stigma, shame, or self-blame Diana may be feeling about binge episodes and (2) set the stage for further work on acceptance, which will, in turn, be followed up with working on action and responsibility for change.

Specifically, the therapist used a *draining* technique, which involves use of open-ended questions and a curious, nonjudgmental MI stance to explore possible contributing factors to a difficult situation (in this case a binge episode). With each patient response, the therapist summarizes and validates and then probes further. This technique is helpful for uncovering functions of behaviors that the patient may not be aware of and allowing the patient and clinician to collaboratively work together on determining what, if any, tools the patient needs in order to have these functions met in other, more adaptive ways. A noteworthy feature of draining is that very often first or second responses are "canned," in that they have been articulated previously. If the therapist perseveres, however, it is common for more sensitive or tender areas that have not been previously discussed to be uncovered, such as Diana's vulnerable feelings about her friends seeing her at this weight.

The session continued with follow-up discussion about increasing awareness of risk factors and acceptance that it is difficult to follow a meal plan when dealing with these challenges. The clinician works with Diana to determine whether she aspires to decrease the impact of these factors on her eating by tackling each (i.e., ensuring that self-care is built into her life, having outlets and alternative skills to manage intense feelings, and strategies to overcoming barriers to sticking with her meal plan) in future sessions.

Chris: Enhancing Self-Acceptance

Chris is a 37-year-old financial consultant who has been struggling with shape and weight concerns and confidence issues. He describes secret eating as a way to cope and self-soothe when he feels overwhelmed. From a young age, Chris recalls sneaking food into his bedroom at night, particularly during his parents' frequent arguments. In grade school he remembers his mother making comments about his eating and body size, which sometimes left him feeling unloved and not good enough. After his parents divorced, Chris struggled to make friends and often ate in secret after school before his mother came home from work. He described these as times that he felt he could most relax and be free from worry about homework and concerns about pleasing his mother or fitting in with his peers.

As an adult, Chris has had times when he was able to stick to a healthy meal plan. During those periods, he reported losing weight and feeling more confident. Recently, however, although he has been working hard at his job and enjoying being a husband and father, he has been getting into arguments with his wife at night, in which they both tend to be critical of one another. Chris noticed that when he feels criticized, he uses his old coping strategies, bingeing at night when his wife and children are asleep. Chris reports feeling depressed about his weight and disappointment and distress over his eating. In previous therapy sessions, he became aware of his tendency to be hard on himself and noticed that eating gives him a break from self-critical thoughts. In the past few weeks he has experimented with distraction, relaxation, mindfulness exercises and self-care before bed, and having only healthy foods in the home to snack on.

CLINICIAN: How did your week go?

CHRIS: Not great. Tracy and I had another fight, and I haven't been doing well. I don't think I lost any weight and may have even gained a couple of pounds.

CLINICIAN: Oh, it's a bummer your week didn't go as you had hoped. It sounds like you and Tracy are having some struggles.

CHRIS: Ya. This last argument was really hard. We just haven't been seeing things eye to eye. An extra contract came up at work, and she wants me to take it so that we have more cash, but for me the most important thing is spending time with her and the kids. I ended up feeling badly afterwards.

CLINICIAN: That sounds like a difficult conversation. How did it end?

CHRIS: Not well. I got the impression that she just sees me as being lazy. She looked flabbergasted and went to bed, and I couldn't sleep. I tried those breathing exercises we did last week, but in the end I went to the kitchen and ate whatever I could find until I passed out on the couch. Thankfully, I had ensured there was no junk food in the house, but I still ate more than I wanted. I don't know what's wrong with me. I just can't get it together.

CLINICIAN: Aw, it sounds like you are being really hard on yourself . . . it is heartbreaking to hear.

CHRIS: Well, I keep doing things I know will only make things worse! I even wondered afterwards if maybe Tracy was right and I should just take the stupid job.

CLINICIAN: Okay, before we go there, would you be okay talking a bit more about what we spoke of last week – about self-compassion, particularly when times are tough?

CHRIS: Okay.

CLINICIAN: Cool. It sounds like you were saying a lot of judgmental things, and I thought we might explore the costs and benefits of being so hard on yourself. What do you think?

CHRIS: Well, okay.

CLINICIAN: Do you remember what feelings you had when you made your way to the kitchen?

CHRIS: I do . . . I felt sad . . . and angry . . . mostly at myself.

CLINICIAN: Do you remember what the feelings were about?

CHRIS: Ya. I felt frustrated with Tracy that she isn't happy with what we have and sad about the possibility of having to give up time with her and the boys.

CLINICIAN: That is understandable. You mentioned how much you missed having your dad around when you were a boy and how important it is for you now to spend time with your own kids. [Chris nods] It speaks to your commitment to the family and to your higher values of wanting to be there for them. Those strike me as wonderful qualities.

CHRIS: That's true. The crazy part is I think Tracy thinks so too, which makes this especially frustrating!

CLINICIAN: Ya, it's a drag when others don't react as we expect and hope. Okay, back to that night . . . I'm curious, what happened when you started eating?

CHRIS: To be honest, I don't remember much after that point. I just felt like I got a break from all the intensity and everything became calm until I passed out.

CLINICIAN: I see, so eating helped settle the feelings of overwhelm.

CHRIS: [Nods] I guess it did help. I was just really hoping that by this time it wouldn't take so little to get me going.

CLINICIAN: It's hard to remember sometimes that recovery is a process and that we all have setbacks, even when we are fully "recovered." From an outside perspective, you have actually come a long way and have made some great headway in taking care of yourself.

CHRIS: Maybe . . .

CLINICIAN: So, in light of this and all the work you have done, I'm curious, do you think that in difficult times, like that night, being self-critical increases or decreases your tendency to overeat?

CHRIS: I know where you're going with this . . . and I know we worked out that overall, when I'm beating myself up for something, I am more likely to get into eating.

CLINICIAN: That's a great observation and true of most of our less healthy behaviors; they often come up when we are being hard on ourselves and are not at our best. In your case, you come by it honestly – when you were growing up, eating was the only way you had to take care of yourself.

CHRIS: Ya . . . it has been helpful realizing here over the past few months that with my parents so focused on their own troubles, being in my room with candy was the best way I had to settle down when I got worked up. I didn't realize until recently that there were other options!

CLINICIAN: Absolutely, it is hard to know when you haven't had exposure to alternatives. I am wondering if you have fully appreciated how difficult it is to change something that has been working and continues, at some level, to work. You have done such a great job the past few weeks experimenting with relaxation and distraction and mindful breathing. In most cases, getting in the habit of using these sorts of alternatives takes time, and there are usually several setbacks until the new ways become part of our regular repertoire.

CHRIS: Ya, I do know that is true and realize I still need to work on this. Maybe I'm not giving myself enough credit.

It should be noted that the components of this dialogue could take place in several sessions over a period of weeks or months. Increasing self-acceptance is especially useful when self-criticism is found to be instrumental to maintaining problematic behavior (in this case, binge eating). As can be seen, the MI therapist used open-ended questioning, highlighting pros and cons, and exploring higher values to address Chris's self-criticism, as opposed to focusing exclusively on his eating.

Frank: Promoting Responsibility for Change

Frank is a single 38-year-old elementary school teacher who has been obese for most of his life. As an adult, one of his major concerns is eating in front of others. He is especially concerned at work because the teachers at his school eat together in the staff lounge. He worries that if his colleagues see him eating, they will think he lacks will power and has given up on himself. Working in education, Frank says he experiences shame because he feels that he should "know better" and be able to control his weight. As a result of his concerns about eating in front of others, his typical eating pattern is to skip or eat a small breakfast, drink coffee throughout the day at work, and then overeat at dinner and binge most evenings. Recently, he consulted with a dietician who advised him that eating regularly throughout the day is a key factor in refraining from overeating at night. With the dietician's encouragement, Frank tried bringing a lunch to the staff lounge for a few days. Although he noted that he was less hungry at night on those occasions, he was so uncomfortable eating in front of his colleagues that he went back to his regular pattern of restricting. Today he tells his therapist that he feels stuck and disheartened about his lack of progress.

CLINICIAN: It sounds like you have been on quite a journey trying to find the best way to address the concerns you have about your weight.

FRANK: Yes, it has been so annoying not being able to get rid of this weight.

CLINICIAN: I'm sorry to hear that it has been such a struggle. Do you have a sense now of what you think will be most helpful?

FRANK: Well . . . I was hoping I would be able to just cut back on my night eating, but that doesn't seem to be happening.

CLINICIAN: Okay, well, let's see if we can come up with some ideas. How about we review in a bit more detail some of the things that you have tried in the past and see if together we can use what we learn to come up with a plan for moving forward?

FRANK: Okay.

CLINICIAN: Great. I was curious about the experiment you did having lunches at school. Can you say what worked and what didn't work about that?

FRANK: Well, what *didn't* work was how awful it was eating with my colleagues! It felt like everyone was watching me, and they were probably all thinking that at my size, I shouldn't be eating like that. It really bothered me and made it hard for me to concentrate on my teaching.

CLINICIAN: That sounds really tough. What was the worst part about having lunches at school?

FRANK: I think it was the anxiety I had each morning, dreading lunch time, and also afterwards worrying about what everyone was thinking about me.

CLINICIAN: That does sound dreadful. Anything else you remember about that time?

FRANK: Well, on the plus side, I was less ravenous when I got home, and I remember feeling I was able to eat more slowly. I noticed that my urge to binge was less.

CLINICIAN: Ah, and how was that, having a less strong urge to binge?

FRANK: It was quite liberating. I remember feeling like I had more control over my food choices. One night I even had a salad for dinner, which never happens!

CLINICIAN: Ah, that sounds pretty different. How often do you feel that sense of liberation and ability to eat more slowly these days?

FRANK: I would say rarely. Even if I pick up a snack on my way home from work, I still feel that when I arrive home, once I start, I just can't seem to stop.

CLINICIAN: Yes, it is very tough to battle hunger and physiology.

FRANK: [Nods]

CLINICIAN: What a tough situation you are in. It's hard to eat lunch during the day when you worry about what your colleagues are thinking, and it's hard to binge most nights knowing that it leads to weight gain. No matter which choice you make, it is going to be hard. How about we go back to our conversation about what your greatest aspirations are and then see if we can work out together the best decision for you moving forward?

In this example, the therapist uses MI techniques to help Frank explore the pros and cons of behavior change. The therapist avoids attempting to "convince" Frank that there is an obvious or preferred course of action. Instead, the therapist focuses on Frank's own experience and higher values to help him come to terms with the costs and benefits of his choices.

Summary

As seen in these vignettes, MI is a valuable approach to use with patients with severe obesity to target self-criticism and shame by enhancing self-awareness, self-acceptance, and responsibility for change. In the case of Diana, the therapist used a draining technique to raise self-awareness of factors contributing to her bingeing. Key to this intervention was maintaining an open and nonjudgmental stance to overcome any barriers (e.g., self-criticism) to identifying the function of her disordered eating. With Chris, the therapist directly tackled self-criticism and shame using MI techniques such as identifying pros and cons of self-criticism and exploring higher values. Finally, in the case of Frank, expressing understanding and validation for the difficulty of his situation both helped to overcome self-criticism and support his autonomy to choose the best course of action for him.

Key Points

- Motivational interviewing aims to develop and foster a trusting, supportive relationship that promotes patient self-awareness, self-acceptance, and responsibility for change.
- Motivational interviewing is useful in identifying factors that contribute to disordered eating in a nonjudgmental manner.
- Self-criticism is one factor that can contribute to disordered eating, and motivational interviewing can be helpful in improving self-acceptance and promoting self-care and health-related behaviors.

References

1. W. R. Miller and S. Rollnick. *Motivational Interviewing: Helping People Change* (3rd edn). New York, NY: Guilford Press, 2013.

2. J. Geller, K. D. Williams, and S. Srikameswaran. Clinician stance in the treatment of chronic eating disorders. *Eur Eat Disord Rev* 2001; 9: 365–73.

3. K. D. Neff. The development and validation of a scale to measure self-compassion. *Self Identity* 2003; 2: 223–50.

Motivational Interviewing for Medication and Vitamin Adherence in Severe Obesity

Marlene Taube-Schiff and Richard Yanofsky

Case Vignette

Jim is a 52-year-old man who underwent bariatric surgery two years ago. He experienced weight difficulties throughout his childhood and as an adult. He made several weight loss attempts before considering bariatric surgery. He has experienced both psychiatric and medical issues, including ongoing symptoms of depression and type 2 diabetes. A multidisciplinary psychosocial team evaluated Jim prior to surgery and considered him to be highly motivated to make the essential dietary and lifestyle changes necessary for bariatric surgery to be successful. For example, the team could see that he was already improving his eating and exercise habits (e.g., he began swimming in his condo building three times per week). Since undergoing bariatric surgery, he has been highly successful in modifying his diet and has lost 65 percent of his excess body weight. However, Jim has not been diligent about adhering to his vitamin supplementation or medication management for his type 2 diabetes, which has not resolved from his weight loss. Furthermore, he recently indicated that it has been difficult to remember to take his antidepressant medication as prescribed. His treatment team was quite surprised by this, given that Jim has been adherent with dietary and lifestyle modifications. When asked about what the difficulties might be, Jim has been vague and indicates, "I just continue to forget" and "My time is so focused on getting in all my meals and the proper nutrients that I can't seem to remember anything else."

The team has become concerned about Jim because his mood seems to be worsening, and he is also noting decreasing appetite and interest in food. Both the dietitian and psychologist from the bariatric team have met with Jim. They have provided further psychoeducation regarding the importance of medication adherence and the challenges that might arise should one cease one's medication. The psychologist has also been using cognitive-behavioral strategies to target some of the negative thinking patterns that have begun to emerge. However, neither healthcare professional is feeling that he is able to enhance Jim's medication adherence. They have also spoken with Jim's family physician, who is feeling quite stuck with respect to getting Jim back on track with his much-needed vitamins and pharmacotherapy.

Introduction

In this chapter, we provide a brief overview of motivational interviewing (MI) and highlight several different MI strategies that can be used to enhance medication adherence for individuals with severe obesity. We then illustrate the strategies using clinical dialogues between a patient and a clinician to demonstrate how they may be applied in clinical practice. Finally, we review the small body of literature that exists regarding the use of MI for medication adherence in individuals with severe obesity.

Overview of Motivational Interviewing

Motivational interviewing can be thought of as a "conversation about change" [1: 12] (see Chapters 2, 5, and 6). This conversation is meant to be collaborative and guiding in order to enable an individual to become intrinsically motivated toward wanting to make a change and then committing to and acting on change talk when it emerges. Throughout the change process, an individual can be overcome by ambivalence – which is a normal part of change but can be difficult to move past [2]. While considering the possibility of change, individuals often voice both *change talk* (i.e., narrative that allows change to emerge) and *sustain talk* (i.e., narrative that supports the status quo and does not favor change) [1]. When using MI, the clinician wants to *evoke* from patients what they might already have within themselves – the desire to become motivated and harness their resources to act according to that motivation [3]. When a clinician begins to argue as to why change is important or the "dangers" of not changing, a patient will often argue that the status quo is actually maintainable, especially if ambivalence is present. When this occurs, the chance of fostering change decreases. Thus MI is used to facilitate a conversation of *genuine curiosity* between clinician and patient, enabling change talk to emerge and ambivalence to decrease. This conversational style will be illustrated throughout the Clinical Dialogues presented in this chapter.

Application of MI Strategies

In order to best understand the use of MI strategies, key skills will be illustrated using Clinical Dialogues.

Core MI Skills

The core skills in MI are often referred to with the acronym OARS (open questions, affirming, reflecting, and summarizing) [1] (see Chapters 2 and 5). The following Clinical Dialogue between Samantha, a woman who had bariatric surgery six months ago, and her bariatric dietitian helps to illustrate some of the core MI skills. Samantha is being seen for a regular six-month follow-up visit, where she presents with low energy and fatigue. Medication adherence issues are explored.

Clinical Dialogue

DIETITIAN: It's really nice to see you, Samantha. I saw that you have now lost 85 pounds when you were weighed today. You have certainly been working hard. [*Affirming*] How are you feeling about this weight loss? [*Open-ended question*]

SAMANTHA: I'm really happy that I have lost so much weight. I don't think I felt this was truly possible! I know the surgery can be very successful – but then when it happens to you and you see these amazing results, it's like having a new lease on life. I am very tired, though, and not sure why. That is something I was hoping we could speak about during our visit today.

DIETITIAN: I'm sorry to hear you've been feeling so tired. That must be difficult, because I know you are very busy with your family. Let's work together today to figure out what might be going on. It would be helpful if you could start by walking me through what you normally eat in a day and when you are taking all your vitamin supplements.

SAMANTHA: I have been sticking to the dietary guidelines to the letter! But I don't have time for all the vitamins … there are so many of them! I find between work and the kids and measuring out and planning all my meals, I just don't have the time.

DIETITIAN: So, it sounds like you have been devoting a great deal of energy to ensuring that all your meals are on target – fabulous! [*Reflecting and affirming*] But then being able to fit in all your vitamins seems to fall by the wayside. Do I have that right?

SAMANTHA: Yes, that is absolutely right. Honestly, I just don't have any time or energy left over to figure out all the vitamins.

DIETITIAN: Perhaps it would be helpful to review the reasons why we need all the vitamins, as time-consuming as they are. Would it be okay if we took a few minutes to go over that information together? [*Asking permission to provide patient education; allows information to be received from an open stance on the part of the receiver*] [*Samantha nods, and the dietitian pulls out a pamphlet on the importance of vitamin supplementation, and the two review this information together.*]

SAMANTHA: That information all makes sense. I see that by not taking the vitamins, I might be putting myself at risk. But normally, other than feeling tired, I think I am doing okay. And I still don't really know how to fit them in and make the time for them. It feels like there are so many pills, and they have to be taken at different times. I'm not sure I can organize it all properly. [*Sustain talk emerging*]

DIETITIAN: So, it sounds like it makes sense to you that the multivitamins are very important to take and that they would likely improve your energy levels, but you are still struggling with how you can fit them in. [*Reflective listening*] I'm wondering how your energy level is affecting you on a day-to-day basis? [*Open-ended question*]

SAMANTHA: Yes, that's exactly how I am feeling. Well, it is hard to keep up with my kids. They have so much energy. Of course, it was hard before my surgery as well. But I guess one of my goals after the surgery was to be able to keep up with my kids. And now I feel a bit stuck because I have lost the weight – so, physically, I can do a lot more – but I still feel tired and need to rest more than I would have imagined. Also, at work I feel wiped out and less efficient. I am not meeting all my deadlines either. Everyone understood when I first went back to work, but now I feel like my boss is having a hard time understanding why I can't always do the job as I should be doing it. Now that you ask, I guess there are a lot of ways in which my low energy seems to be affecting me. I don't know … is there anything we could do to make it easier somehow? [*Change talk now emerging*]

DIETITIAN: Thanks, Samantha, for sharing all that with me. I am thinking we could devote the rest of our time today to figuring out some concrete strategies to help you remember to take your multivitamins so that it fits into your daily routine. I am also wondering if you would be willing to get some blood work done before you leave the hospital today so that I can get a better understanding of any vitamin deficiencies that you might be experiencing.

This dialogue illustrates several skills that are useful when trying to engage a patient in an initial process of understanding an issue that warrants change. The dietitian began with a gentle manner of open-ended questions and reflective listening. This allowed for Samantha to open up about the fact that she was not adhering to her vitamin supplement routine. In doing so, the dietitian then asked permission to review information with Samantha that was likely useful in allowing her to better understand the issues that were arising as a result of her lack of adherence. Importantly, this did not solve the difficulty in Samantha wanting to resume her vitamin intake. She seemed to understand that she needed to take her medications, but she still insisted that it was too difficult for her because her schedule was too busy to fit the regimen in. At this point, it appeared that Samantha was becoming resistant to the idea of change and was exhibiting some ambivalence regarding whether she would be able to make any changes in her schedule. The dietitian then asked her to consider the impact on her life as a result of not taking the vitamins. This appeared to be a turning point for Samantha as she began to reflect on the fact that an important goal for her in undergoing the surgery was to be able to spend time with her children. It was at this point that change talk began to emerge. When Samantha was able to reflect on the fact that she was still feeling very tired and lethargic, likely due to the lack of vitamin adherence, she then began to realize that she was no further ahead in her goal of spending time with her children and having the energy to keep up with them. The dietitian noticed this discrepancy between Samantha's current and ideal functioning with her children and was able to problem solve with Samantha and create a reasonable plan to fit the vitamin regimen into her schedule.

Although this dialogue ended well, with Samantha making a plan to increase her vitamin adherence, she could have continued to resist the idea of taking her vitamins and show very little interest in making a change. In that case, the dietitian would be advised to intervene with other MI strategies – perhaps exploring goals and values more in depth. The following clinical dialogue illustrates MI strategies that could be used if the conversation had taken a different direction. We will return to the previous clinical dialogue at the point where Samantha is asked how the lack of energy is affecting her day-to-day activities.

SAMANTHA: Yes, that is exactly how I am feeling. Well, it is hard to keep up with my kids. They have so much energy. Of course, it was hard before my surgery as well. But I still don't think I can adhere to all the other changes and fit in all the vitamins as well. I'm just not sure that is possible. Things just feel hard enough.

DIETITIAN: I hear that fitting in everything right now feels overwhelming. [*Reflective listening*] I am wondering if we can take a step back from our conversation about the vitamins and explore some other areas of your life. Would that be okay?

SAMANTHA: Sure, that's okay.

DIETITIAN: I would like to hear a bit more about what really matters to you – what do you care most about in life? [*Exploring values*]

SAMANTHA: Well, I would have to say my family matters to me. My children are very important for sure.

DIETITIAN: So, it sounds like being there for your family is important – as a mother and perhaps as a wife, too. [*Complex reflection*]

SAMANTHA: Yes, absolutely those things are very important to me.

DIETITIAN: Samantha, can you share with me some ways in which you feel you are able to achieve being a good wife and a good mother?

SAMANTHA: Well, it *is* harder right now given that I have been feeling more tired. I have to admit that I don't always have the energy to make dinner at the end of the day, and my husband has been picking the kids up more from school as I have been feeling run down.

DIETITIAN: Hmmm . . . it sounds like that must be difficult for you that you can't do those things, especially if they are parts of your life that you value. [*Reflective listening*]

SAMANTHA: Yes, it is difficult. I feel like I am letting people down. When I was first assessed to have the bariatric surgery, I was asked why I was doing it. I said that I wanted to become healthier for my family – spend more time with my children, pick them up from school, go to after-school activities. I feel sad that these things aren't working out.

DIETITIAN: Well, it sounds like, on the one hand, you feel that you are disappointing the people who are important to you, whereas, on the other hand, you don't think that you could alter your lifestyle to incorporate the vitamins – which might then actually allow you to do the things that matter to you the most. [*Complex reflection*] What do you think about that?

SAMANTHA: Wow, I don't know if I had really put it together that way. It's true. I had the bariatric surgery so that I could be there for my family. That is what is important to me. Now I have had the surgery and I could have the energy to do the things I want to do, but I am just feeling zapped of all my energy and motivation. I am not sure what impact it is having on my body – not taking all the vitamins regularly. Do you think that we could somehow figure out a way for me to take the vitamins with everything else that I am trying to juggle? [*Can hear sounds of contemplation in the change talk that is arising*]

DIETITIAN: Absolutely. I can see how important it is for you to have the energy to fully participate in activities with your family and to be the mother and wife that you want to be. Let's spend the rest of our session problem solving how we can make sure that you are able to stay on top of your vitamin regimen.

This alternative dialogue illustrates the use of exploration of values in order to allow the patient to reflect on what is most important to her. Miller and Rollnick speak about the benefit of exploring values with patients [1]. The clinician can begin to understand the patient's motivation in a much richer way when the value framework is used [1]. It can also enhance the engagement and alliance between the clinician and the patient. Furthermore, the expression of positive values can have an affirming impact for the patient when she speaks this narrative [1]. For a more detailed overview of value exploration, the interested reader is referred to Miller and Rollnick [1].

Working with Ambivalence

Ambivalence is a common occurrence when people contemplate change [1]. They might want to make a change, but conflicting emotions or thoughts hold them back. It can be a difficult position to be in, and people will often indicate that they feel "stuck." When an individual experiences ambivalence, it can be useful to explore both the pros and the cons of the change [2,3]. The following dialogue illustrates the use of a decisional or motivational balance exercise.

CLINICIAN: Jon, it's great to see you today. I wanted to begin with a check-in as to how your mood has been since I saw you two weeks ago.

JON: Well, my mood has actually been in what feels like a downward spiral to me. I have started to feel quite down most days, and it seems to last the whole day. I'm not sleeping well, and I can't seem to focus on anything. I've been crying a lot too. It's been really difficult.

CLINICIAN: Hmm, I'm surprised to hear that, given that your mood has been fairly stable over the last few months. Any sense of what might be going on? [*Open-ended question*]

JON: Well, I am really embarrassed to tell you this, but I stopped taking my medication for my mood about one month ago.

CLINICIAN: Thanks very much for sharing that with me, Jon. It's really important information for me to be aware of. I am curious as to why you stopped taking your medication. [*Nonjudgmental exploratory stance taken to learn more about Jon's experience from a place of genuine curiosity*]

JON: Well, this is really embarrassing, and I haven't spoken to anyone about this really . . . but I found that I never wanted to have sex with my wife when I was on the antidepressant. And that was really upsetting for both of us. It was affecting our relationship, and it made me disappointed that I was not able to have a sexual relationship with her.

CLINICIAN: It sounds like your loss of interest in sex was very disappointing for both you and your wife. [*Reflective listening*] That is very difficult. Now that you have stopped your medication, it sounds like your mood is being affected, though. Is that correct? [*Summarizing*]

JON: Yes, unfortunately. I thought because my mood had been really good for awhile, it wouldn't matter. But now my mood is low, so I don't feel like being romantic now anyway! I also wanted to mention that I was gaining weight on the medication, which is really upsetting given how much I struggle with my weight already. [*Note: Jon is currently obese and has been trying to change his diet and lifestyle to manage his weight.*] I don't feel like I am in a better position now without the medication. That being said, I really don't feel like taking it again. Between the weight gain and lack of sexual interest, it just wasn't much fun. [*Sustain talk emerging*]

CLINICIAN: Thanks, Jon. That is a lot of important information for me. As I hear you speak about your difficulties with the medication, which would certainly be upsetting for anyone [*normalizing the experience*], I sense that you are considering not going back on it as well. Is that right? [*Reflective listening*]

JON: Well, I guess that is sort of what I was thinking . . . yeah.

CLINICIAN: I am wondering if I could share some information with you regarding depression? [*Using MI strategy for information exchange referred to as elicit-provide-elicit: after the clinician asks permission to provide psychoeducation (elicit), he or she then provides psychoeducation on depression (provide), and then he or she asks about Jon's understanding and response (elicit).*] So, Jon, what are your thoughts about how depression works and the role of medication in treating depression? [*Open-ended question*]

JON: Well, I understand that my depression is not just going to go away. Given how long I have been depressed, I guess staying on some type of medication is the best thing to do. But I still don't want to continue to gain weight and feel such little interest in being intimate with my wife. That was making me feel terrible.

CLINICIAN: That is totally understandable – it sounds like you're feeling pretty conflicted. Jon, how about we try something out together. Let's take a look at the pros and cons of stopping your medication *and* the pros and cons of staying on your medication. [*This can also be further broken down into short- and long-term pros and cons.*] Then we can take a good look at the overall picture when we finish. How does this sound to you?

JON: Yeah, I like that idea. It will be good to see it all laid out.

Fuller and Taylor outline some key questions that can be asked when creating a decisional balance with individuals [2: 184–85]. When examining reasons for change, the clinician can consider asking the patient: "How would changing your behavior fit with what you want in your life . . . now . . . and in the future?"; "What makes you think that you need to make a change?"; "How would your life be better if this change were made?" For long-term change and goals, the clinician can also ask the individual: "Where do you see yourself in one year's time or five year's time?"; "Would this change be important for that to happen?"; "If things remain the same, what would that be like for you?" When working on a decisional balance, the clinician may also want to probe the reasons for *not changing*. This can sometimes feel like an unusual stance to take, but it can allow the patient to speak to the reasons for remaining where he or she is. If a patient has expressed little ambivalence and is already preparing to change, it may be counterproductive to probe and have patients elaborate on the cons of changing or the pros of remaining the same [1]. In that case, it is best to have the patient elaborate on the reasons for change and proceed to the planning phase.

Within the conversation on the decisional balance, the clinician should be listening for change talk, as indicated in the earlier clinical dialogue [1]. Change talk occurs when an individual begins to express his or her desire for movement within the stuck situation – the desire to begin to make some type of a change, no matter how small that change might be. In Jon's case, the clinician should listen for statements such as: "Well, I would like my mood to improve again" or "I want my sleep to get back to normal and my concentration to be focused again." When a clinician detects a hint of change talk, he or she should work to mobilize it. Jon and his therapist developed a simple decisional balance consisting of his reasons to stay off the medication and his reasons to take the medication again (Table 7.1).

Jon and his therapist spoke about the items in the table, and Jon was asked to put a star next to the most important items – the bigger the star, the more important that item [2]. It is important to note that it is not simply the absolute number of reasons in each column but rather the significance of each reason and how it affects the patient's life. The following dialogue between Jon and his therapist focuses on processing the decisional balance.

Table 7.1 A Simple Decisional Balance Exercise

Reasons to stay off the medication	Reasons to take the medication again
It affects my sexual drive, and I feel badly about myself when I have no sex drive.	Since my mood is worse, I still don't have much sexual interest.
It makes me gain weight, and I struggle with my weight already.	My appetite is now affected by my mood, so it is still hard to keep eating healthy.
	My mood has become much worse; I am crying a lot and feeling down.
	I had the energy to exercise on the medication, and that did help my weight.
	I might be able to problem solve the situation better if my mood is stable again.
	I have had very dark periods of depression in my life; I don't want to revisit those.

Source: Adapted from Fuller and Taylor [2].

CLINICIAN: Jon, what are your thoughts about the items noted in your decisional balance? [*Open-ended question*]

JON: It is actually really helpful. I think what stands out the most for me is when I reflected on how severe my depression had become in the past. I was hospitalized for awhile several years back, and I really don't want to return to that.

CLINICIAN: That does seem to be the most meaningful item, and I see that you've flagged that one with a big star. Any other thoughts about the decisional balance or where you might like to go from here?

JON: Well, after going through the pros and cons, I would actually like to revisit the idea of medication. But I was really hoping we could explore a medication that might not have these kinds of side effects – is there anything like that out there?

CLINICIAN: That sounds very reasonable, and we should do some investigative work together. Let's start by chatting about medications you have tried in the past and then take it from there.

Change Talk

Individuals often experience a mix of emotions when trying to change, and they simultaneously feel uncertain about moving forward while also not enjoying remaining in their current state [1]. Miller and Rollnick discuss the idea of *preparatory change talk*, which refers to self-articulated arguments for change that indicate an individual's desire, ability, reason, or need for change (acronym *DARN*) [1]. Table 7.2 illustrates these types of change talk and provides an example of each type.

Table 7.2 Examples of Preparatory Change Talk

Types of preparatory change talk	Examples
Desire	I *want* to take my medication regularly.
	I *would like* to stick to a proper vitamin regimen.
	I *wish* I was able to remember my medication.
Ability	I *am able to* take my medication regularly; I just need better strategies.
	I *can* take my vitamins every day.
Reasons	If I took my medications regularly . . .
	I would likely have more energy.
	I would probably experience better moods.
	I would control my blood pressure much better.
Need	I *need* to take my medications or my mood is really going to slip
	I *must* take my vitamins because my blood tests show some serious results without them.

Source: Adapted from Miller and Rollnick [1].

Although these factors are all important elements of change, preparatory change talk alone does not necessarily translate directly into change. *Mobilizing change talk* is a key step in making change happen [1]. When this kind of change talk emerges, it often suggests that the ambivalence an individual has experienced is beginning to resolve in the direction of change. Miller and Rollnick speak about "commitment change talk" and how that language can often be the best signal that change is emerging into action [1]. This type of language includes phrases such as, "I *will* begin to take my medications regularly." This type of language could appear in contracts because it suggests firm action that someone is intending to take. Other types of change language can include "activation" language and "taking steps" language [1]. These two types of change talk are not necessarily as clear as commitment language is in terms of suggesting that action is likely. Activation language often sounds as though the person is moving toward change but perhaps not as committed (e.g., "I *am prepared* to take my medication on a regular basis"). Finally, "taking steps" change talk can sound as though the individual has begun to take some concrete actions that indicate change is on the way – perhaps not as strongly, though, as if one were committed (e.g., "I went to the pharmacy and bought my medication"). Miller and Rollnick suggest that a clinician does not need to be overly concerned with the exact change talk that emerges [1]. However, understanding what it sounds like and exploring it when it occurs can be important to ensure that it continues to be fostered and action ensues. We will use a complex Case Vignette and clinical dialogue to illustrate change talk in an individual experiencing medical complications following surgery.

Case Vignette

Joan is a 65-year-old woman who underwent Roux-en-Y gastric bypass six years ago. Her bariatric surgery was relatively uncomplicated, and she has been successful at maintaining a weight loss of 60 percent of her excess weight. She is well known to her clinical team because she attends a monthly bariatric surgery support group offered within the clinic where she received her surgery. Furthermore, she acts as a mentor for early-stage bariatric surgery patients. However, she presents today in follow-up one month after discharge from the hospital where she underwent an elective hysterectomy. She appears somewhat out of sorts and complains of feeling "just not myself." She endorses an ongoing struggle with postoperative pain, and her discharge summary refers to a brief episode of postoperative delirium. As she attempts to review her medications, she admits to being confused about new treatments and expresses uncharacteristic exasperation with her entire medication regimen. She confesses that in her frustration and discomfort she has been more lackadaisical than usual, even when it comes to taking her long-standing medications and vitamin supplementations. When the clinician asks to examine her medications, she pulls out two large plastic zipper bags containing a multitude of different pill bottles and boxes. There is, in fact, a significantly greater supply than merited given the time since medication renewal. She has duplicates of several medications, filled on separate occasions with different prescribing physicians, including individuals she does not recognize as part of her healthcare team. She confesses to feeling discouraged with the recent challenge to her health and is looking for support to "get me back on track."

A best possible medications history reveals the following current prescribed medications:

- Synthroid 0.125 mg every morning
- Atorvastatin 40 mg daily
- Metformin 500 mg three times per day before meals
- Quetiapine XR 150 mg at 8 PM (new in hospital)
- Amitriptyline 25 mg before bed
- Calcium citrate 500 mg three times per day
- Vitamin B_{12} 1,000 µg every other day (Tuesday, Thursday, and Saturday)
- Vitamin D 1,000 IU three times per day
- Multivitamin-mineral 2 tablets daily
- Risedronate 35 mg on Monday (new in hospital)
- Hydromorphone contin 3 mg twice per day (new in hospital)
- Hydromorphone 1 mg twice per day as needed (PRN) (new in hospital)

When approaching Joan's case, it is important to keep in mind that she has experienced numerous risk factors for nonadherence to medications. Data from the general medical literature indicate that recent hospital admission, changes to medications, increasing number of daily doses, total number of medications, and central nervous system depressing agents are all independent risk factors for nonadherence [8,9]. It is worthwhile to consider that, as in Joan's case, these risk factors often cluster together in an aging population facing recurrent medical admissions. Patients leaving hospital may not have had the opportunity to review all new medications, their indications, and plans for follow-up with relevant healthcare providers. While judicious use and timely discontinuation of medications are emphasized by attentive inpatient care providers, decisions regarding pain medications, hypnotics, and antipsychotic medications are often necessary to defer to family doctors or outpatient specialists as reasonable pressures to discharge patients prevail. It is important for MI practitioners to be aware of these risk factors of medication nonadherence in order to optimally serve as empathic partners and engage patients in a pragmatic discussion about change. These points are illustrated in the following clinical dialogue:

PHYSICIAN: Joan, it's nice to see you today. How have you been doing since your surgery?

JOAN: Not well. I don't feel like my usual self. I have a great deal of pain, and I'm confused about all the medications I have to take. I already had so many medications to take due to my gastric bypass surgery, and now so many others have been added on. I can't stay on top of the pain or my medications!

PHYSICIAN: Hmm. Why don't you tell me about your current medication regimen? [*Open-ended question*]

JOAN: Well, I don't know. I can't take everything anymore. I can't keep it straight. I'm embarrassed to admit this, but I seem to have so many medications right now that I just stopped taking many of them, and the ones I do take I'm not sure if I'm taking them at the right time of day.

PHYSICIAN: I can see that this is frustrating for you. [*Reflective listening*] Is it okay if I share some information with you regarding the difficulty in having multiple surgeries and needing to take so many medications? [*Asking permission to provide patient education*] [*The physician then spends some time reviewing with Joan the difficulty when patients are taking so many medications and have had multiple surgeries. The physician then reviews how taking so many medications and having recent changes to the medication can also result in individuals not taking their medications regularly.*]

JOAN: So, are you saying that having so many medications might actually result in me not taking them?

PHYSICIAN: Well, I do think you have a very complicated medication regimen. And yes, you are right, sometimes that can result in individuals not taking all of them because it can become so complicated. Let me ask you . . . do you feel that taking all this medication is making your life better . . . or worse?

JOAN: Well, I know that I need to take the medication. I *want* to be able to stick to it because I felt better while I was on it before . . . [*change talk beginning to emerge*], but I can't seem to keep it all straight. But yes, [*sigh*] I do want to get back on track.

PHYSICIAN: Well, I'm hearing that you want to get back on track [*reflective listening*] and take the medications you need [*validating the change talk*]. I want to work with you on that. Before we get started with that, I'm curious to know how confident you feel that you can begin to take your medications again. [*The physician is now using the technique of the confidence ruler to better understand how Joan is feeling about the possibility of making change.*] On a scale from 1 to10, how confident would you say you feel right now?

JOAN: Well, I would say that I feel 6 out of 10.

PHYSICIAN: Great, that's above the midpoint. I am wondering why you put yourself at a 6 and not a 4? [*By asking the patient why she did not rate herself lower, this allows the patient to begin to discuss her reasons for wanting to change and for believing that she can change, and the clinician can strengthen the change talk.*]

JOAN: Well, I know that I have been able to handle taking a lot of medications before. In fact, not only was I taking a complicated regimen of medications, but I was also on a strict routine with respect to my food and liquids and the supplements. So I'm thinking that if I could do all that back then, I should be able to get back on track with my new medications now. [*More change talk emerging as Joan reflects on why she rated herself as a 6 out of 10 and not a lower number.*]

PHYSICIAN: Well, that is great news, and I agree that you have been on very complicated schedules before. So why don't we bring in the pharmacist, and she can sit down with you and review all your medications, and we can figure out when best to take them all and in the most convenient way possible. I am also happy to speak with clinicians from your bariatric team to see if they might have any further suggestions. How does this plan sound to you, Joan?

JOAN: It sounds great. Thank you so much!

Further MI-informed inquiry by other healthcare providers reveals that Joan is excessively sedated in the morning, and she is embarrassed to admit that she has often been sleeping through her Synthroid dose and morning medications. Moreover, she reports that her husband was recently ill himself, and therefore, he has been less able to support her as she struggled to adjust to her new medication regimen following discharge. She endorses misgivings about some of her newer medications, citing gastric pain following her weekly Risedronate dose (of particular concern in light of ulcer risk associated with the medication possibly exacerbated by Roux-en-Y gastric bypass history). She notes that she is now taking two extended-release formulations of medications and wonders if she may be experiencing side effects from these medications with limited efficacy. She feels tired and frustrated with healthcare providers whom she experiences as frequently dismissive when she expresses concerns regarding medication absorption given decreased gastrointestinal transit time after bariatric surgery.

A closer inspection of Joan's medications with the pharmacist reveals a regimen that calls for at least six to seven discrete medication administration points over the course of the day (not including as-needed prescriptions). Furthermore, she is tasked with very specific instructions surrounding the dosing of many of her medications: Synthroid must be taken first thing in the morning on an empty stomach at least 30 minutes before food and cannot be coadministered with any other medication; metformin must be taken with meals; quetiapine XR is commonly prescribed after dinner but two to three hours before bed; multivitamins must not be taken together with calcium and vitamin D; vitamin B_{12} is taken every other day (or every Tuesday, Thursday, and Saturday); risedronate is taken weekly after an overnight fast on a completely empty stomach with 6 to 8 ounces (200 to 250 ml) of water, in an upright position, with no other food, pills, or beverages for at least 30 minutes. Needless to say, Joan's frustration and overwhelmed feelings regarding medication changes become very understandable in light of these significant additional burdens imposed on her by virtue of dosing schedule and instructions.

While Joan appears quite lucid, the MI practitioner must also maintain awareness that minor deficits in cognitive function may be affecting Joan's adherence. In addition to the deleterious impact that pain has on concentration and energy, opioid pain medications themselves (as well as quetiapine and amitriptyline) have central nervous system depressing properties that interfere with complex tasks, attention, executive function, and working memory. Moreover, the occurrence of an episode of delirium in an inpatient setting may merit subsequent assessment of cognitive functioning. Delirium is a complex neuropsychiatric syndrome characterized by a sudden disturbance of cognition and attention marked by a fluctuating course and due to an underlying medical illness. Delirium may be relatively brief, well circumscribed, and resolve without residual deficits in individuals with significant cognitive reserve. However, in individuals with prior episodes of delirium or underlying cognitive dysfunction, delirium often resolves much more slowly, and patients may experience some degree of ongoing confusion and attention difficulties well after discharge. Antipsychotics are often initiated in hospital for the treatment of delirium, and quetiapine is frequently encountered due to sedating and hypnotic properties that are important in managing agitation and insomnia, which are prevalent and contribute to the risk in delirium. New-standing antipsychotic medications in an individual (especially aged 65 or over) with no history of psychosis or bipolar disorder should prompt further inquiry into their indication and the need for continued use. Quetiapine is commonly prescribed in its XR formulation, which should be avoided in bariatric surgery patients.

Joan's case highlights the strengths of using an MI approach for patients struggling with medication adherence. Motivation, persistence, and resolution may wane in the face of accumulating biological, psychological, and social stressors, even in the most committed and reliable patients. Open questions create a nonjudgmental context that affords patients the opportunity to clearly articulate and self-reflect on factors that are interfering with optimal adherence. Affirmations validate the patient's experience and facilitate communication about the patient's values and goals. Reflective listening creates a supportive environment where the MI practitioner is a partner in care while simultaneously reinforcing the patient's autonomy and self-direction in the discussion about changing behaviors. While the true strength of the MI approach lies in untangling and addressing the multitude of psychological factors contributing to suboptimal adherence to medications, biological and environmental risk factors must not be discounted. Not discussed in Joan's case are the effects that mood disorders, anxiety disorders, or other mental health disorders may have on motivation and adherence. Motivational interviewing can be helpful for collaboratively brainstorming a variety of strategies for optimizing medication adherence, including thoroughly reviewing medications with relevant healthcare providers with an eye toward minimizing unnecessary dose divisions and eliminating unnecessary central nervous system depressing agents. In addition, there is some evidence that simple tools such as dosette boxes, blister packs, and construction of a clear weekly grid noting each individual medication and timing may increase medication adherence [10]. A detailed weekly medication grid was constructed based on Joan's current medications (Table 7.3), and she was referred back to her family doctor to address ongoing medications of concern.

Empirical Evidence for the Effectiveness of Motivational Interviewing for Promoting Medication Adherence

A few studies exist regarding the use of MI to enhance medication adherence in individuals with severe obesity and/or related diseases. For example, a randomized, controlled trial (RCT) examined the impact on "quality-of-care measures" in patients with type 2 diabetes who received up to three MI consultations from their general practitioners (GPs) compared with those who did not [4]. Outcome measures included metabolic status as well as medication adherence. At the one-year follow-up, both groups had improved metabolic status and high medication adherence. The authors hypothesized that this finding might have been due to the GPs in both the control and intervention groups receiving intensive training to treat type 2 diabetes and being encouraged to "act as counselors" with their

Table 7.3 Sample Weekly Medication Grid

Time	Monday	Tuesday	Wednesday	Thursday	Friday	Saturday	Sunday
7 AM	Risedronate						
8 AM	Synthroid	Synthroid	Synthroid	Synthroid	Synthroid	Synthroid	Synthroid
8:30 AM (breakfast)	Metformin Atorvastatin MVI HM Contin	Metformin Atorvastatin MVI HM Contin Vitamin B_{12}	Metformin Atorvastatin MVI HM Contin	Metformin Atorvastatin MVI HM Contin Vitamin B_{12}	Metformin Atorvastatin MVI HM Contin	Metformin Atorvastatin MVI HM Contin Vitamin B_{12}	Metformin Atorvastatin MVI HM Contin
12 noon (lunch)	Metformin Calcium Vitamin D	Metformin Calcium Vitamin D	Metformin Calcium Vitamin D	Metformin Calcium Vitamin D	Metformin Calcium Vitamin D	Metformin Calcium Vitamin D	Metformin Calcium Vitamin D
6 PM (dinner)	Metformin Calcium Vitamin D HM Contin	Metformin Calcium Vitamin D HM Contin	Metformin Calcium Vitamin D HM Contin	Metformin Calcium Vitamin D HM Contin	Metformin Calcium Vitamin D HM Contin	Metformin Calcium Vitamin D HM Contin	Metformin Calcium Vitamin D HM Contin
8 PM	Quetiapine	Quetiapine	Quetiapine	Quetiapine	Quetiapine	Quetiapine	Quetiapine
10 PM (bedtime)	Amitriptyline Calcium Vitamin D	Amitriptyline Calcium Vitamin D	Amitriptyline Calcium Vitamin D	Amitriptyline Calcium Vitamin D	Amitriptyline Calcium Vitamin D	Amitriptyline Calcium Vitamin D	Amitriptyline Calcium Vitamin D

Source: Adapted from Muir et al. [10].

patients. Further, both groups were encouraged to allow a "mutual understanding" to emerge between the GP and patient with respect to illness management. Rubak and colleagues described these components as being some of the key components of MI, potentially resulting in the enhanced adherence found in both groups [4]. Another recent study investigated whether the provision of information regarding medication adherence, with or without MI, improved diabetes and lipid control in individuals who were using medications for diabetic control and lipid level reductions [5]. Results indicated that outcomes were not different between those who received adherence information only or MI and adherence information compared with usual care. The authors noted that lack of impact was potentially attributed to poor patient participation in the MI arm of the study, suggesting that those who could have benefited the most appeared to be the least likely to partake in the intervention [5].

A systematic review and meta-analysis examined the use of various psychological interventions, including MI, to enhance glycemic control in individuals with type 2 diabetes [6]. Although an insufficient number of studies examined MI as a stand-alone psychological intervention, a few of the 25 studies included elements of MI, such as "cognitive motivational therapy" or individual MI sessions combined with another treatment. Most of the psychotherapies incorporated elements of cognitive-behavioral therapy, and a few cited "behavior modification." Control groups within this review included "usual care" as well as "education" [6]. Overall, the use of psychological interventions significantly enhanced glycemic control [6]. Therapies were not found to have an impact on blood glucose concentrations or weight management. It was concluded that although it appears that psychological interventions are able to enhance some elements of control for type 2 diabetes, the types of treatments offering the greatest benefit and the types of patients who would benefit the most are not yet well understood. However, the authors did indicate that the approach of MI to help counsel individuals with unhealthy lifestyles would suggest that it could extend into help for individuals with type 2 diabetes [6].

Relatively few empirical studies conducted to date have examined the efficacy of MI for improving medication adherence specifically in individuals with severe obesity; however, there is a body of research in health-related fields more broadly demonstrating that MI can be beneficial for improving medication adherence. For example, a recent systematic review and meta-analysis examined the impact of MI on medication adherence across various medical issues [7]. Literature databases were searched to assess the effect of several variables on adherence, including the format in which MI was delivered, the "dose" of MI provided, and the backgrounds of individuals delivering the intervention [7]. Seventeen RCTs were included. Motivational interviewing was delivered either by telephone or in person (i.e., individual, group, or combination). Most of the studies reported that 24 hours of training was provided to the counselors delivering the intervention, although the range was from 4 to 40 hours. A number of methods were used to assess medication adherence, including objective adherence measures, self-report measures, and a combination of both. Results of the systematic review and meta-analysis indicated that MI interventions did improve medication adherence. Although the specific MI characteristics that were associated with the improvements were not consistent [7], this evaluation provides some evidence that MI can be used to support medication adherence in a variety of medical populations.

Summary

The clinical dialogues presented in this chapter illustrate a variety of MI strategies that can be useful when working with individuals with severe obesity who are having difficulty with medication adherence. The Case Vignettes were relatively complex in that the patients had undergone gastric bypass or had multiple surgeries. However, these MI strategies can be employed within any situation related to medication adherence. Although formal training in MI would be beneficial for any clinician, the strategies illustrated in this chapter can be easily integrated within the natural dialogue that may occur within a healthcare provider's office during routine follow-up visits. Motivational interviewing can be conceptualized as a language in this regard and not necessarily a set of tools that need to be implemented in a specific manner. By using the MI strategies discussed in this chapter and elsewhere [1–3] and remaining sensitive to the complex realities of medication adherence in patients with severe obesity, the clinician may engage his or her patients directly in the face of medication nonadherence.

Key Points

- Medication and vitamin adherence is important for the physical and mental health of individuals with severe obesity, including bariatric surgery patients.
- Motivational interviewing strategies can be used by clinicians to open up dialogue surrounding complicated medication and vitamin adherence issues, even during routine, brief follow-up visits.
- Although specific MI tools exist, MI can be thought of as a language to decrease defensiveness and create an open conversation in which adherence issues can be explored.
- Little research has examined MI for medication adherence specifically in individuals with severe obesity, but MI has been shown to be effective in promoting adherence in a variety of medical populations.

References

1. R. Miller and S. Rollnick. *Motivational Interviewing*, vol. 3: *Helping People Change*. New York, NY: Guilford Press, 2013.

2. C. Fuller and P. Taylor. *A Toolkit of Motivational Skills*. Chichester: Wiley, 2008.

3. S. Rollnick, W. R. Miller, and C. C. Butler. *Motivational Interviewing in Health Care*. New York, NY: Guildford Press, 2008.

4. S. Rubak, A. Sandbaek, T. Lauritzen, et al. Effect of "motivational interviewing" on quality of care measures in screen detected type 2 diabetes patients: A one-year follow-up of an RCT, ADDITION Denmark. *Scand J Prim Health Care* 2011; **29**: 92–8.

5. M. Pladevall, G. Divine, K. E. Wells, et al. A randomized controlled trial to provide adherence information and motivational interviewing to improve diabetes and lipid control. *Diabetes Educ* 2015; **41**: 136–46.

6. K. Ismail, K. Winkley, and S. Rabe-Hesketh. Systematic review and meta-analysis of randomised controlled trials of psychological interventions to improve glycaemic control in patients with type 2 diabetes. *Lancet* 2004; **363**: 1589–97.

7. A. Palacio, D. Garay, B. Langer, et al. Motivational interviewing improves medication adherence: A systematic review and meta-analysis. *J Gen Intern Med* 2016; **31**: 929–40.

8. A. J. Claxton, J. Cramer, and C. Pierce. A systematic review of the associations between dose regimens and medication compliance. *Clin Ther* 2001; **23**: 1296–310.

9. M. D. Murray and K. Kroenke. Polypharmacy and medication adherence: Small steps on a long road. *J Gen Intern Med* 2001; **16**: 137–9.

10. A. J. Muir, L. L. Sanders, W. E. Wilkinson, et al. Reducing medication regimen complexity: a controlled trial. *J Gen Intern Med* 2001; **16**: 77–82.

Cognitive-Behavioral Therapy for Behavioral and Lifestyle Changes in Severe Obesity

Aliza Friedman and Stephanie E. Cassin

Case Vignette

Sarah is a 40-year-old registered nurse who lives with her husband of 10 years and their son (age five). Sarah was previously employed as a surgical nurse, but about a year ago she decided to take a job as an intake nurse at a hospice care facility due to chronic knee pain and considerable difficulty standing for extended periods of time during surgical procedures. Sarah reports a long-standing history of obesity since early adolescence and is especially distressed that her weight has steadily increased over the past year since starting her position as an intake nurse (current BMI = 40 kg/m^2). Sarah also reports a recent diagnosis of hypertension, for which she has been prescribed blood pressure medication.

When questioned about her current patterns of eating and activity, Sarah describes her patterns as "chaotic." She states that she is very busy in the morning trying to get her son ready for school, which often results in her not having enough time to pack a lunch and snacks for herself. Accordingly, Sarah describes going for long hours at work without eating, as well as struggling to "resist the temptation" of baked goods often available in the staff lunchroom. When returning home from work, Sarah describes feeling "famished" and overeating at dinnertime. She also states that her current position at work is primarily sedentary, which has been helpful with respect to better managing her knee pain but has resulted in a substantial reduction in overall physical activity.

With respect to weight and exercise history, Sarah describes repeated attempts of "yoyo dieting" and difficulty sustaining weight loss for longer than a few months at a time. She also expresses an interest in starting a regular exercise routine but notes that each time she commits to a more structured exercise regime, she stops exercising within a few days of starting the program. Sarah has recently presented to her primary care physician with concerns about recent weight gain, hypertension, and chronic pain. Her physician recommended a course of cognitive-behavioral therapy with a mental health clinician to help promote more sustained behavioral and lifestyle changes.

Introduction

In this chapter, we provide an overview of cognitive-behavioral therapy (CBT) and the rationale for using CBT to promote behavioral and lifestyle changes in individuals with severe obesity. We then discuss a selection of CBT strategies that may be helpful in promoting behavioral and lifestyle changes. We return to the Case Vignette throughout the chapter using clinical dialogues to illustrate the application of select CBT strategies. We also review the empirical evidence regarding the effectiveness of CBT in patients with severe obesity.

Overview of Cognitive-Behavioral Therapy

Cognitive-behavioral therapy is a short-term, skills-based intervention that is based on the theory that thoughts, emotions, and behaviors mutually influence one another [1] (see Chapter 2). In other words, the way in which an individual perceives a situation can influence his or her emotional and behavioral responses. According to cognitive theory, patients often demonstrate systematic errors in their thinking patterns, commonly referred to as *cognitive distortions* or "thinking traps." For example, if after missing one scheduled workout (*situation*) an individual has the thought, "I am a failure for not working out today" (*cognition*), this self-appraisal could contribute to negative affect, including shame, disgust, or sadness (*emotions*), as well as potentially avoidance of exercise the following day or emotional overeating (*behaviors*). In turn, these behaviors often provide confirmatory evidence for the negative self-appraisals such that by avoiding exercise or engaging in emotional overeating, the individual continues to view himself or herself as a failure. Similarly, negative affect such as sadness or shame can increase one's vulnerability for engaging in maladaptive behaviors and experiencing negative automatic thoughts. Accordingly, an individual's maladaptive thoughts, behaviors, and emotions are maintained through a negative-feedback cycle. The goal of CBT is therefore to target the mechanisms that are maintaining this unhelpful feedback cycle, specifically by teaching patients cognitive skills to identify and challenge their negative thought patterns, as well as behavioral techniques aimed at reducing avoidance and increasing health-promoting behaviors.

Cognitive-behavioral therapy is present focused such that patients are encouraged to focus on how their current maladaptive thought and behavioral patterns *maintain* psycho-pathology rather than a more in-depth focus on the origins of these thoughts or behaviors. Given that CBT is short term and skills based, most sessions are spent actively engaging in skills practice, in addition to encouraging patients to practice those skills between therapy sessions (often referred to as *homework* or an *action plan*). Cognitive-behavioral therapists adopt a collaborative stance whereby they work with patients to challenge the accuracy and utility of their negative thought patterns through a process referred to as *guided discovery* [2]. Therapists train patients to gradually apply these skills independently, with the goal of sustaining more long-term behavioral change and emotional well-being.

Cognitive-Behavioral Therapy for Severe Obesity

Severe obesity has a significant psychological impact within a variety of domains, including decreased quality of life, chronic pain, and higher prevalence of psychological conditions such as mood and anxiety disorders [3–5] (see Chapter 1). Individuals with severe obesity similarly demonstrate a high prevalence of disordered eating behaviors (e.g., feeling a loss of control when eating, emotional overeating, grazing, or picking at food), as well as eating disorder diagnoses [6,7]. Given that disordered eating behaviors such as binge eating and emotional eating are associated with greater negative affect, as well as difficulty identifying and regulating emotions [8,9], teaching patients more effective coping skills is an important weight management intervention.

Clinical guidelines for the management of obesity recommend that the following components be included in interventions: goal setting, self-monitoring, physical activity, stimulus control, problem solving, cognitive restructuring (i.e., modification of maladaptive thoughts), relapse prevention, and strategies for dealing with weight regain [10]. The following section will focus on reviewing the practical application of core CBT skills and illustrating the skills using clinical dialogues, with a specific focus on increasing physical activity and promoting regular eating (i.e., eating meals/snacks every three to four hours). The authors of this chapter adopt the position that all food can fit within a healthy lifestyle in moderation, and accordingly, this chapter will not use such words as *healthy/unhealthy* and *good/bad* to describe certain food choices. If a patient chooses to participate in a weight loss program, the skills presented in this chapter could be used as an adjunctive treatment to surgical or medical weight loss interventions. For more detailed descriptions of the use of CBT to promote weight loss in individuals who are overweight or obese, please see Fabricatore [11] or Dalle Grave et al. [12].

Introducing the CBT Model

The first component of most cognitive-behavioral protocols involves introducing patients to the CBT model and developing a personalized formulation (Figure 8.1 provides a visual depiction of a personalized formulation and its relation to core CBT skills). This process helps to orient patients to the treatment being delivered, as well as provide them with a clear framework outlining the interactions between their thoughts, behaviors, and emotions.

The following dialogue illustrates how to collaboratively build a personalized CBT formulation with a patient.

CLINICIAN: Sarah, I'd like to start by introducing you to the cognitive-behavioral model. This framework suggests that our thoughts, behaviors, and emotions are interconnected and mutually influence one another. I find it's easiest to illustrate this model using a relevant example for you. Can you start by sharing with me some of the eating challenges you've been encountering lately?

SARAH: I just can't seem to get it together! I start off every morning telling myself to avoid eating junk food, but I always fall off the wagon by the end of the day! I end up eating leftover junk food in the lunchroom at work or overeating at dinner. I also am trying to start a regular exercise routine but can't seem to stick to one consistently. And sure enough, I keep on gaining weight!

CLINICIAN: That sounds very frustrating. I'm hearing that you're motivated to make some changes in your life, and yet it sounds like you're caught in this vicious cycle between telling yourself to avoid eating certain foods and feeling distressed about some of your choices at the end of the day. Does that fit for you?

SARAH: Exactly. I keep just getting stuck in that cycle. It's so exhausting. It makes me just want to give up on all of my goals.

CLINICIAN: That makes sense. It's so hard for us to keep pushing forward to meet our goals when we're feeling exhausted or defeated. I'm wondering if maybe we could start mapping this example onto the CBT model to give us a better sense of how you're getting stuck in this cycle.

SARAH: Well, like I said before, I start each day thinking, "I have to avoid eating junk food today." And I guess "eating junk food in the lunchroom" and "overeating at dinner" would be behaviors.

CLINICIAN: Okay, let's add those thoughts and behaviors to the diagram (Figure 8.1). What about emotions?

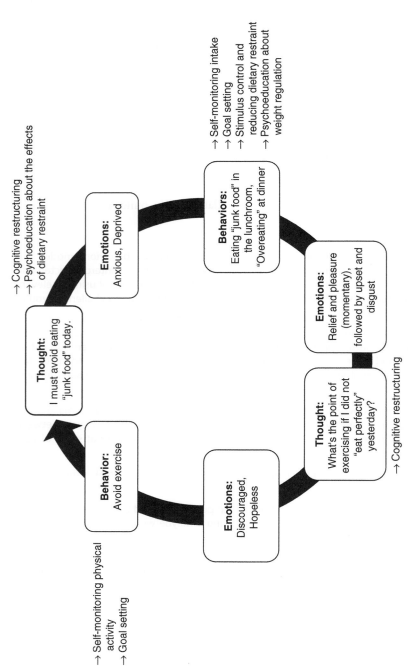

Figure 8.1 Sample personalized CBT formulation and its relation to core CBT skills.

SARAH: I feel so upset and disgusted with myself after eating junk food. I don't know why I keep getting stuck in this cycle.

CLINICIAN: Let's add those emotions to the diagram to see if we can gain a clearer understanding together. [*Note: The clinician collaborates with the patient here to facilitate guided discovery, as opposed to adopting a didactic stance.*] It sounds like some time after eating the food you're trying to avoid, you're feeling upset and disgusted with yourself. [*Note: The clinician should avoid reflecting back words like junk and unhealthy food in order to remain consistent with future messaging.*] Do you have a sense of how you feel when you're actually eating the food, or perhaps just afterwards?

SARAH: Hmm . . . I guess I am a bit relieved right afterwards. And the food does taste good when I'm eating it.

CLINICIAN: That makes a lot of sense. It sounds like initially the food tastes good and you're feeling a bit relieved to have eaten some of the food you're avoiding. We sometimes forget to highlight the positive emotions given how quickly they can shift to disgust or feeling upset, but they can actually provide us with some important information about this cycle. In this context, it sounds like food is making you feel good temporarily and also taking away some of the distress associated with having to avoid certain foods. Both of these can be very powerful motivators to keep engaging in a behavior. [*Note: Accordingly, food functions for this patient as both a positive and negative reinforcer such that it temporarily provides pleasure and also relieves the distress associated with attempts to avoid "junk food."*]

SARAH: I guess that makes more sense. I hadn't thought about how food does make me feel good for a short period of time.

CLINICIAN: That sounds like an important observation. How do you think exercise would fit into this formulation?

SARAH: I've also noticed that after eating junk food, I'm less likely to exercise the following morning. It's almost like if I've eaten junk food the night before, what's the point of exercising the next morning?

CLINICIAN: I'm glad you mentioned that as well. You've identified another way our thoughts and emotions can interfere with our behaviors: we often fall into the trap of being very "all or nothing" with our food and exercise. It sounds like in this situation, eating "treat" food you've been avoiding contributes to some additional negative thoughts of "What's the point of exercising if I did not eat 'perfectly healthy' the day before?". Would you say that these thoughts lead to avoiding exercise?

SARAH: Absolutely. I've noticed that I'm always either "on track" or "falling off the wagon."

CLINICIAN: That's a very common experience reported by people with a history of chronic yoyo dieting. The goal of CBT is to disrupt this cycle. We'll work together to learn techniques to help you identify and challenge some of these thinking traps, as well as help you introduce such behaviors as eating regularly throughout the day to help you best meet your goals.

Setting SMART Goals

Goal setting can help to ensure that patients and therapists are working collaboratively toward an agreed-on desired outcome. In addition, given that patients with a history of yoyo dieting may have a tendency to evaluate their success in treatment based on weight loss, goal setting can also help patients to brainstorm additional ways to measure their success in treatment. The SMART goals technique originated in management settings [13] but over the past four decades has been applied to facilitating behavioral change more generally. Although there has been some discrepancy across papers with respect to defining the SMART acronym [14], the most prevalent definition proposes that an effective goal must satisfy the following criteria: it must be *specific, measurable, attainable, relevant,* and *time bound.*

The following clinical dialogue provides a more detailed description of how to introduce goal setting to a patient.

CLINICIAN: Sarah, it sounds like one of your goals for treatment is to increase your physical activity.

SARAH: Yes, I really want to start exercising more consistently. I've noticed that since I switched to a more sedentary nursing position, I'm feeling even more lethargic during the day. I've also developed some chronic knee pain over the past few years, and I'm worried that it could worsen if I continue to gain weight. My husband keeps telling me that I might feel more energetic if I was more active, but every time I try to make an exercise plan for myself, I never stick with it for more than a few days at a time.

CLINICIAN: What do you think has gotten in the way of exercising more consistently in the past? [*Note: Addressing past barriers to behavior change can help the clinician develop individualized solutions for patients.*]

SARAH: Well, I've noticed that I tend to get really eager when I first decide to start an exercise program, and I set goals to walk outside every morning at 6 AM before I start work. After a few days, I become exhausted and end up sleeping through my workout. Before I know it, weeks have gone by, and I haven't exercised once.

CLINICIAN: You've identified a very common pattern, Sarah. Often when we're first setting a new goal, we have the tendency to want to change our behavior really quickly, and we end up setting goals that might not be the most sustainable for us long term. Does this pattern resonate with you?

SARAH: Absolutely. I think that's one of the main reasons why I stop going to the gym after a few days or weeks. I don't want to keep falling into that trap.

CLINICIAN: That makes a lot of sense. It sounds like developing a more sustainable exercise plan for you might be more helpful. Keeping that in mind, I'd like to introduce you to a goal-setting acronym that I find helpful in working with patients ... and in setting personal goals for myself, too. We aim to set goals that are SMART, which stands for specific, measurable, attainable, relevant, and time bound. In other words, we want our goals to be clearly articulated, and we need to know how we will measure our progress toward those goals. In addition, we want these goals to be attainable given our life circumstances, relevant to our long-term goals and values, and time bound to ensure we are working toward meeting our goals within a specific time period. Does this make sense?

SARAH: It does. *But,* I'm concerned that if I set more realistic goals, I'll end up just being complacent with only minor progress, and I'll stop pushing myself to keep working harder.

CLINICIAN: Sarah, I really appreciate you sharing that concern because it's actually a very common misconception about goal setting. Although we might intuitively think that setting more realistic goals will prevent us from continuing to push ourselves harder, it's often the opposite that occurs: the more realistic a goal, the greater is the sense of mastery we feel after achieving it, and the more likely we are to keep pushing ourselves to continue working toward our goals. Have you ever experienced this pattern before in other domains of your life? [*Note: Encouraging patients to consider past successes in other life domains can help to build mastery, as well as highlight important information that could assist them with setting new goals.*]

SARAH: I've definitely noticed that at work. When I'm feeling really overwhelmed with paperwork, I find it helpful to set small goals to finish a certain amount of work before lunch. Completing those smaller goals does help keep me motivated.

CLINICIAN: That's a great example – it sounds like you've definitely seen the benefit of setting SMART goals at work. With respect to your physical activity goals, let's start by evaluating your original goal of "going to the gym every weekday at 6 AM." How SMART is that goal?

SARAH: Well, it's definitely specific and relevant to my long-term goal of having more energy throughout the day, and perhaps helping to better cope with the chronic knee pain. It's also measurable because if I were attending the gym every weekday morning, I would know that I'm meeting my goal. That being said, I don't think it's the most attainable. Between getting ready for work and helping my kids get ready for school, there just isn't enough time in the morning to fit in a workout. I also never considered making a goal time bound.

CLINICIAN: Okay, so keeping in mind that you want to make your goal more attainable and time bound, how might you modify it?

SARAH: I think using part of my lunch break to exercise would be more realistic. Now that it's getting warmer outside, I think I'd like to try walking outside for about 20 minutes during my lunch break.

CLINICIAN: That sounds like a great idea! How many times a week do you think you'd like to start with? [*Note: Clarifying questions can help coach the patient to make his or her goals more specific.*]

SARAH: I think walking for 20 minutes on my lunch break three times a week is a realistic place to start. I'd like to evaluate my progress on this goal by the end of the next two months.

CLINICIAN: Good work incorporating the SMART goals criteria. Can you anticipate any barriers that might get in the way of you meeting this goal? [*Note: Encouraging patients to anticipate and problem solve potential barriers ahead of time can increase the likelihood of them meeting their goals.*]

SARAH: Hmm . . . it could rain on my lunch break. I also sometimes end up working through lunch. If it's raining most of the week, maybe I'll walk for 20 minutes at the shopping mall across the street, and if I do have to work some days through lunch, I can definitely fit in some walking over the weekend.

CLINICIAN: Those ideas sound great. What about your knee pain? Do you think that could interfere with you meeting your goals? [*Note: It is important to address pain in the context of severe obesity because pain can interfere with adherence to a regular exercise program.*]

SARAH: It definitely could, but I do typically find walking to be low impact on my knees. If I do experience pain, maybe I'll replace walking with some lighter stretching on those days.

CLINICIAN: That sounds like a good solution. At the start of our next session, I'll check in with you regarding your progress over this next week. Does that sound okay?

SARAH: Yes, I'd like that. I think that might help me to stay more accountable.

Self-Monitoring Dietary Intake and Activity

Self-monitoring of dietary intake and activity patterns has been described as the most important behavioral skill when working with individuals with obesity [11]. Patients are instructed to record their daily dietary intake and activity patterns in real time to ensure accurate recall either using a written monitoring record or a mobile application. Within a cognitive-behavioral framework, there are three main goals for self-monitoring intake and activity: (1) to identify patterns in eating and activity, (2) to help facilitate changes in eating and activity, and (3) to assist patients with staying on track with their goals [15]. Given that the purpose of self-monitoring is to assess and modify eating and exercise patterns rather than explicitly reducing caloric intake, patients not engaging in an adjunctive weight loss program should be encouraged to include general measurements of intake instead of counting calories (i.e., about half a cup of rice, half a family-sized bag of chips). Accordingly, a CBT monitoring record (Figure 8.2) includes space to record daily intake and activity, as well as thoughts, feelings, and behaviors. Self-monitoring records can also help to provide more objective evidence of the

CBT Self-Monitoring Record							
Date	Time	Location and People You Were With	Description of Food & Liquid & Amount Consumed	Thoughts	Emotions	Behaviors	Physical Activity
Wednesday	9:00 am	Alone at work	1 Granola bar 1 Banana Greek Yogurt (1 container) Coffee with milk and sugar	I know this day is going to be really busy and stressful.	Anxiety		
Forgot to pack my lunch!! I didn't have time to buy any food at work either.				I am so hungry!	Disappointment		Went for a short walk during work (10 minutes)
Wednesday	6:00 pm	Eating dinner with my husband and son	1 beef hamburger with bun 2 servings roasted potatoes with butter 1 serving roasted vegetables 1 serving chocolate cake	I am overeating. I failed my goal.	Disappointment Shame	I didn't write down everything I ate for dinner.	I am definitely not exercising tomorrow.

Figure 8.2 Sample CBT self-monitoring record for dietary intake and physical activity.

patient's patterns over the past week, which can be helpful in the context of cognitive restructuring. For example, patients might present with thoughts such as, "I completely failed my workout plan this week"; however, their records demonstrate that they only failed to meet their exercise goal one day this past week.

Cognitive-behavioral therapy may also include monitoring weight on a weekly basis. Weekly in-session weighing can help to reduce both avoidance of the scale and frequent weight checking, both of which can increase weight preoccupation and distress [16]. The following dialogue includes detailed descriptions of introducing self-monitoring records, as well as reviewing a record following completion.

Introducing Self-Monitoring Records

CLINICIAN: Now that you've set your goals for the week, I'd like to introduce another skill we refer to as *self-monitoring*. Have you ever recorded your eating and activity patterns before?

SARAH: So many times! I find it really annoying to keep writing out what I eat and how much I exercise on a daily basis. I always lose the forms midday, and by that time, I've completely forgotten what I ate earlier in the day.

CLINICIAN: That makes a lot of sense. Many patients report some difficulty with completing their self-monitoring records on a regular basis. Why do you think it might be important for us to problem solve how you can complete these records regularly, despite how challenging it's been in the past? [*Note: Clinician uses Socratic questioning and a collaborative approach to facilitate the process of guided discovery.*]

SARAH: Maybe it's to help get a better sense of what my actual week looks like with respect to eating and exercise. There's no way I'd remember all of that at our next appointment a week later.

CLINICIAN: That's a great point. Self-monitoring definitely helps us evaluate more accurate patterns in our eating and activity. We also know that our thoughts can sometimes color the way we remember the past week – for example, we might have the tendency to hyperfocus on one day that we did not meet our goals and label the whole week as a "terrible week" instead of noticing the days in which we did meet our goals.

SARAH: I've definitely done that before.

CLINICIAN: When we're falling into those traps with our thinking, self-monitoring records can help to provide us with more objective evidence to challenge some of those thoughts. They can also help to identify some places where you may want to make changes in your eating or activity patterns and keep you motivated to stay on track with these goals. Does this reasoning make sense?

SARAH: Yes, it does. But I still can't see myself carrying around those paper records everywhere.

CLINICIAN: What about using a mobile application? Some patients find it easier to report what they're eating and how much they're exercising in real time when using their cell phones.

SARAH: I could try that.

CLINICIAN: That's great. Do you think you could commit to recording everything you eat and drink over the next week, in addition to your physical activity? The goal is not to specifically count calories or measure out every meal but rather to describe your intake in more general patterns, such as a palm-sized amount of chicken or one chocolate bar.

SARAH: That sounds a bit less daunting than what I've tried in the past. I find it exhausting to count every single calorie I've consumed in a day.

CLINICIAN: That would be very exhausting indeed. It's also possible that counting calories could make you more focused on the specific amount of energy you're taking in rather than on including a variety of food groups for more nutritionally balanced meals. Instead of focusing on calorie counting, our goal is to get a sense of your eating and activity patterns, as well as how they're related to your thoughts and feelings.

SARAH: Okay.

CLINICIAN: For example, you've mentioned going for long hours at work without eating, as well as feelings of disappointment after overeating in the evenings. We want to have the best understanding of the factors that contribute to going long hours without eating, as well as the consequences. On this self-monitoring record, we have included a space for your "situation, thoughts, feelings and behaviors" to ensure that you have space to record some information about the particular context when you were eating or exercising. [*Note: This exercise is most helpful if the patient and clinician can both look at a self-monitoring paper record or mobile application together.*] Would that be something you would be willing to experiment with?

SARAH: Definitely. I've never tried recording my thoughts or feelings when I'm eating.

CLINICIAN: I think it's definitely worth an experiment then to see whether certain patterns of eating are connected to your thoughts and feelings. Another important component to remember is to focus on updating the application with what you've eaten and how much you've exercised as close to the meal or activity as possible. This can help to ensure that we get the best overall representation of your weekly patterns. Are there any strategies you've found helpful in the past when trying to remember to complete a task?

SARAH: I could try setting an alarm on my cell phone to remind me to update my application at lunchtime. I'm usually better at remembering to record after eating breakfast and dinner, but I tend to forget more when busy at work during the day. I have an alarm set to remind me to take my blood pressure medication, and it usually helps me remember to take my medication on time.

CLINICIAN: That sounds like a really good idea. Let's add "set cell phone alarm for self-monitoring records" to your weekly homework to ensure that you remember to try that strategy this week.

Reviewing Self-Monitoring Records

CLINICIAN: Thank you for completing your self-monitoring record over this past week, Sarah [*Note: If the patient is using a mobile application, it can be helpful to use an application that allows for viewing the full week's intake/activity pattern within the screen.*] Let's take a look at it together (Figure 8.2).

CLINICIAN: Would you say that this record is an accurate representation of your eating and activity over the past week?

SARAH: Overall, I'd say it is pretty accurate. It was definitely easier recording my intake and activity using the app.

CLINICIAN: I'm glad to hear that! Did you try setting the alarm as a reminder to record in real time? [*Note: Clinician checks in about homework completion from a nonjudgmental stance.*]

SARAH: I did. It didn't work every single time, but I found it pretty helpful actually.

CLINICIAN: It's great that you've identified a helpful strategy. Are there any instances this week when you forgot to include, or decided not to include, some of your intake or activity? Were there any examples of eating that were more atypical for you? [*Note: It can also be helpful to query about portion sizes and timing of meals when reviewing food records. Clinicians should be encouraged to continue to maintain a nonjudgmental stance when reviewing food records because patients with obesity may present with significant shame or embarrassment about particular food choices perceived to be "bad" or "unhealthy."*]

SARAH: There was one night this past Wednesday when I felt like I was overeating at dinner and didn't record everything I ate.

CLINICIAN: Let's take a look at that night on your record together. I'm hearing that on Wednesday night you had a thought of "I am overeating." Do you think this thought may have contributed to not wanting to record everything you ate? What types of emotions did you identify? [*Note: Clinician separates thoughts, feelings, and behaviors.*]

SARAH: Definitely. I hate recording what I eat when I think I've eaten too much. I also wrote down that I was feeling really disappointed in myself.

CLINICIAN: Okay . . . It sounds like the thoughts of overeating contributed to some disappointment in yourself, as well as deciding not to write down everything you ate at that meal. Were there other thoughts or emotions in addition to thinking "I am overeating" and feeling disappointed? How did you know you were overeating? [*Note: Clinician is evaluating the potential for additional negative automatic thoughts, as well as objective evidence for "overeating."*]

SARAH: Well, I remember feeling so sick to my stomach afterwards, which makes me think I was eating too much. I remember I also had another two servings of potatoes after recording my meal on the app, and I just couldn't bring myself to enter those two servings into the program. I also remember feeling ashamed of what I had eaten. And I definitely didn't exercise the next day.

CLINICIAN: It sounds like we've identified a bit of a pattern here. You described overeating during the meal and feeling sick to your stomach afterwards, which contributed to the feeling of disappointment and shame, thoughts of "failing" your goal, as well as deciding not to exercise the next day. Does that pattern resonate with you?

SARAH: Definitely. It just keeps on happening.

CLINICIAN: Taking a look at this self-monitoring record. What do you think might have made you vulnerable to overeating on Wednesday night? What might be leading to getting stuck in this cycle?

SARAH: I'm not sure.

CLINICIAN: What was going on earlier in the day?

SARAH: I was so busy at work, and I didn't have time to pack a lunch that day, so I ended up going most of the workday without eating a full meal. I was so hungry by the time I got home.

CLINICIAN: That sounds like another important observation. We know that more chaotic eating patterns throughout the day can increase our vulnerability to overeating. Do you understand how your low intake throughout the day may have increased your vulnerability to overeating that evening?

SARAH: I do. But I still just think I should be better able to resist the temptation to overeat.

CLINICIAN: That makes sense – if you learned more skills, you might be better able to prevent yourself from overeating. That being said, if you're spending many consecutive hours per day when at work without eating, you are biologically vulnerable to overeating when you return home from work. [*Note: Distinguishing between biological and psychological vulnerability to overeating is paramount at this point in treatment; although patients may want to focus on learning skills to "resist temptation" or "avoid sweets," the most important protective factor for reducing overeating or emotional overeating is regular eating throughout the day. Once patients are eating regularly and have reduced their biological vulnerability, they can begin to learn cognitive skills to help them reduce their psychological vulnerability as well.*] We want to first start by reducing your biological vulnerability to overeating by encouraging you to eat regular meals and snacks throughout the day every three to four hours (i.e., three meals and two to three snacks per day) in order to best regulate your blood sugar and satiety. We want to focus on including a variety of food groups at each meal [*Note: Patients are encouraged to consult national food guides to better assess serving sizes. They would also be encouraged to meet with a registered dietitian if they desire a more specific dietary plan.*] Do you think that this is something you can try?

SARAH: I could do that. I'd just have to do some more problem solving to ensure that I pack my lunch for work.

CLINICIAN: That's a great plan. Once we've reduced your biological vulnerability to overeating by encouraging regular eating patterns and reducing feelings of hunger throughout the day, we can work on introducing some of the cognitive skills as well.

Stimulus Control and Dietary Restraint

Stimulus control can be particularly important in the beginning phases of treatment. Rooted in both classical and operant conditioning, implementation of stimulus control strategies in the context of obesity typically involves weakening the associations between environmental stimuli (i.e., watching television) and unhealthy eating behaviors (i.e., emotional overeating). Similarly, by limiting purchases of "treat food" within their homes or work settings, individuals may reduce the likelihood of consuming these foods, as well as potentially working toward weakening the association between food and pleasurable outcomes such as reward or relaxation. Stimulus control can also be used to increase the likelihood of individuals engaging in more adaptive behaviors [12]. For example, to increase adherence to activity goals, patients could choose to change into their gym clothes prior to leaving work that day in order to strengthen the association between changing into workout clothing and exercising. Participants are also often encouraged to start engaging in pleasurable activities that are enjoyable but incompatible with unhealthy eating behaviors in order to enhance their behavioral repertoire and increase pleasure derived from sources other than food [12].

However, clinicians should be cautioned about recommending stimulus control for eating behaviors as a stand-alone intervention because it can also reinforce messaging to patients around *dietary restraint*, defined as setting conscious limits around intake or holding dietary rules about food [16]. Dietary restraint has long been proposed to be a predictor of unhealthy eating behaviors, but it is important to note that the restraint proposition has been contested by some researchers [17,18], with some longitudinal data suggesting that restraint can be protective with respect to long-term weight maintenance [19]. Although these perspectives may appear to be conflicting, it is important to understand that treatments aimed at encouraging patients to eat (rather than entirely avoid) "treat foods" (e.g., sweets or exceptional meals) do so within moderation, as well as with the goal to reduce any fear associated with the potential of overeating certain treat foods. This messaging helps to inform patients that all foods fit within a healthy lifestyle and may also be protective for reducing emotional overeating or binge eating. Accordingly, clinicians should also refrain from using terms that promote dietary restraint. For example, such words as *healthy* versus *unhealthy, good* versus *bad, junk foods*, and *clean eating* undermine the premise that *all* food can fit within a healthy lifestyle. Instead, clinicians should focus on encouraging more *balanced* eating patterns, which include eating a variety of food groups regularly throughout a day. Accordingly, thoughts such as "I ate so badly today" or "I need to get back on track tomorrow and only eat healthy foods" should be countered with statements like "*All* foods can fit within a healthy eating plan when consumed in moderation." Similarly, if patients do choose to participate in an adjunctive weight loss program, focusing on a specific *goal weight* is discouraged given that it may influence patients to solely measure their successes according to weight loss rather than implementation of healthy behavior change (e.g., increasing exercise, increasing fruit and vegetable consumption). For example, consider the following dialogue in which the clinician encourages Sarah to start incorporating treat food in a planned manner.

CLINICIAN: Sarah, you've mentioned a number of times feeling distressed about eating some of the leftover treat food in the staff lunchroom.

SARAH: Absolutely. It happens way too often.

CLINICIAN: Given that we've already started working on reducing your biological vulnerability to overeating or feeling out of control around food [*by incorporating regular eating*], the next step is to see how you might incorporate these foods into your lifestyle in a planned way.

SARAH: You mean, actually *planning* to eat a treat food?

CLINICIAN: Exactly. Why do you think that might be important?

SARAH: Well, I guess my attempts to "resist temptation" aren't actually working. I end up eating the cookies anyway and feeling disappointed with myself.

CLINICIAN: What would it look like if you were to incorporate eating a cookie without feeling disappointed or out of control? Is there a particular setting that you would feel the least vulnerable to overeating or feeling disappointed with yourself?

SARAH: I guess I could take one cookie from the lunchroom and eat it back at my desk or during my walk on my lunch break. I don't think I could eat the cookie in the lunchroom just yet without feeling out of control.

CLINICIAN: Those sound like great ideas. What about also ensuring that you try eating this cookie on a day when you've eaten regularly that morning?

SARAH: Sure. I'd probably be less hungry then.

CLINICIAN: This sounds like a good experiment with respect to testing whether you can have a different experience with treat food, one in which you're feeling more in control of your choices.

By encouraging patients to incorporate treat foods in a planned way, these experiences help to break the associations between these foods and feeling out of control or disgusted or disappointed with oneself. Eventually, it would be advantageous for patients to not solely rely on stimulus control as a strategy such that they are able to consume treat foods in their homes or other desired settings in moderation.

Psychoeducation about Weight Regulation

It is important to provide patients with psychoeducation about how bodies regulate weight and shape. Patients are often unaware that weight is under strong biological control and may instead strongly endorse the belief that they need to control their weight and shape. Psychoeducation about weight control is often perceived as being countercultural, such that messaging encouraging individuals to focus on living a healthy lifestyle and accepting their natural weight (i.e., an individual's body weight when following national food guides and engaging in regular eating patterns and recommended levels of activity) goes against diet culture, as well as much of the messaging provided by healthcare professionals. Similarly, Laliberte and colleagues found that beliefs of needing to control one's weight were associated with more disordered eating patterns, greater body dissatisfaction, and lower self-esteem within a nonclinical sample of female participants [20]. Conversely, believing that individuals should focus on controlling their lifestyle and accepting their natural weight was not associated with maladaptive eating behaviors, lower self-esteem, or body dissatisfaction, suggesting that focusing on lifestyle management can be beneficial for improving eating behaviors and emotional well-being [20].

CLINICIAN: Sarah, I'd like to start off today's session with a discussion about how our bodies regulate weight and shape. What types of factors do you think influence our body weight?

SARAH: Hmm ... definitely our environment. Processed foods are so accessible, whereas foods such as fruits and vegetables can be more expensive and more time-consuming to prepare.

CLINICIAN: Absolutely. Our environment certainly plays a role in determining our weight and shape. What about additional factors aside from the environment?

SARAH: Maybe our genes? I'm not entirely sure.

CLINICIAN: That's a great guess! In fact, our body weight is actually under very strong biological control. When reviewing how our body regulates weight and shape, we often cite research studies comparing identical twins raised together in the same home with identical twins raised apart. Given that identical twins share the same genetic makeup, this paradigm provides us with a method by which we can separate out some of the effects of genes from environment. [*Note: See Silventoinen and colleagues* [21] *for a systematic review of twin and adoption studies on childhood and adolescent obesity and Min et al.* [22] *for a systematic review of heritability of BMI within twin studies.*]

SARAH: That makes sense.

CLINICIAN: Taken together these research studies demonstrate that our weight is strongly influenced by our biological makeup, with some studies demonstrating that up to 90 percent of the variability in weight can be attributed to our genes. Our genetics also interacts with our lifestyle choices, as well as some of the factors you mentioned earlier, such as increased access to processed foods. Are there other members in your family who are overweight or obese?

SARAH: Ya, both my parents and my younger sister are obese. I just always figured it's because we don't exercise enough or eat too many processed foods.

CLINICIAN: That's a really common belief. Certainly our environment and lifestyle choices do affect our weight and shape, and that's why we've been focusing on goal setting and recording your dietary intake and physical activity. However, it's important to remember that genetics plays a strong role. The second important piece of information I'd like you to consider is that there are data to suggest that our body has multiple systems that regulate our weight and shape. In other words, our muscle metabolism, body fat, brain, and stomach work together to defend our weight, even if our weight is not in a "healthy" BMI range according to the BMI charts. This defense system is often activated after individuals lose about 5 to 15 percent of their body weight. [*Note: Laliberte et al.* [23] *recommend using a thermostat as an analogy to illustrate how a body regulates its weight within the context of a healthy lifestyle such that just as a thermostat regulates the temperature within a home, so too does the body adjust to occasional overeating or undereating within a small weight range.*]

SARAH: *But,* I'm obese! How could my body be defending a weight that is not considered to be healthy?

CLINICIAN: That's a great question. Although our body can adjust to occasional overeating, sustained patterns of overeating do lead to weight gain over time. Once the body has been at that weight for an extended period of time, it will work to defend it.

SARAH: This is so discouraging.

CLINICIAN: I hear that this information is disappointing. I do want to reinforce that living a healthy lifestyle can prevent you from continuing the upward trajectory of weight gain you've been describing over the past year, as well as work toward greater acceptance of your natural weight range. That being said, if you are interested in weight loss, we can also discuss some of the pros and cons of behavioral and surgical weight loss options.

At this stage in treatment, patients may also be considering behavioral, medical, or surgical weight loss interventions. If patients do choose to engage in a behavioral weight loss program, they should be informed that modest weight loss of 5 to 10 percent can provide health benefits for individuals with obesity [24], but maintaining this weight loss long term does require significant long-term lifestyle changes. Data from the National Weight Control Registry demonstrate that behaviors including limiting intake (e.g., caloric intake of fewer than 1,400 calories per day), significant weekly energy expenditure, as well as weighing oneself at least once per week are associated with better weight maintenance over a 10-year period [19], which are not often behaviors that patients expect within a weight "mainte-nance" (i.e., rather than a weight "loss") program. Similarly, for patients with BMIs in higher classes of obesity (i.e., BMI $\geq$ 40 kg/m^2), the amount of weight loss potentially achievable within a behavioral weight loss program may be significantly lower than patients' weight loss expectations. Accordingly, it is important to remind patients that the primary focus of treatment is changing health behaviors (i.e., regular eating, physical activity) as opposed to weight loss per se and that these behaviors alone can improve their overall health. Patients who identify weight loss as their only (or even their primary) goal may feel hopeless if weight loss is not substantial enough and may subsequently return to previous maladaptive health behaviors.

Behavioral weight loss programs would not be appropriate for patients who have a history of more restrictive eating or exercise patterns, as well as for those who are solely looking to improve their body image [23]. Patients expressing interest in surgical weight loss interventions should be informed that bariatric surgery can provide a more sustainable option for long-term weight maintenance and be provided with information regarding typical long-term weight loss outcomes following various bariatric surgery procedures.

Cognitive-Therapy Strategies

Once patients have begun to reduce their biological vulnerability to unhealthy eating behaviors such as emotional overeating, they may benefit from an introduction to cognitive skills. These skills are aimed at helping individuals develop more adaptive thinking patterns, with the goal of reducing their psychological vulnerability to unhealthy lifestyle behaviors. Basic cognitive skills include helping patients to identify cognitive distortions in their thinking, as well as guiding them to use challenging questions to counter their negative automatic thoughts [1]. Some examples of cognitive distortions common among individuals with obesity include "all-or-nothing" or "black-or-white" thinking ("I've *totally* blown my diet, so I might as well really overdo it"), overgeneralization ("I *always* gain weight"; "I'm *never* able to stick to my exercise goals"), discounting the positive ("I'm more physically active now, but I still haven't lost much weight"; "I walk to work, but do not do any real exercise"), fortune-telling errors ("I will not be able to keep the weight off"), labeling ("I'm lazy"; "I'm undisciplined"), *should* statements ("I *should* have reached my goal weight by now"; "I *should* not eat any junk food"), and mind reading ("Everyone is judging me") (see Chapter 2). The following dialogue provides a short explanation of how to introduce cognitive distortions to a patient, followed by an example of how to restructure a patient's negative automatic thoughts.

CLINICIAN: Sarah, let's take a look at this list of cognitive distortions [*showing a sheet with a list of cognitive distortions and some examples*]. Cognitive distortions can be best understood as "thinking traps" that we all fall into, especially when we're feeling more down or anxious. One of the goals of CBT is to help you identify when you might be falling into one of these thinking traps and how to use countering questions to jump out of these traps. Do any of the thinking traps on this list resonate with you?

SARAH: Hmm . . . I'm definitely a very all-or-nothing person. For example, this past week, I was going to pack my lunch for work on Monday, Wednesday, and Friday. I forgot to pack my lunch on Monday, which meant I had already failed my goal.

CLINICIAN: It sounds like this is another example of oscillating between "being on track" and "falling off the wagon" like you described a few sessions ago. Do you have a sense of how these thoughts affect your emotions and behaviors?

SARAH: Definitely. I didn't pack my lunch for the rest of the week and just felt more and more disappointed with myself. If I failed on the first day, why bother continuing for the rest of the week? I also notice labeling myself as a "failure" or "incompetent" when I don't meet my goals.

CLINICIAN: That sounds really challenging. It would be so hard to keep working toward your goals when you're using such harsh language to describe yourself.

SARAH: It is, and then I just think of myself as more and more of a failure as the week goes by, and I continue to not pack my lunch.

CLINICIAN: That makes sense. We often end up unintentionally confirming our negative beliefs about ourselves by continuing to engage in unhelpful behaviors. Before we work on learning to challenge some of these thoughts, let's add them to this worksheet. We call this worksheet a *thought record* (Figure 8.3).

CLINICIAN: Taking a look at this worksheet, we've identified the following thoughts: "I didn't pack my lunch on Monday, so I failed my goal"; "I didn't pack my lunch on Monday, so why bother continuing for the rest of the week?"; "I am a failure"; and "I am incompetent," as well as cognitive distortions of "all-or-nothing thinking" and "labeling." [*Note: Clinicians may need to probe for additional automatic thoughts. Some sample questions include: "What does that thought mean or say about you?"; "What is the worst thing that could happen?"; "What types of thoughts were going through your mind prior to feeling sad or discouraged?"*] When did these thoughts first come up, and what types of emotions did you notice?

SARAH: I started feeling really sad and disappointed with myself after sitting at my desk on Monday morning thinking about how I didn't pack lunch for work.

CLINICIAN: Okay, so it sounds like the situation was "sitting at my desk on Monday, thinking about how I didn't pack my lunch," and some of the emotions were sadness and disappointment. Could you rate how strongly you experienced these emotions in that moment, on a scale from 0 to 100 (with 100 referring to really strong feelings of sadness or disappointment)?

SARAH: Probably about a 70 for sadness and an 80 for disappointment. [*Note: Patients are encouraged to identify and rate multiple emotions if present in an individual situation.*]

CLINICIAN: Okay, now that we have a sense of what was going on at the time and some of the traps you were falling into with your thinking, we want to do our best to start challenging your thoughts. Is there a particular thought that you think was really driving the emotion in that moment? [*Note: This is commonly referred to as the "hot thought"* [25].]

SARAH: Yes, "I didn't pack my lunch on Monday, so I failed my goal."

CLINICIAN: Okay, let's call this your "hot thought," or the thought that was really contributing to the sadness and disappointment in the moment. Let's start by evaluating the evidence for and against your hot thought, which refers to the specific facts you have to support your conclusion, as well as some of the facts that might indicate that your automatic thoughts are not 100 percent accurate.

SARAH: Okay. Well, I guess "not packing my lunch on Monday" is one piece of evidence supporting my negative automatic thought. Also, I didn't pack my lunch on Wednesday or Friday either.

CLINICIAN: Remember, we're focusing on the experience you had on Monday. Did you have information at the time about what happened on Wednesday or Friday?

SARAH: Oh, right. Okay, then I guess just "not packing my lunch on Monday."

CLINICIAN: Let's add that to the list. What about any evidence against this negative automatic thought?

SARAH: Hmm . . . well, I guess it's not as black and white as I thought. I'm basing that conclusion on only one day this past week.

CLINICIAN: That's right. Let's add that point to the "Evidence Against" column. I wonder, Sarah, is there potentially a gray area between "meeting a goal" and "failing"?

SARAH: Yes. I didn't really give myself a chance to meet the goal on the other days. I could have potentially met the goal on the other two days. Or at least one.

CLINICIAN: That's right – there are in fact other options other than just "failing" or "meeting a goal." What do you think you would say to a friend in this situation?

SARAH: I would be so much more encouraging to a friend than I am to myself . . . just the other day, my friend was telling me that she was struggling to exercise regularly, and I encouraged her to be proud of herself for the days she did exercise this past week as opposed to beating herself up for the days she didn't.

CLINICIAN: I'm hearing that when a friend is in this situation, you find it a lot easier to be compassionate. That's a really common experience – we're unfortunately often much less compassionate with our selves than we are with our friends. To sum up the "Evidence Against," I'm hearing that "my conclusion was based on only one day"; "there is a gray area between 'failing' and 'meeting a goal'"; and "if I were speaking to a friend, I would encourage them to focus on the days in which they did meet the goal." Is that a fair summary?

SARAH: Yes. I never really thought about it like that.

CLINICIAN: Taking an assessment of both the evidence for and against this automatic thought, can you come up with a more balanced thought that would more appropriately reflect all the pieces of evidence? Often a balanced thought takes the form of "Even though ..." in order to incorporate both the evidence for and against.

SARAH: Hmm ... what about "Even though I didn't meet my goal on Monday, that doesn't mean I completely failed. Monday was just one setback."

CLINICIAN: I agree! Looking at this balanced thought, can you rerate your current levels of sadness and disappointment?

SARAH: My sadness would probably be at about a 30 and disappointment at a 50. I'm still feeling upset that I did not meet my goal on Monday but not quite as sad and disappointed with myself.

It is important to note that when engaging in cognitive restructuring with individuals with severe obesity, patients often do have some evidence to support their negative automatic thoughts. For example, consider a situation in which our patient Sarah suggests, "Everyone was staring at me at the gym because I am fat." Given the widespread prevalence of weight-based stigma and discrimination [26] (see Chapter 3), it is likely that at least some individuals in the gym were in fact judging Sarah's weight and shape. If a clinician were to ignore this evidence and solely focus on challenging the accuracy of this statement, he or she could risk invalidating Sarah's experience as a woman with obesity living within a diet-obsessed culture. Instead, a clinician could still help Sarah identify the cognitive distortions of *mindreading* (i.e., how did Sarah know they were staring at her? Is it at all possible that some people were staring off to the distance, or distracted, rather than judging her for her weight?) and *overgeneralization* (i.e., How does Sarah know *everyone* was staring at her? Did she notice *every* face in the room, or is she basing this conclusion off of one or two negative or ambiguous glances?), while also validating how deeply upsetting it is that many individuals continue to hold the belief that weight-based stigma and discrimination is socially acceptable.

In addition to identifying cognitive distortions and using cognitive restructuring skills, patients may also benefit from a greater understanding of their core beliefs and assumptions, which can be understood as the driving forces behind individuals' negative automatic thoughts. Automatic thoughts are the most superficial level of cognitions (i.e., "everyone was staring at me at the gym because I'm fat"), followed by intermediate assumptions or rules (i.e., "I need to lose weight in order to be worthy"), and lastly, by core beliefs (e.g., "I am worthless") [1]. These core beliefs and assumptions are influenced by a number of factors, including societal messages, personal expectations, and experiences throughout one's developmental history.

CBT Thought Record

Situation	Emotions (Rate 0–100%)	Negative Automatic Thoughts	Type of Cognitive Distortion	Evidence Supporting the Negative Automatic Thought	Evidence Not Supporting the Negative Automatic Thought	Balanced Thought	Re-rate Emotions (0–100%)
Sitting at my desk on Monday, thinking about how I did not pack my lunch.	Sadness (70%) Disappointment (80%)	*I didn't pack my lunch on Monday, so I failed my goal.* I didn't pack my lunch on Monday, so why bother continuing for the rest of the week? I am a failure. I am incompetent.	All-or-nothing thinking Labeling	Not packing my lunch on Monday.	My conclusion was only based on one day. There is a grey area between failing and meeting a goal. If I were speaking to a friend, I would encourage them to focus on the days in which they did meet the goal.	Even though I didn't meet my goal on Monday, that doesn't mean I completely failed. Monday was just one setback.	Sadness (30%) Disappointment (50%)

Figure 8.3 Sample CBT thought record.
Note: Sarah's "hot thought" is in italicized font.

In working with Sarah, a clinician would want to further explore what it means to Sarah that others judge her for her weight and shape. For example, Sarah could be strongly attached to the rule that "I am only worthy if I am on a diet and trying to lose weight," in which case being stared at while exercising at the gym could activate more entrenched core beliefs and assumptions about self-worth. In this context, a clinician may want to engage in more extensive core belief work in order to help Sarah start experimenting with building up her self-worth beyond weight, shape, and dieting. Potential behavioral experiments could include engaging in, rather than avoiding, activities an individual is waiting to participate in "until they lose weight" or perhaps engaging in regular eating for a week to challenge the rule that "one should always be dieting." Behavioral experiments can also be especially helpful for improving body image and reducing body dissatisfaction among individuals who are overweight or obese. For a more detailed explanation of implementing core belief work, see Beck [1] or Laliberte [23].

Relapse Prevention

Once patients have grasped the core CBT skills and have demonstrated behavior change, clinicians are encouraged to work collaboratively with patients to develop a personalized relapse prevention plan. Relapse prevention plans typically include a review of patients' goals at the outset of treatment and their assessment of their progress to date, discussion about any additional goals moving forward, and identification of a few key skills they found to be particularly helpful within treatment [1,15,27]. Patients are also encouraged to consider behaviors that may signify a setback (i.e., for Sarah, this could include not packing her lunch or walking during her lunch hour for a few days), as well as a specific plan if setbacks do arise. This plan could include rereading some of the materials and skills learned during treatment, reconnecting with a therapist, or perhaps seeking additional support from friends and family. Clinicians may also want to consider tapering sessions (i.e., seeing patients on a biweekly or monthly basis) toward the end of treatment in order to enhance the patient's confidence in implementing the skills independently before discontinuing treatment [1].

Modifications for Patients Undergoing Bariatric Surgery

The CBT skills described in this chapter can also be applied to working with patients either before or after bariatric surgery. Among both pre- and postoperative patients, behavioral skills such as goal setting and self-monitoring intake and physical activity can be used to help them prepare for the lifestyle changes required postoperatively. Self-monitoring has also been found to reduce the likelihood of weight regain postoperatively [28]. With respect to cognitive restructuring skills, clinicians should be aware of some concerns that are prevalent in the context of bariatric surgery, in particular, worry about weight regain and concerns about excess skin [27]. Patients should be informed that bariatric surgery is considered to be a sustainable form of weight loss, but at least some weight regain can occur following the "honeymoon period," typically referring to the first 6 to 12 months after surgery. Some behaviors associated with greater weight regain include higher levels of "picking" and "nibbling" at food [29], increased mental health concerns such as depression [30], and sedentary behavior [31]. Furthermore, patients may also experience a significant delay between their physical weight loss after surgery and the reconfiguring of their cognitive perception of their bodies, referred to as the *mind-body lag* [32]. Bringing awareness of this concept to patients can help to validate their experiences.

Empirical Evidence for the Effectiveness of CBT for Behavioral and Lifestyle Changes in Severe Obesity

Current clinical guidelines recommend multicomponent lifestyle interventions as the treatment of choice in the management of adult obesity [10,33]. The lifestyle modification programs for obesity that have been examined in the empirical literature have been quite heterogeneous, making it difficult to directly compare results across studies. However, they typically include cognitive and behavioral strategies to increase physical activity, improve eating behavior and food quality, and decrease energy intake and sedentary behavior [11]. The interventions have been delivered in a variety of settings, including clinical research settings, primary care settings, residential programs, private clinics, and remotely through telecommunication [12]. Regardless of the setting, it is recommended that the interventions be delivered by multidisciplinary teams, including physicians, dietitians, behavioral health specialists (e.g., psychologists, behavioral therapists), and exercise physiologists [12,33]. According to a review of lifestyle modification programs for obesity, the programs typically consist of an intensive weight loss phase (approximately 16 to 24 weekly sessions) lasting approximately six months, followed by a weight maintenance phase that varies substantially across studies with respect to the intensity and duration [12].

A randomized, controlled trial (RCT) comparing CBT, behavioral therapy, and guided self-help found that 24 sessions of CBT and 24 sessions of behavioral therapy both resulted in a mean weight loss of 10 percent of initial body weight after the intervention; however, the majority of participants regained their weight over a three-year follow-up period [34]. These results indicate that longer-term maintenance sessions are likely required to sustain weight loss over time, consistent with the idea of obesity being managed as a chronic disease. A recent study that randomized patients with obesity who lost weight during a 16-week group-based weight loss program to either a telephone-based weight maintenance intervention focused on relapse prevention and self-monitoring or to a control group found that the intervention significantly reduced the rate of weight regain [35].

The Look AHEAD study is a large RCT that assigned 5,145 participants with excess weight (mean BMI = 36 kg/m^2) and type 2 diabetes to either an intensive lifestyle intervention or a diabetes support and education group [36]. The lifestyle intervention focused on decreasing caloric intake and increasing physical fitness using a variety of cognitive and behavioral techniques, including self-monitoring, stimulus control, cognitive restructuring, and relapse prevention. On average, participants receiving the intensive lifestyle intervention lost 8.3 percent of their initial body weight at 12 months compared with 0.7 percent in the support and education group. Regarding clinically significant weight loss, 38 percent of participants receiving the intensive lifestyle intervention lost more than 10 percent of their body weight, and 30 percent of participants lost 5 to 10 percent of their body weight [36,37]. At 10 years, participants receiving the intensive lifestyle intervention maintained an average weight loss of 6 percent of their initial body weight [38].

To examine whether intensive lifestyle interventions are effective in individuals with severe obesity, the Look AHEAD Research Group compared 12-month outcomes across different BMI groups: overweight (BMI = 25–29.9 kg/m^2), class I obesity (BMI = 30–34.9 kg/m^2), class II obesity (BMI = 35–39.9 kg/m^2), and class III obesity (BMI > 40 kg/m^2) [39].

Individuals with class III (severe) obesity lost a greater percentage of their initial body weight than individuals who were overweight (9.1 versus 7.4 percent), with a comparable percentage for individuals with class I obesity (8.7 percent reduction) and class II obesity (8.6 percent reduction). Moreover, all BMI groups demonstrated comparable improvements in physical activity, fitness, blood pressure, and cholesterol, triglycerides, and fasting glucose levels. The researchers concluded that intensive lifestyle interventions are an effective option for individuals with severe obesity.

A study examining CBT in individuals with excess weight (mean BMI = 36 kg/m^2) and nonalcoholic fatty liver disease found that a 13-session group intervention focused on weight loss and increased physical activity was effective in reducing weight across a two-year follow-up period [40]. On average, those in the CBT group reduced their initial body weight by 5.6 percent, whereas those in the control group (who received only recommendations for diet and physical activity) reduced their weight by 1.4 percent. The study operationalized clinically significant weight loss as a 7 percent reduction in initial body weight, and the CBT group was 2.5 times more likely to achieve this outcome at two-year follow-up than the control group. Moreover, CBT was associated with improvements in liver enzymes, insulin sensitivity, and metabolic syndrome scores. Based on the encouraging findings, the authors recommended that CBT should be routinely offered to individuals with nonalcoholic fatty liver disease.

The National Weight Control Registry is a large longitudinal study of adults who have successfully lost at least 30 pounds and maintained the weight loss for at least one year. Individuals in the registry have lost 66 pounds on average and have maintained the weight loss for more than five years [41]. They report using a number of strategies to maintain their weight, including regular physical activity (1 hour/day), consuming a diet low in calories and fat, maintaining a consistent eating schedule, and self-monitoring their weight [41]. A follow-up study of 2,668 participants reported that 87 percent of participants were maintaining a 10 percent weight loss at 5- and 10-year follow-up. Increases in dietary disinhibition and fat consumption and decreases in physical activity and frequency of self-weighing were associated with weight regain [19]. Members of the National Weight Control Registry research team have concluded that although long-term weight control is difficult, it is possible and requires sustained behavioral changes, most notably ongoing adherence to diet and physical activity recommendations [19,41]. Although the National Weight Control Registry is not an intervention study, the findings regarding the maintenance of weight loss have implications for CBT given that ongoing adherence to diet and physical activity recommendations is a focus of treatment. Given the variability in weight loss outcomes both within and across studies examining CBT interventions for obesity, additional research is warranted to compare individuals who successfully maintain 10 percent weight loss and those who regain their weight and to examine predictors of successful weight maintenance following CBT.

Difficulties achieving and sustaining changes to dietary intake and physical activity also account for some of the variability in weight loss outcomes following bariatric surgery, and a number of review articles suggest that CBT interventions targeting diet and physical activity are beneficial for bariatric surgery patients [42–45]. A systematic scoping review examining the impact of preoperative behavioral lifestyle interventions reported that the interventions facilitated weight loss in five of the eight studies reviewed [43]. The duration of the interventions included in the review ranged from one to 15 months. They were delivered in a variety of formats, including face-to-face individual sessions, group sessions, telephone coaching, and some combination thereof. Although the results appear promising, it is worth noting that the studies reporting the greatest benefit assessed weight loss outcomes immediately following the preoperative behavioral intervention. Preoperative weight loss alone can be a positive outcome for individuals who are required to lose some weight prior to undergoing surgery, but the data regarding the impact of preoperative behavioral interventions on postoperative weight loss are mixed [42,43]. The few studies included in the systematic review that assessed weight loss outcomes following surgery either lacked a control group or did not find evidence for a significant benefit of preoperative behavioral interventions in comparison with a control group [43]. Similarly, another review examining psychosocial interventions for bariatric surgery patients concluded that preoperative lifestyle interventions have a positive short-term impact on diet, physical activity, and weight, but the available evidence challenges the long-term utility of preoperative interventions. Specifically, the studies included in the review found that interventions that improved weight loss immediately after the intervention did not confer additional benefits over bariatric surgery alone when reassessed up to two years postoperatively [42].

A systematic review of eight studies examining the impact of postoperative behavioral lifestyle interventions concluded that individuals receiving these interventions lose more weight on average than those receiving standard care or no treatment [44]. A meta-analysis of the five RCTs included in the review demonstrated that postoperative behavioral lifestyle interventions resulted in 2 percent greater excess weight loss in comparison with usual care. Although the average additional weight loss was modest, significant heterogeneity existed regarding the intensity and duration of the interventions across studies, and greater benefit was reported in studies examining intensive lifestyle interventions delivered over a longer period [44].

One RCT included in the meta-analysis by Rudolph and Hilbert examined the efficacy of an intensive lifestyle intervention rooted heavily in CBT delivered over a three-year period in comparison with the usual postoperative care [46]. Those in the lifestyle intervention received 40-minute sessions at each of their routine postoperative clinic visits, for a total of 30 sessions. The lifestyle intervention focused on adopting healthier eating habits and a more active lifestyle using strategies such as goal setting, self-monitoring, reinforcement, stimulus control, and relapse prevention. The lifestyle intervention resulted in greater weight loss and maintenance over the three-year postoperative period. Specifically, those receiving the lifestyle intervention experienced 75 percent excess weight loss at three years after surgery compared with 50 percent in the usual care control group. They also increased their consumption of fruit and vegetables, decreased their consumption of sweets, increased their physical activity level, and decreased their TV watching to a greater extent than the control group. The results suggest that an intensive lifestyle intervention delivered over an extended period can improve weight loss and maintenance postoperatively.

A more recent systematic review identified 11 RCTs that examined the effectiveness of pre- and/or postoperative behavioral lifestyle interventions with an explicit focus on changing diet and/or physical activity [45]. A meta-analysis was conducted using eight of the studies, and behavioral interventions were found to improve weight loss. Specifically, percentage excess weight loss was greater in the intervention groups than in control groups at one year after surgery (mean difference = 10.8 percent) and two years after surgery (mean difference = 14.0 percent). However, similar to the aforementioned review [44], findings were limited by small sample sizes, methodological heterogeneity, and methodological quality. Although behavioral lifestyle interventions appear promising, additional RCTs are required with adequate sample sizes, standardized treatment protocols, follow-up periods extending beyond two years, and comprehensive assessment of outcomes including weight loss and improvements in diet, physical activity, fitness, medical comorbidities, and psychosocial functioning.

Clinicians and researchers who work with bariatric surgery patients have contemplated the ideal timing of behavioral interventions, specifically whether they should be offered preoperatively to help patients prepare for bariatric surgery or postoperatively to help them adjust to surgery and maintain long-term changes. Although no RCTs have directly compared the efficacy of a preoperative versus postoperative behavioral intervention, it has been recommended that behavioral lifestyle interventions be delivered early in the postoperative period before significant weight regain has occurred [42,44]. Another review acknowledged that the evidence base is currently stronger for postoperative interventions than preoperative interventions but stated that "robust" conclusions could not be drawn to recommend postoperative over preoperative interventions due to the limited research conducted to date and a number of methodological issues [45]. Finally, another suggested that in the absence of sufficient objective evidence regarding the optimal timing of intervention, both preoperative and postoperative interventions should be promoted to help support bariatric surgery patients [33]. However, given that few bariatric surgery programs have the resources to provide psychosocial interventions both preoperatively and postoperatively, those resources would likely be best used by offering preoperative lifestyle interventions specifically to bariatric candidates who are required to lose some weight and improve their mobility prior to surgery and offering postoperative interventions routinely to all bariatric patients to improve long-term outcomes.

Summary

Severe obesity has a significant impact on psychological health and well-being, thereby underscoring the importance of the development and implementation of psychological treatments for this population. This chapter provided an overview of cognitive-behavioral therapy (CBT), a skills-based psychological intervention that has been found to be both efficacious and effective among individuals with severe obesity. Using a clinical vignette format, this chapter presented a number of core CBT skills, including goal setting, cognitive restructuring, and relapse prevention, as well as modifications for individuals both before and after bariatric surgery. Within the implementation of each of these CBT skills, this chapter emphasized the importance of improving health behaviors (i.e., increasing physical activity, eating regularly throughout the day) rather than a sole focus on weight loss. However, the majority of research studies conducted to date do focus primarily on weight loss outcomes following CBT (i.e., typically resulting in approximately 5 to 10 percent weight loss). Accordingly, more research is needed to evaluate the impact of CBT on health behaviors in the context of severe obesity, as well as whether improvement in health behaviors is maintained over time.

Key Points

- Cognitive-behavioral therapy is a present-focused, skills-based psychological treatment that has been found to be efficacious among individuals with severe obesity and has also been modified for individuals both before and after bariatric surgery.

- Cognitive-behavioral therapy focuses on the interaction between an individual's thoughts, feelings, and behaviors and is often delivered as part of a multicomponent lifestyle intervention for obesity.
- Key components of CBT for severe obesity include presenting the CBT model, goal setting, self-monitoring intake and activity, stimulus control, providing psychoeducation about the regulation of body weight, cognitive restructuring, and relapse prevention.
- Clinicians working with patients with obesity should be mindful of the language they use in session when describing food choices in order to emphasize the message that *all* food can fit within a healthy lifestyle (e.g., avoiding such words as *healthy* versus *unhealthy* and *junk foods*).
- Following CBT treatment for obesity, weight loss outcomes are typically in the 5 to 10 percent range.

References

1. J. S. Beck. *Cognitive Behavior Therapy: Basics and Beyond* (2nd edn). New York, NY: Guilford Press, 2011.

2. C. A. Padesky. Socratic questioning: Changing minds or guiding discovery? Presented at the European Congress of Behavior and Cognitive Therapies, September 24, 1993. Available at https://padesky.com/newpad/wp-content/uploads/2012/11/socquest.pdf (accessed May 1, 2017).

3. J. Collins, C. Meng, and A. Eng. Psychological impact of severe obesity. *Curr Obes Rep* 2016; 5: 435–40.

4. G. Gariepy, D. Nitka, and N. Schmitz. The association between obesity and anxiety disorders in the population: A systematic review. *Int J Obes (Lond)* 2010; 34: 407–19.

5. F. S. Luppino, L. M. de Wit, P. F. Bouvy, et al. Overweight, obesity, and depression: A systematic review and meta-analysis of longitudinal studies. *Arch Gen Psychiatry* 2010; 67: 220–9.

6. M. A. Kalarchian, G.T. Wilson, R.E. Brolin, et al. Binge eating in bariatric surgery patients. *Int J Eat Disord* 1999; 24: 89–92.

7. R. Saunders, L. Johnson, and J. Teschner. Prevalence of eating disorders among bariatric surgery patients. *Eat Disord* 1998; 6: 309–17.

8. A. A. Haedt-Matt, P. K. Keel, S. E. Racine, et al. Do emotional eating urges regulate affect? Concurrent and prospective associations and implications for risk models of binge eating. *Int J Eat Disord* 2014; 47: 874–7.

9. U. Whiteside, E. Chen, C. Neighbors, et al. Difficulties regulating emotions: Do binge eaters have fewer strategies to modulate and tolerate negative affect? *Eat Behav* 2007; 8: 162–9.

10. National Institute for Health and Care Excellence. Obesity: Identification, Assessment, and Management (Clinical Guideline 189), 2014. Available at www.nice.org.uk/guidance/cg189/resources/obesity-identification-assessment-and-management-pdf-35109821097925 (accessed May 1, 2017).

11. A. N. Fabricatore. Behavior therapy and cognitive-behavior therapy of obesity: Is there a difference? *J Am Diet Assoc* 2007; 107: 92–9.

12. R. Dalle Grave, S. Calugi, and M. E. Ghoch. Lifestyle modification in the management of obesity: Achievements and challenges. *Eat Weight Disord* 2013; 18: 339–49.

13. G. T. Doran. There's a S.M.A.R.T. way to write management's goals and objectives. *Manag Rev* 1981; 70: 35–6.

14. R. S. Rubin. Will the real SMART goals please stand up? *TIP* 2002; 39: 26–7.

15. R. F. Apple, J. Lock, and R. Peebles. *Preparing for Weight Loss Surgery: Workbook*. Oxford: Oxford University Press, 2006.

16. C. G. Fairburn. *Cognitive Behavior Therapy and Eating Disorders*. New York, NY: Guilford Press, 2008.

17. F. Johnson, M. Pratt, and J. Wardle. Dietary restraint and self-regulation in eating behavior. *Int J Obes (Lond)* 2012; **36**: 665–74.

18. K. Schaumberg, D. A. Anderson, L. M. Anderson, et al. Dietary restraint: What's the harm? A review of the relationship between dietary restraint, weight trajectory and the development of eating pathology. *Clin Obes* 2016; **6**: 89–100.

19. J. G. Thomas, D. S. Bond, S. Phelan, et al. Weight loss maintenance for 10 years in the National Weight Control Registry. *Am J Prev Med.* 2014; **46**: 17–23.

20. M. Laliberte, M. Newton, R. McCabe, et al. Controlling your weight versus controlling your lifestyle: How beliefs about weight control affect risk for disordered eating, body dissatisfaction and self-esteem. *Cogn Ther Res* 2007; **3**: 853–69.

21. K. Silventoinen, B. Rokholm, J. Kaprio, et al. The genetic and environmental influences on childhood obesity: A systematic review of twin and adoption studies. *Int J Obes (Lond)* 2010; **34**: 29–40.

22. J. Min, D. T. Chiu, and Y. Wang. Variation in the heritability of body mass index based on diverse twin studies: A systematic review. *Obes Rev* 2013; **14**: 871–82.

23. M. Laliberte, R. E. McCabe, and V. Taylor. *The Cognitive Behavioral Workbook for Weight Management: A Step-by-Step Program*. Oakland, CA: New Harbinger Publications, 2009.

24. M. D. Jensen, D. H. Ryan, C. M. Apovian, et al. 2013 AHA/ACC/TOS guideline for the management of overweight and obesity in adults: A report of the American College of Cardiology/American Heart Association Task Force on Practice Guidelines and the Obesity Society, 2013. Available at http://circ.ahajournals.org/content/circulatio naha/early/2013/11/11/01.cir.0000437739.71477.ee.full.pdf (accessed May 1, 2017).

25. D. Greenberger and C. A. Padesky. *Mind over Mood: Change How You Feel By Changing the Way You Think*. New York, NY: Guilford Press, 1995.

26. T. Andreyeva, R. M. Puhl, and K. D. Brownell. Changes in perceived weight discrimination among Americans, 1995–1996 through 2004–2006. *Obesity (Silver Spring)* 2008; **16**: 1129–34.

27. S. E. Cassin, S. Sockalingam, S. Wnuk, et al. Cognitive behavioural therapy for bariatric surgery patients: Preliminary evidence for feasibility, acceptability, and effectiveness. *Cogn Behav Pract* 2013; **4**: 529–43.

28. J. Odom, K. C. Zalesin, T. L. Washington, et al. Behavioral predictors of weight regain after bariatric surgery. *Obes Surg* 2010; **20**: 349–56.

29. E. Conceicão, J. E. Mitchell, A. R. Vaz, et al. The presence of maladaptive eating behaviors after bariatric surgery in a cross sectional study: Importance of picking or nibbling on weight regain. *Eat Behav* 2014; **15**: 558–62.

30. B. R. Yanos, K. K. Saules, L. M. Schuh, et al. Predictors of lowest weight and long-term weight regain among Roux-en-Y gastric bypass patients. *Obes Surg* 2015; **25**: 1364–70.

31. K. M. Herman, T. E. Carver, N. V. Christou, et al. Keeping the weight off: Physical activity, sitting time, and weight loss maintenance in bariatric surgery patients 2 to 16 years postsurgery. *Obes Surg* 2014; **24**: 1064–72.

32. K. Lyons, B. A. Meisner, S. Sockalingam, et al. Body image after bariatric surgery: A qualitative study. *Bariatr Surg Prac Patient Care* 2014; **9**: 41–9.

33. D. C. W. Lau, J. D. Douketis, K. M. Morrison, et al. 2006 Canadian clinical practice guidelines on the management and prevention of obesity in adults and children (summary). *CMAJ* 2007; **176**: S1–13.

34. Z. Cooper, H. A. Doll, D. M. Hawker, et al. Testing a new cognitive behavioural

treatment for obesity: A randomized controlled trial with 3 year follow-up. *Behav Res Ther* 2010; **48**: 706–13.

35. C. I. Voils, M. K. Olsen, J. M. Gierisch, et al. Maintenance of weight loss after initiation of nutrition training: A randomized controlled trial. *Ann Intern Med.* 2017; **166**: 463–71.

36. Look AHEAD Research Group. Reduction in weight and cardiovascular disease risk factors in individuals with type 2 diabetes: One year results of the Look AHEAD trial. *Diabetes Care* 2007; **30**: 1374–83.

37. J. G. Christian, A. G. Tsai, and D. H. Bessesen. Interpreting weight losses from lifestyle modification trials: Using categorical data. *Int J Obes (Lond)* 2010; **34**: 207–9.

38. Look AHEAD Research Group. Cardiovascular effects of intensive lifestyle intervention in type 2 diabetes. *N Engl J Med* 2013; **369**: 145–54.

39. J. Unick, D. Beavers, J. M. Jakicic, et al. Effectiveness of lifestyle interventions for individuals with severe obesity and type 2 diabetes: Results from the Look AHEAD trial. *Diabetes Care* 2011; **34**: 2152–7.

40. S. Moscatiello, R. Di Luzio, E. Bugianesi, et al. Cognitive behavioural treatment of non-alcoholic fatty liver disease:

A propensity score adjusted observational study. *Obesity (Silver Spring)* 2011; **19**: 763–70.

41. R. R. Wing and S. Phelan. Long-term weight loss maintenance. *Am J Clin Nutr* 2005; **82**: 222S–5S.

42. M. A. Kalarchian and M. D. Marcus. Psychosocial interventions pre and post bariatric surgery. *Eur Eat Disord Rev* 2015; **23**: 457–62.

43. R. H. Liu. Do behavioural interventions delivered before bariatric surgery impact weight loss in adults? A systematic scoping review. *Bariatr Surg Prac Patient Care.* 2016; **11**: 39–48.

44. A. Rudolph and A. Hilbert. Post-operative behavioural management in bariatric surgery: A systematic review and meta-analysis of randomized controlled trials. *Obes Rev* 2013; **14**: 292–302.

45. F. Stewart and A. Avenell. Behavioural interventions for severe obesity before and/or after bariatric surgery: A systematic review and meta-analysis. *Obes Surg* 2016; **26**: 1203–14.

46. A. Papalazarou, M. Yannakoulia, S. A. Kavouras, et al. Lifestyle intervention favorably affects weight loss and maintenance following obesity surgery. *Obesity (Silver Spring).* 2010; **18**: 1348–53.

Chapter

9 Cognitive-Behavioral Therapy for Disordered Eating in Severe Obesity

Alexis Fertig and Wynne Lundblad

Case Vignette

Allison is a 38-year-old divorced woman with a history of severe obesity (body mass index [BMI] = 43 kg/m²), hypertension, seasonal allergies, and major depressive disorder that was self-referred to the Eating Disorders Clinic for management of her "out of control" eating behaviors. On intake, she reports that she had been slightly overweight as a child and was teased by her classmates. In an attempt to help, her mother placed her on a series of diets (calorie counting, low-carb, low-fat, meal replacement), all of which resulted in short-term weight loss. However, her weight usually increased past its previous level after she stopped the diet. In college, she decided to stop dieting and tried to "eat intuitively." Although she was overweight at the time (BMI = 26–28 kg/m²), she felt healthy and noted that this was a happy time in her life. She began to gain weight steadily during her first pregnancy at age 28, and she began to eat for energy and comfort when her daughter was an infant. This resulted in her gaining a significant amount of weight, and her BMI was 34 kg/m² when her second daughter was born five years ago. She feels that the transition from information technology professional to stay-at-home mother was difficult for her, and she comforted herself with food. She and her husband divorced two years ago, and she returned to work for financial reasons. This has resulted in her becoming more sedentary and relying on fast and prepackaged foods for her meals. Several nights per week she comforts herself by eating large amounts of "junk food" after her daughters have gone to bed. She often skips breakfast because she still feels full from eating the previous night. She eats very little during the day and tends to have a reasonable dinner on the nights when her daughters are with her. On the nights when they are with their father, she starts eating when she gets home, usually high-sugar snack foods, and eats chaotically until she falls asleep.

She did not endorse any alcohol use, noting that her father is an alcoholic and she does not want to end up like him. Her father was emotionally abusive to her when she was growing up and would call her "Fattie" regardless of her weight. She was diagnosed with major depressive disorder after graduating from college, when she found herself in an unhappy romantic relationship that she subsequently ended. She saw a counselor a few times and did not want to try medications.

Introduction

In this chapter, we discuss the rationale for using cognitive-behavioral therapy (CBT) to improve disordered eating in individuals with severe obesity. We then discuss a number of CBT strategies that may be helpful in improving eating behaviors such as binge eating, emotional eating, and grazing. We return to the Case Vignette throughout the chapter using clinical dialogues to illustrate the application of select CBT strategies and some of the challenges encountered when using CBT in patients with severe obesity. We also review the empirical evidence regarding the effectiveness of CBT for improving disordered eating in patients with severe obesity.

Cognitive-Behavioral Therapy for Disordered Eating
Psychoeducation and Goal Setting
The initial step when working with patients with severe obesity involves educating the patient about the theory behind CBT and the connection between thoughts, feelings, and behaviors (see Chapters 2 and 8). It is helpful for patients to know that CBT is a time-limited therapeutic approach that will help with recognizing and understanding patterns and factors that contribute to disordered eating. The goal is to identify and challenge automatic thoughts and behaviors that keep the patient stuck in a pattern of disordered eating and weight gain. To this end, an illustration of this cycle may help patients recognize how this pattern may play a role in their lives (Figure 9.1).

Clinical Dialogue

The clinician reviews the theory behind CBT and some basic examples with Allison, and she agrees that the theory makes sense. A cognitive-behavioral conceptualization of binge eating can then be used to guide the discussion (see Figure 9.1).

CLINICIAN: Can you think of a time in the past week when this feedback loop may have occurred for you? Let's focus on the psychological and behavioral factors for your food intake and eating patterns.

ALLISON: Let's see . . . I think the dietary restriction part is something I do. I had a really big project at work this week and spent a lot of time on it. I would even use it as an excuse to skip lunch so that I didn't stop working. I was really proud of myself for being able to do this and thought "maybe I'll lose some weight working on this project." By midafternoon, I could barely focus on the project and would go to the staff lounge to see if anyone brought in "treats." Someone always brings in some kind of pastry or something. I found a box of cookies and took half of one back to my desk to eat while I kept working. About 15 minutes later I was even hungrier, so I went back for the other half. It was gone, and I figured I may as well take a whole cookie because I haven't eaten anything else today. Thirty minutes later I had four more cookies in my pocket and ate them in my car in the parking lot so that no one would see. I was so ashamed and disgusted with myself. I went home two hours later and thought, "Well, I might as well just go for it now."

CLINICIAN: Go for it?

ALLISON: Yeah, I mean when I got up in the morning I decided that on my way home from work I would stop and get stuff to make a healthy salad for dinner. Then I was going to go for an hour-long walk and make the salad after that. After eating all those cookies, I figured, "Why bother? I already blew it. Might as well sit in front of the TV and have some comfort food." So I stopped at the grocery store and got a frozen pizza, some ice cream, and some more cookies. And then I ate most of that when I got home, and I felt awful. My stomach hurt and I was so disappointed. I went to bed and thought, "I'll never do that again. Tomorrow I'm not eating anything but fruits and vegetables."

Allison's report indicates that she has the potential to benefit from CBT targeting her binge eating. Next, the clinician proceeds with collaboratively setting appropriate treatment

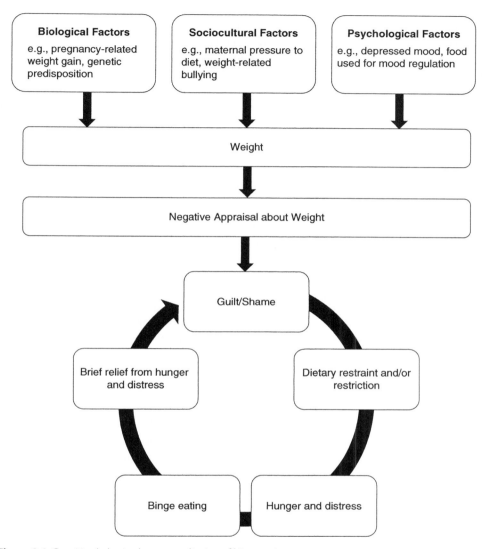

Figure 9.1 Cognitive-behavioral conceptualization of binge eating.

goals with Allison. Many patients focus on weight loss as a primary goal for treatment, and often their expectations are unrealistic. This is an opportunity to direct the patient to think of ways in which being overweight, and continuing to gain weight, has had a negative impact on his or her life. This may include physical and psychological effects, such as chronic pain, sleep apnea, fatigue, mobility issues, depression, anxiety, and shame (see Chapter 1). This is by no means an exhaustive list, and other related problems have been described in detail in the literature [1–7]. While often focused on weight loss, significant psychological distress accompanies disordered eating behaviors at any weight, and patients are eager to relieve the distress.

When asked about her goals for treatment, Allison explains that she feels "out of control" in relation to food, and she is unhappy with her body and weight. She would like to learn how to stop binge eating and to lose weight because she has been unable to maintain her weight loss with previous diets. She is hoping to get back down to the weight she was at in college (BMI = 26–28 kg/m^2). This is a perfect opportunity for the clinician to review realistic expectations regarding weight loss while receiving CBT for disordered eating and also the potential consequences of further weight gain.

> CLINICIAN: Thank you for sharing your goals. I want to make sure we are on the same page about what this type of treatment can do. While there is good evidence that CBT will help with your sensation of loss of control around food, there is no guarantee that you will lose weight. It is likely that your binge eating plays a role in your weight, and if we can improve that, you may see some weight loss. However, the amount of weight you are hoping to lose would be unlikely to occur even with a surgical procedure. A reasonable goal would be to lose about 5 percent of your current weight.
>
> ALLISON: You did mention earlier that I wouldn't lose a lot of weight. I guess I didn't think that 70 pounds was a lot to lose, but I guess it is. That's pretty disappointing to hear.
>
> CLINICIAN: Yes, that's hard for a lot of people to learn. I have found that people tend to feel much better physically and emotionally when they lose some weight, even if they don't lose the amount of weight they had been hoping to lose. I know you mentioned that you have hypertension. That amount of weight loss can certainly help lower your blood pressure. Some people also say they have an easier time doing things they enjoy and even that they find that they enjoy more activities.
>
> ALLISON: Yeah, I guess that would be nice. I do have a tough time exercising, and I know that I'm happier when I am able to be more active. When I was in college, I would go for walks with friends and do yoga. Maybe another goal can be to increase my physical activity.

Allison seems to be agreeable to using CBT to address her binge eating. She did initially have unrealistic goals about her potential weight loss. It is important to address expectations early in treatment, and this discussion may need to be revisited throughout treatment as well. It is also important to help patients focus on what they can improve, such as learning and practicing coping skills to reduce vulnerability to binge eating. Allison's homework is to spend more time reviewing the cognitive-behavioral conceptualization of binge eating and considering how it applies to her.

Self-Monitoring and Planning Regular Meals

Behavior change of any kind requires an awareness of current behaviors. In order to understand the relationship between thoughts, feelings, and behaviors, it is important to monitor all these factors. In working with individuals with severe obesity, *self-monitoring* is a critical step in identifying patterns in eating behaviors, and this information can be used to help regulate eating patterns. The importance of this step cannot be overemphasized and is described in detail in Chapter 8. Patients often eat in response to cravings, emotions, or availability of palatable food and no longer recognize their hunger cues. Regulating meals and snacks helps draw attention to urges to eat for reasons other than hunger, keeps the body and brain appropriately nourished, and allows the patient to redevelop recognition of hunger cues.

When Allison comes in for her next session, she has developed a personalized model of her binge eating based on Figure 8.1. While reviewing this model with the clinician, she provides more examples of "dieting" during the day and binge eating in the evening. The pattern she has identified will be useful in explaining the importance of eating regularly scheduled meals, monitoring her eating behavior, and weighing herself regularly.

CLINICIAN: The goal is to eat three meals and two to three small snacks per day, and the meals and snacks should be about three to four hours apart. It is important that you track everything you eat and drink on a self-monitoring record, also known as a *food record* (see Figure 8.2). Please record the type of eating episode, such as a snack, meal, binge, or grazing episode. You should record the time and location as well and be specific about the location. If you are at work or at home, write exactly what room you are in – for example, "At my work desk" or "In front of the TV in the living room." It is also important to record your thoughts and your feelings at these times to help us understand the context. Does this make sense?

ALLISON: Yes, that seems easy enough.

CLINICIAN: Great. The log will be most useful if you carry it with you and fill it out while you are eating. If you notice an urge to eat between scheduled meals and snacks, write down when and where that happens along with what thoughts and feelings you're having. If you eat outside of your scheduled meals or snacks, it's important to track that too. This is how we learn your patterns and track your progress. Finally, it's important to weigh yourself regularly – once a week is an appropriate frequency. It's important to remember that there are normal fluctuations in weight, and any short-term changes are likely due to fluid shifts rather than changes in fat or muscle. Sometimes it can be hard to make yourself eat at scheduled times. It can also be difficult to make yourself fill out the monitoring log. Is there anything you think might get in the way of your being able to do these things?

ALLISON: No, I don't think so. This seems like an important starting point, so I will do my best to eat regularly and complete these forms every day.

CLINICIAN: It is great to hear that you're eager to get started on this! Some people find that it's difficult to complete these records when they're busy at work or out with friends or if they've had an eating binge. Do you anticipate any of those things being difficult for you?

ALLISON: No. Those things shouldn't be too difficult for me.

When Allison returns next week, the form is sparsely filled out. She explains that she had a busy week and was not able to complete it. She realizes that it is important and says that she will complete it for next week. In the meantime, she does not think she has been able to decrease her binge eating, and her mood is still really low. She also had an argument with her mother that she wants to discuss.

Patients are often reluctant to record what they are eating, and it is necessary to explore this reluctance gently and firmly. Sometimes there is a tendency to focus on another "crisis." It can be helpful to validate their struggle, acknowledge competing priorities, and return to the goals of your work together.

CLINICIAN: It sounds like that interaction with your mom was difficult for you. It's important that we spend a little time on it, but I wouldn't be doing my job if I don't make sure that we keep track of the goals we set when we started. Let's look back at what we wrote down as your goals. We were aiming to decrease your sense of feeling out of control while eating, learn more about the relationship between eating and your mood, and increase your activity level. Let's start by taking a look at your food record together.

ALLISON: So I did really well during the day, eating small meals with a lot of protein and fiber. I probably wasn't very mindful because I was busy and ate at my desk. I got home around 6 PM and had some grapes and cheese slices while I figured out what I wanted for dinner. I was feeling pretty tired, so I just decided to have some cereal instead of a proper dinner, even though it's sugary and I usually binge on sugary foods. I ended up having about two bowls of cereal and then just decided that since I'd started, there was no reason to stop. I'm fat already, right? So I kept going . . . [*at this point Allison becomes flushed and tearful and stops speaking*].

CLINICIAN: I can see that it's really painful to talk about this. I wonder if you can step back and identify what feelings are coming up as you talk about this.

ALLISON: I feel so disappointed in myself and so embarrassed. I never really talk about this. Honestly, I am disgusted with myself.

CLINICIAN: Is it okay with you if I share some thoughts about this?

ALLISON: Yes.

CLINICIAN: I hear a lot of very powerful negative emotion when you talk about binge eating. I think it would be worth looking at the automatic negative thoughts associated with these emotions and whether there are more useful thoughts you could come up with. [*Allison and the clinician proceed to fill out a thought record related to her binge* (see Figure 9.2).]

CBT Thought Record

Situation	Negative Automatic Thoughts	Rate Emotions	Type of Cognitive Distortion	Balanced Thought	Re-Rate Emotions
I binged after coming home from work yesterday	I am disgusting	Shame(100%) Anger(70%)	Labeling	One binge does not determine my worth as a person	Shame(30%) Relief(20%)
	I am totally out of control	Anxiety(90%) Anger(90%)	All-or-Nothing Thinking	I lost control when I ate last night but I don't always lose control	Anxiety(40%) Anger(70%)
	No one will want to date me if they see how I eat	Sadness(80%)	Mindreading	I have no evidence that someone wouldn't date me because of my eating habits	Sadness(10%)
	I should be able to stop eating once I start	Anxiety(70%) Anger(40%) Hopelessness (70%)	"Should" statements	I was hungry when I got home and that set me up to lose control	Anxiety(40%) Relief(20%)

Figure 9.2 Sample CBT thought record.

Alternatives to Overeating

Once Allison is on track with self-monitoring, she can start to recognize the brief periods of pleasure she gets from binge eating and to understand how that feeling maintains her pattern of binge eating and weight gain. It is important to help her build skills and increase her repertoire of pleasurable activities. It is usually easier to replace one behavior with another than to simply stop a behavior. This is especially true for behaviors that are enjoyable, even if the positive feeling is not long lasting.

There are several important considerations when brainstorming alternative behaviors. For example, it is important to have a variety of options that can be used in different settings, for different periods of time, and at different times of the day. Some will be meaningful activities that help with progress toward other goals, such as increasing social interactions or one's sense of mastery in some area, whereas other activities may help to distract during an acutely challenging time.

Marsha Linehan provides a list of over 150 activities in her *Skills Training Manual* [8]. The clinician can provide a list of examples of alternative activities and work with Allison to develop her own list of activities to try. The activities should be practical, affordable, realistic, and require varying time commitments. In addition, a number of the activities should be incompatible with eating. Allison's list consists of the following 10 activities:

1. Calling a friend. She writes down the phone numbers for three good friends, all of whom are helpful in different ways. One makes her laugh, one is a good listener, and one will meet her for a walk.
2. Going to a yoga class at the studio in town. She downloads the schedule on her phone.
3. Coloring. She thinks this is for kids but has seen adult coloring books, so she plans to look at some this weekend and will consider trying it with her kids.
4. Deep breathing for three minutes.
5. Listening to music. She will work on making a playlist that she finds energizing and another one that she finds soothing.
6. Playing a board game with her kids.
7. Giving herself a manicure.
8. Going to a movie with a friend.
9. Going to the playground with her kids.
10. Doing a crossword puzzle. She will carry an easy one with her so that it's always available.

CLINICIAN: It's important to note that it's unlikely any of these activities will work as well, or as quickly, as food does in soothing you or bringing you pleasure. Persistence is the key, and you'll need to practice these activities when you are relaxed rather than waiting until you are trying to resist an overwhelming urge to binge. It's also important to keep adding new activities to this list. During the week, please think of 10 more activities you could potentially try. For now, pick two activities that you will practice between now and our next session. Remember, you should continue to self-monitor, have regular meals and snacks, and weigh yourself weekly. We will check in on all of those items when we meet next week.

Problem Solving

Problem solving provides an opportunity to look at the food records more closely and observe patterns related to binge eating. These patterns can include certain days of the week or times of the day, being around certain people or at certain places, or attending particular events. Once these patterns are identified, problem solving can begin.

CLINICIAN: Let's look at your food record for the past week and see how things are going.

ALLISON: Overall, the week went well, but I really struggled on Friday night with the urge to binge. I was supposed to go for coffee after work with a colleague, and she ended up canceling at the last minute, so I just went home. The kids were with their dad, and I was tired and hungry, so my defenses were down.

The clinician can use a six-step problem-solving approach to help Allison identify solutions to reduce her vulnerability to binge eating.

1. Identify the problem as early as possible.

ALLISON: I knew that I was tired, hungry, and feeling lonely, all of which are triggers to binge.

2. Specifying the problem accurately.

ALLISON: I was tired, hungry, and lonely and wanted to binge after Carol canceled our coffee date.

3. Considering as many solutions as possible.

ALLISON: I could . . .

Call Mary and see if she is available for a walk.
Watch the new season of my favorite show on Netflix.
Continue to work on the project that is due next week.
See if one of my friends is interested in going to dinner or getting takeout.
Go to bed as soon as I get home.

4. Thinking through the implications of each solution.

ALLISON: Calling Mary to see if she is available for a walk would get me outside and help with loneliness.
Watching the new season of my favorite show on Netflix is not going to help with loneliness, and TV has been a trigger for bingeing in the past.
Continuing to work on the project that is due next week is likely to increase my anxiety, and I need a break from working for a little bit. It might increase my sense of mastery but not address loneliness, hunger, or fatigue.
Seeing if one of my friends is interested in going to dinner or getting takeout would provide me with company and a positive mealtime experience.
Going to bed as soon as I get home tends to be a way for me to avoid feelings, and it usually disrupts my sleep.

5. Choose the best solution or combination of solutions.

ALLISON: Looking at these options, I think the best solution would be to call Mary and ask if she would like to go for a walk and have some takeout.

6. Act on the solution.

ALLISON: If I find myself feeling this way again, I will call Mary and ask if she would like to go for a walk and have some takeout. That will give us a chance to connect and talk about our weeks and share a meal together.

Challenging Counterproductive Thoughts

Challenging problems can lead to binge eating, emotional eating, and grazing because eating is gratifying and serves as a distraction from the problem at hand. Learning problem-solving skills can help tackle the problem head-on instead. Another challenge area is counterproductive thoughts. Clinicians can use thought records to help patients reframe automatic negative thoughts, as demonstrated in the CBT thought record in Figure 9.2. The goal is to help patients to recognize their cognitive distortions and begin to challenge them (see Chapters 2 and 8).

After a few weeks of therapy, Allison is in the habit of completing thought records and challenging her thoughts. She shares the following example with her therapist.

ALLISON: So last night my ex-husband and I were arguing about the custody schedule for the upcoming school holiday. I went to the kitchen after we got off the phone, but before I started eating, I recognized some automatic thoughts and challenged them.

CLINICIAN: That's wonderful. Can you give me an example?

ALLISON: Well, I started to think that I was a bad mother and that he and I will never stop fighting, but then I realized that there is a lot of evidence that I am a good mother, and I reminded myself about this – the kids are happy and thriving socially and academically, and we have a great relationship. As far as the fighting, I realized that was a pretty catastrophic interpretation of just one fight! Most of the time we are pretty civil, but it was easy to feel panicked about going back to nonstop fighting in that moment.

CLINICIAN: How did it feel to challenge those thoughts?

ALLISON: Good. I felt like I was really getting better at recognizing how my thoughts can get out of control and really affect my mood. Previously, I probably would have binged in response to having conflict with him. Oh, and once I worked through it, I decided to call a friend instead to chat about the conflict with my ex, and that was much healthier than overeating.

Relapse Prevention

Patients will undoubtedly experience triggers for disordered eating during and after therapy, and helping them to anticipate triggers is a crucial element in relapse prevention. The clinician should review skills and problem-solving strategies with patients and encourage them to develop coping plans for a variety of situations. It is also important to educate patients that they are likely to reexperience disordered eating behaviors at some point following treatment and that this experience provides an opportunity to implement the skills and problem-solving strategies detailed earlier. As they are terminating therapy, Allison and her therapist spend several sessions discussing relapse prevention.

CLINICIAN: Last week I had asked you to think about possible triggers for binge eating in the future. Were you able to think of any triggers?

ALLISON: Yes. I think the biggest trigger for me is stress at work. It's hard for me to make time to eat a proper meal, and I tend to let myself get too hungry, which I know sets me up for a binge. This will probably be something I have to stay mindful of. And, of course, anything bad happening could really set me off – if I lose my job or something happens to a family member . . . Oh! And the holidays are hard. My aunt hosts Christmas, and she tends to push food on people.

CLINICIAN: That's a good list. It sounds like you recognize the importance of eating regularly, particularly when you have a big deadline at work. That will be important in your recovery, and that is something within your control. We can't necessarily control outside events, like illness or other adverse events, but you can take care of yourself if they do happen. Do you have any thoughts about how to approach the holidays?

ALLISON: Well, my cousin knows that I am getting help for binge eating, and she is very supportive of me. I can ask her for support when my aunt is pushing treats. I'm not sure I want to tell everyone why I am not eating as much. And I will try to stay mindful and focused on enjoying time with my family. I can always step outside for a quick walk or call a friend if I need a break.

Case Vignette Revisited

Allison participated in 15 sessions of CBT focused on her binge eating. By the end of treatment, she noticed a significant decrease in binge episodes and in the feeling that she was "out of control" with her eating. Additionally, she began to experience a greater sense of mastery and self-esteem around her ability to better manage her eating. As expected, her weight decreased by a small amount, which she acknowledged was frustrating to her because she had hoped to lose more weight. She felt that the best part of the therapy was learning how to cope with stressors and incorporate a greater variety of activities into her daily life.

Empirical Evidence for the Effectiveness of CBT for Disordered Eating in Severe Obesity

The rate of binge eating disorder (BED) in people with severe obesity is significantly higher than in the general population [9], and 40 to 80 percent of people with BED or bulimia nervosa (BN) are obese [10]. Patients with obesity and binge eating have greater psychopathology than those without binge eating [11]. There is a very strong evidence base for CBT in the treatment of eating disorders, and it is the most studied intervention in patients with obesity and eating disorders [12–14]. Cognitive-behavioral therapy leads to a decrease in binge eating episodes in the short term, and this decrease is sustained for many people. There is little evidence for long-term weight loss following CBT interventions focused on binge eating, but weight loss is significantly greater in those who sustain abstinence of binge eating. Weight loss does occur with behavioral weight loss programs alone, although it is rarely sustained in patients with binge eating [15]. While Grilo and colleagues did not show a benefit from CBT combined with other behavioral weight loss therapies, there has been some suggestion that this may be an effective route [11,13–16].

Agras and colleagues followed 93 women with obesity (mean BMI = 36.7 kg/m^2) with BED who received group CBT followed by weight loss treatment for one year after treatment [16]. At the end of the CBT component, 72 percent of participants had reduced binge eating, and 41 percent had completely stopped binge eating. By one-year follow-up, the rates were 64 and 33 percent, respectively. Those who stopped binge eating after CBT lost 4.0 kg by the end of the one-year follow-up, whereas those who did not gained 3.6 kg over the same period. Weight loss was 6.4 kg at one-year follow-up for those who continued to refrain from binge eating after the CBT component.

Vanderlinden and colleagues evaluated CBT alone for patients with obesity and BED and followed participants for 3.5 years [11]. The CBT program was attended for one eight-hour day per week for 24 to 48 weeks, with an average of 29 weeks of treatment. In addition, physical activity for 30 minutes at least five days per week was promoted. Participants experienced significant improvements in binge eating episodes, psychological measures, and BMI (11-kg weight loss on average). For all areas, the majority of improvement occurred during treatment, but it persisted for up to 3.5 years afterwards. It is important to note that this CBT program differs from most in terms of the amount of treatment and the addition of a physical activity component [11].

With increasing numbers of people experiencing both obesity and binge eating, there is an increased demand for access to treatment. As a result, increased efforts are being made to develop and evaluate additional methods of offering CBT using various forms of technology [12,17–18] (see Chapters 14 and 15), to combine CBT with behavioral weight loss therapies with a goal of decreasing eating disorder behaviors while encouraging weight loss [10], and to evaluate different levels of care [19].

Summary

Severe obesity has a significant impact on physical and psychological health, and the presence of binge eating tends to make treatment more challenging. This chapter provided an overview of a psychological treatment called *cognitive-behavioral therapy* (CBT), a skills-based intervention that has been found to be effective in decreasing binge eating behaviors. Using a clinical vignette format, this chapter reviewed the essential features of CBT for binge eating while highlighting that weight loss is not the primary goal. Given that improvements in binge eating and relatively small amounts of weight loss can lead to significant improvements in physical and mental health, more research is warranted to evaluate the role of CBT in decreasing binge eating in individuals with severe obesity.

Key Points

- Cognitive-behavioral therapy is an effective and durable treatment for disordered eating.
- Cognitive-behavioral therapy alone is unlikely to lead to weight loss in patients with obesity and disordered eating, and it is important to set realistic expectations with patients at the beginning of treatment.
- Food records and self-monitoring are an essential part of CBT for disordered eating.

- Many patients struggle with self-monitoring, and this provides an important opportunity to explore any barriers to change during treatment.
- Patients with severe obesity and significant disordered eating have unique treatment challenges; thus further research is warranted in this population.

References

1. W. T. Garvey, J. I. Mechanick, E. M. Brett, et al. American Association of Clinical Endocrinologists and American College of Endocrinology comprehensive clinical practice guidelines for medical care of patients with obesity. *Endocr Pract* 2016; **22**: 1–203.

2. K. M. Carpenter, D. S. Hasin, D. B. Allison, et al. Relationships between obesity and DSM-IV major depressive disorder, suicide ideation, and suicide attempts: Results from a general population study. *Am J Public Health* 2000; **90**: 251–7.

3. L. T. Goldstein, S. J. Goldsmith, K. Anger, et al. Psychiatric symptoms in clients presenting for commercial weight reduction treatment. *Int J Eat Disord* 1996; **20**: 191–7.

4. F. S. Luppino, L. M. de Wit, P. F. Bouvy, et al. Overweight, obesity, and depression: A systematic review and meta-analysis of longitudinal studies. *Arch Gen Psychiatry* 2010; **67**: 220–9.

5. K. M. Scott, M. A. McGee, J. E. Wells, et al. Obesity and mental disorders in the adult general population. *J Psychosom Res* 2008; **64**: 97–105.

6. G. E. Simon, M. Von Korff, K. Saunders, et al. Association between obesity and psychiatric disorders in the US adult population. *Arch Gen Psychiatry* 2006; **63**: 824–30.

7. S. Z. Yanovski, J. E. Nelson, B. K. Dubbert, et al. Association of binge eating disorder and psychiatric comorbidity in obese subjects. *Am J Psychiatry* 1993; **150**: 1472–9.

8. M. M. Linehan. *DBT Skills Training Manual.* New York, NY: Guilford Press, 2014.

9. V. Abiles, S. Rodriguez-Ruiz, J. Abiles, et al. Effectiveness of cognitive-behavioural therapy in morbidity obese candidates for bariatric surgery with and without binge eating disorder. *Nutr Hosp* 2013; **28**: 1523–9.

10. M. A. Palavras, P. Hay, S. Touyz, et al. Comparing cognitive behavioural therapy for eating disorders integrated with behavioural weight loss therapy to cognitive behavioural therapy-enhanced alone in overweight or obese people with bulimia nervosa or binge eating disorder: Study protocol for a randomised controlled trial. *Trials* 2015; **16**: 578–67.

11. J. Vanderlinden, A. Adrianensen, D. Vancampfort, et al. A cognitive-behavioural therapeutic program for patients with obesity and binge eating disorder: Short- and long-term follow-up data of a prospective study. *Behav Modif* 2012; **36**: 670–86.

12. G. Castelnuovo, G. Pietrabissa, G. M. Manzoni, et al. Cognitive behavioural therapy to aid weight loss in obese patients: Current perspectives. *Psychol Res Behav Manag* 2017; **10**: 165–73.

13. P. Hay. A systematic review of evidence for psychological treatments in eating disorders: 2005–2012. *Int J Eat Disord* 2013; **46**: 462–9.

14. M. A. Palavras, P. Hay, C. A. dos Santos Filho, et al. The efficacy of psychological therapies in reducing weight and binge eating in people with bulimia nervosa and binge eating disorder who are overweight or obese: A critical synthesis and meta-analyses. *Nutrients* 2017; **9**: 299–317.

15. C. M. Grilo, R. M. Masheb, G. T. Wilson, et al. Cognitive-behavioural therapy, behavioural weight loss, and sequential treatment for obese patients with binge eating disorder: A randomized controlled trial. *J Consult Clin Psychol* 2011; **79**: 675–85.

16. W. S. Agras, C. F. Telch, B. Arnow, et al. One-year follow-up of cognitive-behavioural therapy for obese

individuals with binge eating disorder. *Clin Psychol* 1997; **65**: 343–7.

17. M. de Zwann, S. Herpertz, S. Zipfel, et al. Effect of internet-based guided self-help vs individual face-to-face treatment on full or subsyndromal binge eating disorder in overweight or obese patients: The INTERBED Randomized Clinical Trial. *JAMA Psychiatry* 2017; **74**: 987–95.

18. S. E. Cassin, S. Sockalingham, C. Du, et al. A pilot randomized controlled trial of telephone-based cognitive behavioural therapy for preoperative bariatric surgery patients. *Behav Res Ther* 2016; **80**: 17–22.

19. G. R. Dalle, M. Satirana, M. El Ghoch, et al. Personalized multistep cognitive behavioural therapy for obesity. *Diabetes Metab Syndr Obes* 2017; **10**: 195–206.

10

Mindfulness-Based Therapies in Severe Obesity

Jean Kristeller, Susan Wnuk, and Chau Du

Case Vignette

Linda is a 52-year-old married professional African-American woman with type 2 diabetes, osteoarthritis, and hypertension. At 5 feet, 2 inches and 230 pounds, her body mass index (BMI) is 42 kg/m². Her physician recommended bariatric surgery due to her health problems. However, she was concerned about doing so because she has lost and regained weight multiple times due to "out of control" eating, and a friend of hers regained most of his weight following bariatric surgery. She had heard that mindfulness-based eating awareness training (MB-EAT) could be helpful for such issues.

On initial evaluation, she met criteria for binge eating disorder and subclinical depression. Her current weight had been stable for several years. She had no history of regular exercise, acknowledging that she had always avoided exercise, including walking ("I was one of those kids who always tried to get out of gym class"). Both parents were heavy, as were her husband, adult children, and most friends. She was an active member of a local church. When she first understood that the MB-EAT program entailed learning to meditate regularly, she expressed some concern from a religious perspective. However, this concern was alleviated by framing the program as influenced by Buddhist psychology rather than Buddhism as a religion.

She was asked to describe an ideal eating pattern during the MB-EAT orientation, and she provided a response consistent with a low-calorie (approximately 1,200 calories) structured diet. Given her plans for bariatric surgery, this was realistic in the short term but also reflected a common pattern of "all or nothing" thinking, without flexibility and lack of knowledge of how to eat even small amounts of higher-calorie foods. Therefore, the value of the MB-EAT program was framed for her in two ways: (1) to help her bring her binge eating under control in the short term to prepare for surgery and (2) to help her create a new relationship to eating and food by learning to attend to both physical hunger and satiety cues, to recognize her other common triggers for eating, and to gain pleasure from smaller, rather than larger, amounts of foods. Even though she would not be able to eat any sweets for a while after surgery, she would become more confident that when she was able to eat them again, she could better resist eating large amounts of those foods. She was also informed that the program would encourage everyone to become more physically active in order to help them prepare for surgery and recover afterward. She was intrigued that although she would be asked to reduce her caloric intake, the primary goals were to incorporate flexibility and find ways to eat her favorite foods at a lower but sustainable level. By the end of the orientation, her enthusiasm was evident for beginning MB-EAT.

Introduction

Mindless eating is rampant in our society. Eating out of habit because food is available or eating as a favored way to seek pleasure or deal with stress often leads to weight gain, obesity, and a lifelong struggle with how and what to eat. Mindfulness is being increasingly recognized as a way to counter such patterns and, as a component of therapy, is broadly applicable and can be linked with a range of other approaches [1,2].

What Is Mindfulness?

Mindfulness is the practice of "bringing one's complete attention to the present experience on a moment-to-moment basis" [3: 68]. Another often-cited definition is "paying attention in a particular way: on purpose, in the present moment, nonjudgmentally" [4]. Mindful awareness can be brought to any aspect of experience, such as thoughts, emotions, sensations, external objects, sounds, and events. Mindfulness instructions involve directing attention to a particular experience or process, such as the breath, physical hunger, walking, or the sensations of an emotion.

Often perceived as a type of "relaxation training" or, alternatively, an esoteric practice linked to Buddhist religious beliefs and training, mindfulness is both – and neither. Mindfulness practice does indeed induce a sense of relaxation in most people because focus is shifted gently onto the breath, engaging both a physiologic relaxation process [5] and disengagement from intruding concerns or worries. It also has its roots in Buddhism, in both Buddhist psychology and spiritual practice [6]. Buddhist psychology frames distress and dysfunction as associated with excessive attachment and avoidance (consistent with contemporary conditioning theory), with practice providing a means to diminish such struggle and engage alternative feelings, actions, or thoughts.

Mindfulness practice is a path to growth because attention is shifted away from struggling with desires toward a healthier, wiser perspective of choices, a flexibility in the face of challenges, and a greater understanding of one's own goals and resources. In relation to eating, engaging mindfulness heightens awareness of long-standing conditioned patterns; facilitates awareness of physical hunger, taste, and satiety cues; and allows access to alternative, healthier choices. At the simplest level, in relation to eating and food, engaging mindfulness may mean realizing that the last bite of a favorite food is "enough," leading to a comfortable decision to stop eating, rather than forcing oneself to clean the plate. At a more substantive level, it may facilitate rewiring the neurocircuits of the brain as highly conditioned reactions are weakened and food preferences change in pervasive ways, leading to a healthier diet and sustainable weight loss.

Many mindfulness practices also encourage acceptance and self-compassion [7,8] (see Chapter 11). A common misunderstanding of acceptance is that it involves passivity or even approval of harmful behavior. Instead, acceptance refers to experiencing events fully, without denial, suppression, or amplification. Acceptance also means avoiding ruminating about events, instead allowing the experience of the associated emotions and bodily reactions to arise and dissipate. Afterward, decisions can be made about what action, if any, to take. Defined this way, mindfulness involves a set of skills designed to encourage deliberate, nonevaluative engagement with events that are here and now [9]. Mindfulness can also be conceptualized as a human capacity that can be cultivated to be used more effectively with practice [10]. The relationships between various aspects of internal and external experience, which may previously have been out of awareness and operating automatically, can be more clearly observed. With this new information, individuals can more easily make substantive changes in their behavioral responses.

Third-Wave Psychotherapies for Eating and Weight Problems

Contemporary mindfulness training, while informed by Buddhist psychology, was first secularized by Jon Kabat-Zinn in an eight-session mindfulness-based stress-reduction (MBSR) program for medical patients with chronic pain or serious illness [11,12]. The MBSR program incorporates breath-awareness meditation, body-awareness practices including yoga, and substantial instruction/discussion to help patients adjust to the physical and psychological challenges of their medical conditions. Variations and extensions of the MBSR program have since emerged, including mindfulness-based cognitive therapy (MBCT) [13] for decreasing relapses in individuals with past episodes of major depression [14,15], mindfulness-based relapse prevention (MBRP) [16] for substance-use disorders, and MB-EAT [17].

These mindfulness-based programs and psychotherapeutic treatments incorporating mindfulness, including dialectical behavior therapy (DBT) and acceptance and commitment therapy (ACT), have been termed *third-wave psychotherapies* [18] to distinguish them from the first two waves (behavior therapy and cognitive therapy). According to Hayes [18], the primary difference between these and third-wave therapies relates to the aspects of human functioning that are to be addressed. First- and second-wave therapies aim to change the *content* of problematic aspects of experience, especially thoughts and emotions. Third-wave therapies aim to change one's *relationship* to those problematic thoughts and emotions. For example, instead of seeking to find evidence for and against a problematic thought and restructure it into a balanced thought, as would be typical in traditional cognitive-behavioral therapy (CBT; see Chapter 8), the goal of a third-wave therapy would be to identify the thought as a thought, regardless of content, and help the person choose skillful behavior in line with his or her values without needing to change the thought itself.

Eating is an ideally suited context for cultivating and applying mindfulness approaches. As Wansink's work has so creatively shown [19], virtually everyone is susceptible to "mindless" eating, whether as a reaction to subtle contextual cues or to long-conditioned habits, thoughts, feelings, and situations. Wansink has also documented that, on average, people make approximately 200 decisions per day about their eating: when to eat, how much to eat, what to eat next, and when to stop. This increases to approximately 300 decisions per day for individuals with obesity [20]. It could be argued that one of the appeals of many structured diets is the reduction in this complexity of choice. Unfortunately, artificially limiting choices is unlikely to help people retrain themselves to more effectively handle these challenges once the structured diet is over.

Decisions regarding eating also require a constant balance between body-based signals to eat – or to stop eating – and the multitude of other triggers or cues that become conditioned triggers for eating behavior, overriding physical hunger cues, taste, and satiation signals. Research clearly demonstrates how easily these signals are overridden and that this is particularly true of individuals with obesity [21]. A core reason for learning mindfulness is to increase one's capacity to attend to such signals and then use them to inform decisions to initiate or stop eating. Many of these elements overlap with the principles informing "intuitive eating" programs [22,23], which, although developed independently of MB-EAT, also draw on the core value of cultivating awareness of inner experiences of hunger and satiety but do not engage formal mindfulness meditation practice. Intuitive eating will not be explored in this chapter because its origins are in dietetics rather than Buddhist psychology or psychotherapy.

Many individuals with obesity also experience very high levels of self-criticism, guilt, shame, and embarrassment. This experience varies considerably depending on the social norms of an individual's family and community, of course, but with the pervasive perception that weight is under one's personal control, it becomes part of one's identity. Helping people negotiate the dichotomy between complete acceptance of current weight versus the legitimate need, for many, of weight loss/management for health reasons, mindful approaches can help to promote greater self-acceptance regardless of current weight, nonjudgment to interrupt the reactivity that arises to deeply embedded self-critical thoughts related to weight and social evaluation, and self-compassion in the midst of these challenges. While mindfulness-based approaches may vary in the ways in which they promote nonjudgment, self-compassion, and self-acceptance, these values are part of all mindfulness-based therapies.

One consideration in understanding these approaches is the degree to which weight loss, in addition to eating regulation, is explicitly addressed or encouraged. This distinction between improved eating regulation and weight loss as primary goals is applicable at virtually any weight level. There is a tension between the core principles of self-acceptance and nonjudgment emphasized in mindfulness that can be interpreted as far more compatible with "health at every size" [24] than with an explicit goal of losing weight. When self-identity is overly fixated on weight, and when weight per se is not notably interfering with other functioning, there is no question that individuals may become overly concerned with the "number on the scale." Yet mindfulness can also be applied to goals that are undertaken for a variety of reasons and can help to discern between inappropriate reasons or means to attain such goals and more balanced means. This distinction, for example, informs many elements of the MB-EAT program, DBT for binge eating, and ACT for overeating and weight loss. These modalities have in common a "nondieting" approach while at the same time encouraging participants to carefully observe their own eating patterns for ways in which they may choose to remove or limit certain types of foods, but without necessarily restricting themselves entirely from any particular type of food. There may be sound rationales for limiting food in a variety of situations, such as when eating is frequently used to regulate emotions. In these programs, when there is an emphasis on weight loss, it is promoted in terms of sustainable long-term weight management (rather than restrictive dieting and rapid weight loss) along with the cultivation of healthier eating in regard to improving both compulsive overeating and food choices.

In this way, when third-wave therapies are used to address problematic eating, the goal is to balance acceptance of subjective food preferences and hunger and fullness cues with a respect for the real consequences of certain eating patterns and frequent food choices. It is possible to flexibly adhere to basic guidelines about healthy nutrition and caloric intake without excessive preoccupation or guilt. Mindfulness-based interventions, including MB-EAT, ACT, and DBT, are described in more detail below.

Mindfulness-Based Eating Awareness Training

The development of mindfulness-based eating awareness training (MB-EAT) was initially inspired by early models of self-regulation theory [25], linked with models of food intake regulation exploring the interplay of psychological and physiologic control processes [26–28]. Self-regulation theory [29] highlights the importance of intentional interoceptive awareness as a core element of internal regulatory processes, highly pertinent to the dysregulation in eating disorders and the overeating observed in obesity [21], and cultivated through mindfulness practice [30].

Physiologic regulation of food intake and weight is surprisingly complex. Signals most available to interoceptive awareness include physical hunger signals (e.g., low blood sugar, stomach growling), taste (e.g., pleasure, quality, and intensity), and signals to terminate eating a particular food or an entire meal (e.g., decrease in taste, sensation of fullness, rise in blood sugar) [31,32]. Individuals with compulsive eating patterns show a decreased attunement to these "internal" cues and marked oversensitivity to "external" or "nonnutritive" cues to eat (social, emotional, or conditioned craving for certain foods). While structured diets or prescribed eating plans may promote healthier eating/weight loss, they do not help individuals learn to reconnect with these internal regulatory signals. In contrast, self-regulation theory posits that when appropriate internal feedback systems are engaged, even complex systems can be reregulated with relatively little effort or struggle [33,34], in contrast to willpower or self-control models, which entail the need for effortful vigilance of behavioral choices.

MB-EAT is based on the premise that cultivating self-regulation through mindful awareness of internal signals of hunger, taste, and satiety, in conjunction with awareness of competing triggers for eating (e.g., thoughts, feelings, environmental cues), will lead to a more balanced, sustainable, and flexible pattern of eating with less sense of struggle. The evidence for meditation training, particularly mindfulness practices, for improving self-regulatory processes has been steadily growing since the 1970s [2]. Although initial development leading up to MB-EAT incorporated meditation practice, full development was highly influenced by the structure and content of the MBSR program [35]. Sitting practice, often using a focus on the breath, cultivates a more general capacity for engaging mindful attention. Guided practice focuses awareness on a specific targeted experience yet in an observing, stable, nonjudgmental, and curious manner. MB-EAT incorporates both elements, helping people to learn to tune into their patterns of physical versus emotional hunger, taste, and fullness with curiosity rather than self-judgment, thus leading to wiser and healthier food choices.

The concept of "wisdom" or insight, core aspects of traditional meditation practice, is also central to the program. Wisdom, from a psychological perspective, involves exercising good judgment in complex or uncertain situations [36]. Baltes and Staudinger frame wisdom as exercising judgment in the "fundamental pragmatics" of life [37]. Ostafin and Kassman have demonstrated that even novice meditators increase in creative or insight-oriented problem solving [38]. From a neuroscience perspective and within the context of meditation practice, wisdom arises from greater access to and integration of the experience and knowledge that each person already carries within, whether more broadly or in regard in eating [39–41]. The MB-EAT program emphasizes how mindfulness practice can be used to access such "tacit" knowledge and judgment in any situation, useful in making complex decisions regarding food choice and eating.

Substantial research addresses the disordered patterns of both eating initiation and termination observed in individuals with binge eating disorder (BED) and obesity, including higher reactivity to food cues [42] and frequently using eating to manage stress [43]. Paradoxically, little comfort may be derived from the food being consumed, unlike for individuals without eating issues, who may acknowledge using food to manage negative emotions [44]. Eating may also help them to dissociate from overwhelming feelings and/or reflect virtually their only coping mechanism, a significant failure of self-regulation.

Deciding when to terminate food intake is also complex. Individuals who are obese and who eat larger amounts of food tolerate higher levels of stomach fullness and discomfort as a result of both expanded stomach capacity and a failure to attend to distention signals as indicators for stopping eating [47–49]. They may note that they do not stop eating "until the food is gone" or "when they feel too full to eat anymore." They virtually never mention attending to more moderate levels of fullness or gradually becoming less hungry as blood sugar levels rise, creating a sense of satiety.

Tuning into taste is another core component of MB-EAT, drawing on two areas of research: the sensitivity of taste buds to even small variations in the type or intensity of flavor, particularly sweets [45,46], and the process by which food loses its appeal as the taste buds habituate to specific combinations of flavors (sensory-specific satiety [SSS], the most rapid satiety-related feedback system) [50,51]. Sensory-specific satiety may be disrupted in obesity or binge eating [52] but may function more normally when adequate awareness is brought to the process [53]. Ironically, the hedonic value of food is often ignored in the treatment of obesity and/or compulsive eating but often informs addictive models of excessive food intake [54].

As in other mindfulness-based interventions, MB-EAT places an emphasis on the importance of becoming aware of and valuing one's own personal preferences and patterns. People vary considerably in their underlying patterns in regard to whether they initiate eating without being physically hungry, eat in reaction to emotional distress, or continue eating even when sated. These variations occur regardless of weight and eating issues [55]. Again, cultivating an exploratory and self-accepting approach to food choices and eating is core to the MB-EAT program, in contrast to harsh self-judgmental and externally imposed rules.

The MB-EAT program consists of 10 weekly and two monthly follow-up sessions, developed over the course of multiple clinical trials, from primarily addressing BED in individuals with obesity to being more broadly applicable. The program is designed to cultivate both "inner wisdom" and "outer wisdom" in relation to eating and food choice: the inner-wisdom components assist individuals in learning to attend to experiences of physical hunger, taste, and fullness and to differentiate these from other triggers, whether emotional, cognitive, or situational [17,35,56]. The outer-wisdom components address, in ways that are personally meaningful and sustainable, caloric/"food energy" needs, nutritional and health concerns, and increasing physical activity. Participants learn how to "respond," from a range of possible options rather than with highly conditioned "reactions" that leave them feeling helpless and out of control of their own eating.

Mindfulness practice is augmented by drawing on principles from psychophysics using visual analog scales [45]. Individuals learn to identify where their hunger, fullness, and "taste satisfaction" from a particular food lie on a 10-point scale and to be aware of the physical experiences informing that number. One value of such scales is that they move people away from "all-or-nothing" judgments ("I'm hungry/I'm not hungry"; "I love this"/"Yuck"; "I'm full/I'm not full") to more subtle evaluations of physical hunger, fullness, and taste satisfaction. It is also emphasized that there is no "right" point on the scale to decide to eat – or stop eating – but that circumstances can be taken into account (e.g., a light lunch prior to exercising versus an occasional holiday dinner, attending a birthday party versus choosing an everyday snack).

Cultivating taste awareness and taste satiety is a particularly core element of MB-EAT. When mindful awareness is brought to taste experience, people discover how quickly the pleasure of a food can drop, particularly for highly sweet or salty foods. The initial taste practice in MB-EAT involves eating four raisins mindfully. When participants are asked to observe whether they actually want the fourth raisin, many realize that they do not. This experience then extends to other foods: cheese and crackers, chips, chocolate, and cookies. Initial clinical applications revealed that even individuals with marked history of obesity and binge eating could easily tune into these subtle variations when doing so mindfully.

The next step is learning to differentiate physical hunger, taste, and satiety from the complex interplay of feelings, thoughts, and situations that trigger eating. For example, common thoughts include "I deserve this"; "Just one (cookie/doughnut/taste of ice cream) won't hurt"; "I have to clean my plate." Marlatt's classic "abstinence violation effect," as applied to alcohol intake [57], is also a hallmark of compulsive overeating, reworded as the "I've blown it" effect. Many individuals vow every morning "to be good," restricting food intake all day, and then attribute their nightly overeating to stress, when it is as likely to be triggered by hunger flavored with negative self-judgment at their poor self-control. Emphasis is placed on breaking this cycle, first through awareness and then by replacing the guilt with enjoyment of smaller, more appropriate amounts of food. Individuals are also encouraged to expand their coping tools to far more than food – but *not* to remove food/eating, in smaller quantities, from their coping list. For example, one man realized that his regular evenings at "all-you-can-eat" buffets with friends were more a left-over mark of "rebellion" that had begun decades before in high school and that he could still enjoy his evenings out without overeating. A woman realized that boredom, rather than stress, led her to overeat in the evenings and that once she was eating in a more balanced way during the day, she was fine just watching television – and knitting to keep her hands busy.

Additional inner-wisdom components help to cultivate attitudes of self-acceptance and flexibility. Throughout the MB-EAT program, people are encouraged to find more joy and pleasure in their eating and relationship to food. Several practices focus on greater aware-ness and acceptance of the physical body. A powerful practice is a "forgiveness meditation" addressing anger at both oneself and others as a common trigger for overeating. A "values practice" challenges individuals to reconsider how much "worry" time they may be spend-ing focused on eating and weight concerns that would more usefully be spent on other important parts of their lives. This exercise is informed by research showing that mind-fulness practice can help to reduce the tendency of the "wandering mind" to move to negatively charged life issues [58]. Finally, a "wisdom meditation and a self-acceptance practice" further formalize these aspects of self-growth.

Also core to the MB-EAT program are the outer-wisdom components. Checking calories on food choices is so associated with dieting that many individuals completely avoid checking the caloric or nutritional values of richer foods eaten between diets or admit feeling very anxious when doing so. The MB-EAT program emphasizes that outer wisdom entails tuning into and making use of such information in a flexible, accepting, and personalized way. Doing so is modeled as part of the mindful eating practices. For example, at the end of the cheese and crackers practice in the second week (see description of the practice below), the group is asked to guess the caloric value of one cracker topped with cheese. Virtually every one guesses double or more: 40 or 50 calories rather than approximately 18 calories. Participants are then asked to check their own cupboards for foods that are both lower – and higher – than they might have expected to help cultivate an attitude of curiosity rather than anxiety. They are also encouraged to mindfully spread caloric intake out over the day, including moderate snacks, counteracting the very common pattern of being "good" earlier in the day and then overeating later. Conversely, individuals who "graze" throughout the day are encouraged to let themselves become somewhat physically hungry after meals, before eating again.

To address the goal of moderate (and sustainable) weight loss, we introduce the "500-calorie challenge." Although originally based on the now-outdated guideline that this would lead to approximately 1 pound of weight loss per week (500 kcal × 7 days = 3,500 kcal) [59], this challenge still provides encouragement to identify a meaningful amount of food to remove from daily intake. To make it less intimidating, we point out that 500 calories would be about 100 calories from each of three meals and two snacks. Individuals with less weight to lose would adjust this caloric goal accordingly. We also emphasize holding an attitude of exploration and experimentation, but that final changes should be sustainable reductions, ones that they are willing to live with indefinitely, to avoid the common pattern of cutting out food while "dieting" and then returning to those foods (or quantities) later. Common choices include less soda consumption; less butter on side dishes; smaller portions of meat, side dishes, or dessert; and lower-calorie salad dressings. One participant cut out four sodas and then added back in two when he realized that he missed them – only to cut out all of them again a few weeks later as his taste preferences shifted away from highly sugared flavors.

Other outer-wisdom components include working with nutritional information, such as creating meals according to national guidelines and adding healthier food choices to daily eating plans. In week 7, a culminating challenge involves a potluck meal within the session, to which participants contribute one "healthier" dish and one that may be more indulgent but which they wish to continue to include in their regular food choices. This meal is followed by eating out at an "all you can eat" buffet as home practice. Four guidelines are provided: (1) review everything on the buffet table before choosing, (2) savor very small "tastes," (3) go back for the most appealing foods, and (4) leave food on the plate. This exercise is almost always anxiety provoking given memories of overeating at buffets. However, participants find that they do not overeat when using the guidelines and instead enjoy the experience for the variety, rather than the quantity, of food eaten.

Research. The first pilot research with MB-EAT, enrolling adult women with obesity and BED, demonstrated the viability of a seven-session program incorporating mindfulness meditation and most of the current inner-wisdom components [60]. Using an extended baseline/follow-up single-group design, binge episodes decreased from over four per week to approximately 1.5 per week, along with clinical improvement on the Binge Eating Scale [61] and depression. Daily mindfulness practice showed significant correlations with improvement in eating control. This study was followed by a National Institutes of Health (NIH)–funded randomized, controlled trial (RCT) comparing a nine-session MB-EAT program with a psychoeducational control and wait list control in a mixed-gender popula-tion with both obesity and BED [62]. While improvements in frequency of binge episodes and the Binge Eating Scale were generally comparable for the two active intervention groups, the MB-EAT group improved to a greater extent on other measures of self-regulated eating, such as the Hunger Scale of the Three-Factor Eating Questionnaire (TFEQ) [63]. One concern remained: although improvement, including weight loss, was related to the amount of mindfulness practice, there was no average weight loss, with approximately one-third losing weight, one-third remaining the same weight, and one-third gaining weight.

This observation led to further development of the outer-wisdom components of MB-EAT. The outer-wisdom components were incorporated into the next trial, which enrolled patients with a BMI of 35 kg/m^2 or greater with or without BED. An average weight loss of approximately 7 pounds was reported regardless of BED status and was maintained at follow-up, consistent with the "500-calorie challenge." Also consistent with engaging outer wisdom was improvement in "healthy restraint" for both those with and without BED, which was sustained into follow-up [64]. Another trial enrolling individuals with type 2 diabetes also showed significant improvement in weight, eating regulation, and metabolic regulation [65,66]. Finally, a large clinical trial with the University of California San Francisco for individuals without BED and a range of obesity extended both the inner- and outer-wisdom components to 16 sessions, added more stress management, and compared it with a diet/exercise/stress-management program. This study demonstrated more sustained weight loss for the mindfulness-based intervention, with comparable improvement across a range of other measures [67].

MB-EAT also has been adapted for adolescents with a range of weight issues, delivered within a predominantly African-American high school setting [68]. Sessions were shortened to the length of a classroom period and delivered over a semester. Students randomly assigned to MB-EAT showed better nutritional intake and higher exercise levels both at the end of the semester and three months later, compared with students who remained in their regular health course.

MB-EAT also has been adapted for use with bariatric surgery patients. Once patients transition from the active weight loss phase (which lasts for approximately the first postoperative year) to the weight maintenance phase, preoperative eating problems may recur. Suboptimal weight maintenance has been attributed to poor adherence to postoperative dietary advice [69] and disordered eating behaviors, such as lack of control over food urges [70], eating in reaction to painful affect [71,72], regularly eating past the point of fullness, and eating continuously throughout the day [73]. Given that individuals seeking bariatric surgery have higher rates of binge eating and emotional eating [74,75] and that behavioral interventions tend to be more effective delivered after bariatric surgery, there is a rationale for delivering mindfulness interventions to improve eating behavior after bariatric surgery [76]. Introducing patients to mindful eating preoperatively, as illustrated in the Case Vignette, may also be effective as patients develop more confidence in managing their eating prior to surgery.

Although relatively few studies have examined the effectiveness of mindfulness interventions in bariatric populations, the preliminary data are encouraging. One study examined the effectiveness of a 10-week mindfulness group intervention for seven postoperative bariatric surgery patients who reported emotional eating or subjective eating binges [77]. Participants reported improvements in eating behaviors, emotion regulation, and depression following the intervention. In another study, 18 postoperative bariatric surgery patients were randomly assigned to either a mindfulness intervention or an active control group [78]. Participants in the control group received a 60-minute individual counseling session with a registered dietitian. The two groups did not differ with respect to weight loss at 12 weeks and 6 months postbaseline. However, participants in the mindfulness group reported a significant decrease in emotional eating six months after baseline. Finally, a pilot study of MB-EAT adapted for postoperative bariatric surgery patients found that for 22 of the 26 participants who completed the intervention, depression significantly decreased, and there were trends toward statistically significant improvements in binge eating and emotional eating [79].

Dialectical Behavior Therapy

Dialectical behavior therapy (DBT) is an integrative psychotherapeutic treatment originally developed by Marsha Linehan [80] to treat individuals with borderline personality disorder, who exhibit extreme emotional reactivity and frequent self-harming behavior. In addition to drawing heavily from CBT and clinical techniques, DBT combines principles and strategies from person-centered therapy, Buddhist psychology, and mindfulness practice. From the DBT perspective, problematic, impulsive behaviors ranging from self-harm to binge eating stem from deficits in emotion regulation skills. Emotion dysregulation is understood to be difficulty managing painful emotions in adaptive and effective ways. Instead of allowing themselves to experience the aversive emotion directly, individuals engage in problematic impulsive behaviors to avoid their distress. They experience temporary relief, which reinforces the behaviors and increases the likelihood they will recur. The long-term consequences of the behaviors such as distress about episodes of compulsive overeating and weight gain cause more problems. Impulsive behaviors, by their nature, occur quickly and, with repetition, become paired with emotional distress. Over time, the process leading from distress to problematic behavior becomes automatic, and the person may not be aware of specific triggers associated with overeating or binge eating.

The DBT understanding of reality is that opposing forces are always operating and can be synthesized in new ways, a philosophical concept referred to as *dialectics*. The most fundamental apparently opposing forces are acceptance and change. It is through practicing acceptance of difficult or undesired realities that one is freed to change them. For example, instead of ruminating about the difficulties related to or influenced by obesity, such as medical conditions or mobility issues, one would acknowledge and accept these difficulties and problem solve where possible. Problem solving might include changing problematic eating habits related to weight such as binge eating, taking appropriate medications, and engaging in valued activities.

Dialectical behavior therapy is characterized by its strong emphasis on developing mindfulness as the foundation for addressing the emotion regulation skill deficits. The other three key skills are interpersonal effectiveness, distress tolerance, and emotion regulation. This is consistent with models of eating disorders whereby binge eating is viewed primarily as a symptom of poor emotion regulation [81,82]. Because DBT was developed for individuals with impulsive, problematic behaviors, it theoretically and clinically lends itself to the treatment of BED and bulimia nervosa (BN). Standard DBT involves weekly individual therapy, a weekly two-hour skills group, 24-hour access to telephone crisis coaching, and a weekly consultation group for therapists.

The goals of DBT mindfulness skills are to decrease judgment of self and others and to increase awareness and acceptance of experience [83]. Learning to observe and then nonjudgmentally describe sensations, emotions, and impulses helps patients to avoid over-identifying with and magnifying their experience and emotions and thereby improves impulse control. Mindfulness is also taught as a means to reduce secondary emotional reactions such as guilt and shame that are typically fueled by self-judgment. Psychoeducation is provided about urges and cravings as classically conditioned reactions that have been associated with a particular cue or cues. Mindfulness can help to bring awareness to the presence of these cravings and cues as they are happening, thereby helping patients to respond more skillfully.

In DBT, mindfulness is considered to be a set of specific skills that can be learned and practiced. These skills include observing and describing experiences nonjudgmentally and with complete attention. Patients are encouraged to fully participate in each moment and to make effective decisions based on their goals and values. Each group session begins with a brief mindfulness practice regardless of the skill that is the focus of that teaching session. Patients are not expected to commit to extended periods of sitting meditation, but they may choose to do so in discussion with their individual therapists.

The mindfulness skills used in DBT for BED and BN are the same as in standard DBT, except for the addition of mindful eating, *urge surfing*, and *alternate rebellion*. Alternate rebellion was borrowed from a DBT program for substance-use disorders [84], and urge surfing, from a relapse-prevention treatment for substance abuse [85]. Urge surfing involves mindful, nonattached, nonjudgmental observing of urges to binge or eat mindlessly, cultivating awareness that urges, like waves, need not crash down and instead rise and then fall if simply observed rather than reacted to. Alternate rebellion involves satisfying a wish to rebel without binge eating. Individuals with BED may describe the desire to "get back at" society, friends, or family whom they perceive to be judgmental about their eating and weight by consuming even more food or making poor food choices [86]. Patients are encouraged to observe the wish to rebel, label it as such, and find an alternative that does not involve binge eating or other problematic behavior. While in vivo mindful eating practice may be a part of DBT sessions for BED, the program is more focused on understanding and problem solving eating difficulties that occur outside of sessions.

When applied to BED and BN, DBT involves adaptations to standard DBT to reflect the needs of these patient populations. Goals include decreasing mindless eating and binge eating, decreasing preoccupation with food, increasing adaptive options for regulating painful emotions, and avoiding/limiting focus on weight loss and weighing if this is problematic [86]. Relevant thoughts, emotions, and behaviors, including mindless eating episodes, are tracked on a daily diary card. Problematic mindless eating episodes are those deemed inappropriate, but without the sense of loss of control or excessive food consumption that characterizes a binge. Resources detailing DBT for BED and BN include an overview by Wiser and Telch [83] and case reports [87,88].

Several published studies, including RCTs, have examined DBT for disordered eating in individuals with and without obesity [89–91]. One study showed that 16 of the 18 women (89 percent) who received DBT no longer engaged in binge eating at the end of the 20-week treatment compared with 2 of the 16 wait list controls [89]. Safer and colleagues compared a 20-session DBT group to an active comparison group therapy (ACGT) for 101 individuals with BED [91]. The ACGT group used supportive strategies to enhance self-esteem and self-efficacy. Posttreatment binge abstinence and reductions in binge frequency were achieved more quickly for the DBT group than for the ACGT group. The DBT group also had fewer dropouts. However, there was a lack of differential effects between groups at the 3-, 6-, and 12-month follow-ups.

Acceptance and Commitment Therapy

Acceptance and commitment therapy (ACT) is a cognitive and behavioral intervention developed by Hayes, Strosahl, and Wilson [92,93]. It has been used with a variety of health conditions and psychological disorders, including chronic pain, depression, anxiety, psychosis, substance-use disorders, and eating disorders. The overall goal of ACT is to establish greater psychological flexibility [94,95]. Psychological flexibility is the ability to experience and accept the present moment more fully, whether pleasant or unpleasant, and to change or persist with behaviors when doing so serves one's chosen values [95,96]. This is accomplished by promoting acceptance and mindfulness with a commitment to one's values and goals. Values and goals then guide the process of behavior change. Acceptance and commitment therapy was developed within a pragmatic philosophy called *functional contextualism*, and it is centered on *relational frame theory*, a comprehensive theory of language and cognition stemming from behavior analysis [97].

From an ACT perspective, much of human suffering and psychological disorders emerge from the excessive use of language and thought, which produces cognitive fusion and experiential avoidance. Cognitive fusion is the tendency to interpret thoughts literally or stay in a problem-solving mode when it is unhelpful, and experiential avoidance is an attempt to escape or avoid aversive internal events such as unpleasant thoughts, emotions, memories, or physical sensations [93–95]. Overeating and disordered eating patterns are conceptualized in ACT as coping mechanisms that individuals develop to help them avoid distressing thoughts, emotions, or physical sensations. For instance, cognitive fusion may occur when individuals develop rigid dietary rules and are unable to respond effectively to internal cues, like hunger and satiety levels, or physiologic sensations associated with unpleasant emotions (e.g., depression, anxiety, boredom, anger). Experiential avoidance may be reflected in an obsessive focus on calories and food, overeating, loss of control, compensatory behaviors (excessive exercise, fasting, vomiting), or avoidance of difficult emotions or thoughts in the context of body image and weight [98]. When these two processes are present, they contribute to psychological inflexibility, characterized by the individual's inability to moderate various behavioral patterns (e.g., inaction or passivity, impulsivity, avoidance) in achieving valued actions [99]. Treatment in ACT, therefore, aims to foster psychological flexibility through six core processes: (1) acceptance, (2) cognitive defusion, (3) being present (mindfulness), (4) self as context, (5) values, and (6) committed action, which are all overlapping and interdependent [92,93].

In ACT, mindfulness is viewed as a combination of acceptance, defusion, self as context, and contact with the present moment. Mindfulness techniques are used in ACT to target cognitive fusion of thoughts about the body, cultivate moment-to-moment experiences, and increase acceptance of thoughts, feelings, and physical sensations as they arise. Acceptance and commitment therapy trains individuals to observe and notice present external and internal private events and then to label or describe them without overanalyzing, judging, or evaluating. It also teaches individuals to become aware of conditioned chains of behavior, which ultimately allows them to choose behaviors that correspond with their valued actions. Experiential exercises used in ACT to treat obesity and disordered eating include mindfulness of the breath, mindfulness of thoughts, appetite awareness monitoring [100], and mindful eating with raisins, chocolates, carrots, and pretzels [100–102]. The practice of mindful eating is a tool to help patients become aware of the deliberate food choices they make during unpleasant experiences (e.g., whether to eat the food and how much of it to eat). In addition, mindfulness provides an opportunity to engage in a valued action in the present moment. For instance, choosing whether to eat a carrot versus a piece of chocolate [102], rather than mindlessly eating or using food to escape or avoid internal events, is a mindful process.

Recent studies indicate that ACT may be an effective treatment for patients with obesity, BED, BN, and emotional eating. In a RCT, ACT has been shown to be effective for significantly improving disordered eating behaviors, body satisfaction, quality of life, and acceptance of weight-related thoughts in bariatric surgery patients [103]. One-day ACT workshops have also been shown to decrease body-related anxiety and eating pathology among women with body dissatisfaction [100] and to decrease binge eating episodes among adults with obesity [104]. Case-series studies indicated that 10 weekly sessions of ACT can significantly decrease binge eating and emotional eating episodes among individuals with obesity [101]. In addition, preliminary support has been found for the feasibility and effectiveness of acceptance-based behavioral interventions (ABI) for weight loss among adults who are overweight or obese [102–105].

While the literature on ACT for obesity, emotional eating, and binge eating is promising, more research is needed to determine the adequate length and format of ACT (e.g., workshop, short term, long term) for individuals with obesity. It would also be of importance to investigate the mediating effects of mindfulness versus other core processes in ACT in establishing psychological flexibility and increasing valued actions.

Qualities of a Mindfulness Facilitator and Training in Mindfulness-Based Interventions

Given that mindfulness-based interventions emphasize awareness and exploration through experiential learning in the present moment, it is integral that facilitators are able to engage the seven attitudinal characteristics of mindfulness practices. These include (1) nonjudging (being an impartial witness to one's experience), (2) patience (allowing experiences to unfold in their own time), (3) beginner's mind (approaching everything as if for the first time), (4) trust (developing a basic trust in one's own experiences and intuition), (5) nonstriving (allowing things to be as they are, without trying to change them in any way), (6) acceptance (appreciating things as they are in the present moment), and (7) letting go [12,106]. In order to embody these qualities, therapists and facilitators should have personal experience in mindfulness and professional training specific to the approach and be committed to a personal mindfulness practice [107–111]. In addition, clinicians delivering mindfulness-based interventions are expected to have relevant professional-level qualifications in psychology, medicine, or another health-related field. Through their personal practice, facilitators will naturally further develop their own awareness and experience with mindful eating and in everyday life, as well as through the program working with participants.

MB-EAT Practice with Cheese and Crackers: Practical Tips and Mindful Inquiry

Intention of the Practice

This MB-EAT practice was chosen to present a core approach to mindful eating because it illustrates the experiential foundation of helping clients feel more confident about and satisfied with eating richer types of food in small quantities. Many weight loss programs eliminate or greatly restrict high-fat, high-sugar, and processed foods from the diet. An alternative approach is to combine both inner and outer wisdom to decide when, what, and how to eat such foods, cultivating a healthier but flexible relationship with such foods [35]. This practice occurs in Session 2 of MB-EAT – prior to this mindfulness exercise, patients have experienced eating four raisins mindfully in Session 1 and practiced mindful meditation for one week.

Preparation for Group Session

Each participant should be provided with three pieces of cheese and crackers on a small plate. We recommend a small, good-quality wheat cracker and a good-quality commercially sliced cheese cut into small squares approximately the same size as the crackers. Check calories for each to inform the discussion after the practice and have the box/packaging available for the discussion but not visible prior to or during the practice. Mindfulness facilitators can also adapt this practice for individual psychotherapy or select a different type of desired or "trigger" food depending on the target population.

Style of Delivery

Facilitators are encouraged to read the following script slowly, pausing enough between instructions to give participants sufficient time to reflect on their moment-to-moment experiences. After the mindful eating practice, use open-ended questions when eliciting responses, practicing reflection rather than advice giving and adopting a nonjudgmental, accepting, curious, and nonstriving attitude.

Mindful Inquiry

Following the mindful eating practice, it is essential for the facilitator(s) to debrief the exercise with participants by engaging in a process called *mindful inquiry*. Inquiry is a dialogue between a facilitator and a participant that aids in the exploration of direct experiences arising from a mindfulness practice [112]. It overlaps with other techniques of exploration performed in various modes of psychotherapy or counseling, but with clearer intentions for connecting qualities of mindfulness. Furthermore, inquiry helps participants to foster reflecting, curiosity, compassion, and insight toward their experience in the present moment rather than generalized ideas or narratives [106]. Last, the process can build on a participant's inner and outer wisdom as it relates to food and eating and then integrate these insights back to the core themes of MB-EAT.

Facilitators new to MB-EAT can apply three layers or steps of inquiry/questions to a mindful eating practice [110,112,113]. Layer one involves inquiry into what transpired during the mindful eating practice (e.g., bodily sensations, thoughts, emotions). Layer two explores what was noticed in layer one within a wider context of understanding and linking them to habitual behaviors. Finally, layer three is an invitation to explore how experiences of mindfulness/mindful eating (learning from layers one and two) can be integrated into everyday life. An example script is provided below [35] and is followed by a conversation between two mindfulness facilitators and participants following a mindful eating practice with cheese and crackers.

Mindful Eating with Cheese and Crackers: Facilitator's Script

The intention of this meditation is to help you experience mindful eating by savoring a small amount of a more challenging food, and to observe any thoughts, feelings, or sensations that come from eating with curiosity, compassion, and a nonjudgmental attitude. This practice can also help you to cultivate a healthier relationship with food and to become aware of its nourishing and nurturing qualities.

Kindly take a few moments to settle into a relaxed sitting position with your feet placed flat on the floor and uncrossed. I am now going to give you a small plate with three pieces of cheese and crackers. While you are waiting, notice any thoughts or feelings you are having about this food or this practice [*wait to give further instructions until everyone has his or her plate*]. As you feel comfortable, gently close your eyes fully or partially. Take several deep breaths through your nose [*five-second pause*]. With each in breath, become centered and relaxed ... [*pause*]. On your next in breath, quickly scan your body from head to toe, and notice if there are areas in your body where you are holding tension. If so, breathe into these areas ... [*pause*]. Next, notice if there are areas in your body where you feel comfortable or relaxed. If so, breathe into these areas as well ... [*pause*]. Notice, without judgment, other feelings, experiences, or thoughts that are going through your mind, particularly any related to the food in front of you ... [*pause*]. Continue to be aware of any physical sensations in your body, and breathe into them ... [*pause*].

Now open your eyes, and remaining in a mindful space, take one cracker and piece of cheese. First, look at it carefully with fresh eyes ... [*pause*]. Now, closing your eyes, bring it up to your nose and smell it ... [*pause*]. Place it in your mouth or take a bite of it. Notice how it feels in your mouth. Before beginning to chew, move it around for a moment in your mouth, and notice the sensations ... [*pause*]. Now, beginning to chew, notice how the taste changes ... [*pause*]. As you slowly continue chewing this first bite, taking another bite to finish the cracker if needed, see if you notice any changes in the taste or other sensations ... [*pause*]. Resisting the urge to swallow ... [*pause*], savor the experience of this small piece of food ... honoring the satisfaction you experience from it ... [*pause*]. Notice how your body, thoughts, emotions, and mind react to this food ... [*long pause*], choosing to swallow ... [*pause*]. When you finish, notice how you feel ... [*pause*]. Notice any sensations still remaining in your mouth ... [*pause*]. Open your eyes enough to take a second cracker ... looking at this one ... [*pause*]. Now close your eyes, and again, smell it ... [*pause*]. Placing it in your mouth, experience the texture and taste before chewing, and then as you begin to slowly chew it ... [*pause*]. How is it the same, how is it different from the first cracker? ... [*pause*]. Enjoy it as much as possible ... [*pause*]. Notice any thoughts and feelings as they arise ... [*pause*]. Again, choose to swallow, and notice the experience of doing so ... [*pause*]. As you are ready, bring your awareness back to your breath ... [*pause*]. Does your body or mind want another cracker? ... [*pause*]. If so, help yourself to the last one, and lead yourself through eating it mindfully. If you are not eating, return your awareness to your breath ... [*pause*]. If you are eating, does this cracker taste or feel any different from the first two? ... [*pause*]. Whether you are eating the third cracker or not, notice your thoughts and your emotions ... [*pause*]. If you are eating, how is your body responding? ... [*pause*]. What are your thoughts now? ... [*pause*]. As you decide to swallow, appreciate that you are feeding your body a complex food to provide energy and create well-being ... [*pause*]. Appreciate for a moment the many hands that contributed to creating these little bites of food, growing and harvesting the ingredients, creating the food, even moving it to the stores ... [*pause*]. As you're finishing the third cracker, consider whether you would want a fourth one if it were available ... [*pause*]. What does that feel like? [*Wait to continue when everyone is finished.*] Now bring your awareness back to your breath ... back to your body ... back to the room ... and when you are ready, gently open your eyes.

Mindful Inquiry Dialogue

FACILITATOR 1: Let us start off by sharing what you noticed while eating the cheese and crackers mindfully, including any thoughts, emotions, or physical sensations. [*Layer one*]

PARTICIPANT 1: Well, my mind was racing with a lot of thoughts . . .

FACILITATOR 1: Would you be able to say what kinds of thoughts went through your mind?

PARTICIPANT 1: I thought about how crackers are bad for me . . . I remember having a bad binge three weeks ago where I ate most of a box of crackers with a brick of cheddar cheese . . . I couldn't stop eating . . .

FACILITATOR 1: It sounds like the thoughts and that memory made it hard for you to stay in the moment with the practice.

PARTICIPANT 2: I felt the same way, too! I couldn't focus on eating because I was worried that afterwards I was going to buy crackers and cheese on my way home and eat them all tonight.

FACILITATOR 1: So there were worries about something that might happen later. This is a nice example of how the practice was to eat the cheese and crackers mindfully in the present moment, yet the mind goes elsewhere, as in the future when you are on your way home or in the past with a bad binge eating episode. It is normal for the mind to jump to worries and to notice them when they come up. What did others notice?

PARTICIPANT 3: I enjoyed this exercise. I tasted the cheese, and it was very flavorful, and I also loved the crunch of the cracker. I was satisfied with the first piece, which lead me to eat the second piece, but the second piece didn't taste as good as the first one.

PARTICIPANT 4: For me, the two pieces were enough. I thought they were both delicious, but when I asked myself how much I wanted the third piece, I was really surprised that I didn't want it. I realized that I wasn't hungry, so I decided to stop eating. I don't think I've ever done that before!

FACILITATOR 1: These are lovely examples of how we can have similar and different experiences with the same type of food. For one person, the cheese and crackers might be really anxiety provoking, another person might enjoy it, and others still might have a mixture of emotions and thoughts. The intention of the mindful eating practice is to be open to whatever arises and to rely on your inner wisdom when it comes to food and eating, including your likes, dislikes, hunger levels, and satiety cues.

FACILITATOR 2: Can all of you use your outer wisdom to estimate the number of calories or nutritional content in each piece of cracker and cheese?

PARTICIPANT 1: Each piece must be at least 50 calories!

PARTICIPANT 2: I think it is closer to 40 calories.

PARTICIPANT 4: I am going to guess that it is 45 calories.

FACILITATOR 2: Each cracker is 9 calories; the piece of cheese is about 11, so the total is 20 calories [*whole group looks surprised*].

PARTICIPANT 1: I was worried over 20 calories!?

FACILITATOR 2: How was eating cheese and crackers in this way different from how you normally eat this type of food. [*Layer two*]

PARTICIPANT 5: If I were at home, I probably would have eaten a whole roll of crackers within 10 minutes without really tasting them . . . so just eating one piece was interesting.

FACILITATOR 2: What was interesting about it? What did you notice when you ate one piece versus eating a roll of crackers?

PARTICIPANT 5: Well, for starters, I tasted the flavor of the cheddar and the saltiness of the cracker. Slowing down made a difference. Looking back, I thought I enjoyed eating all those crackers, but I was eating too fast to even taste them, whereas I enjoyed eating just the two pieces today.

PARTICIPANT 7: I love cheese, and I always eat a plateful of assorted cheeses with crackers and grapes at dinner parties. But when we did the exercise, I didn't really like it. I don't know if it is this type of cheese, but when I paid attention to the flavor, I found the cheese very fatty and the cracker wasn't crunchy enough.

FACILITATOR 2: That sounds like a new experience for you, and once you paid attention, you didn't enjoy the food as much as you expected. By practicing mindful eating, you may notice that certain foods are no longer as enjoyable, and it is also possible to develop a relationship with food where you still eat the foods you like but enjoy them even more. We call it "cultivating your inner gourmet!"

FACILITATOR 1: How might eating in this way help you make better eating choices in the future or prevent overeating? [*Layer three*]

PARTICIPANT 5: I think just eating more slowly is a big takeaway for me. Really taking the time to taste what I'm eating will help me to stop eating sooner and maybe enjoy my food more. I'd probably eat less but feel more satisfied.

PARTICIPANT 6: I agree – eating slowly will be huge for me because right now I eat so fast that I don't realize I've eaten too much until afterwards when I feel stuffed.

PARTICIPANT 4: Paying attention to how hungry I am before and during eating will be a good tool for me. I think it will help me with portion control and knowing when to stop eating.

PARTICIPANT 1: Well, for now, I think I'll continue not having cheese and crackers in the house because it's preventing me from binging, but I think the next time I'm at a party where they have cheese and crackers, I'll eat a few pieces mindfully and see what that's like.

FACILITATOR 1: Okay, so we have some similarities and differences in how you want to incorporate mindful eating into your daily lives. It's going to take some time to figure out ways to make changes with this new skill that you are learning, and as with any other skill, it can take trial and error and patience. As best as you can, be curious, accepting, and compassionate with yourself as you continue to explore these mindfulness practices.

Case Vignette Revisited

Linda did very well in the program and was able to stop binge eating entirely. She also markedly reduced her scores on the Binge Eating Scale and increased her scores on a measure of "healthy" restraint. She was pleased with her weight loss of approximately 15 pounds. She noted that her husband had also lost some weight and had become comfortable with the healthier foods she was preparing and the smaller serving sizes. The hardest part for him was her refusal to bring full boxes or bags of snacks into the living room in the evening while they were watching TV. She noted that although she'd tried to get him to "mindfully" taste even very small amounts like she did, he didn't have the mindfulness training and so found it much harder to do. She did note that he had begun to talk more about not being "hungry" or not wanting to be too "full." Linda had also become aware of some of the very common triggers for her overeating, which included very large family meals, pressure to "clean her plate" as well as the serving bowls and platters, and using food both for handling emotional stress and for celebrating with her family. She had begun talking to a close sister about wanting her support in resisting some of these patterns when they were together. She had also begun bringing healthier foods to church events and was surprised to find that others appreciated this gesture. She had a more difficult time increasing her physical activity because she had little opportunity to walk at work or elsewhere during most days. But as she began using the pedometer and trying to meet the goal of increasing her steps just 10 percent per week, she gradually found more ways to do so. By the end of the program, she was climbing the two flights of stairs to her office instead of taking the elevator.

After surgery, Linda was surprised to discover how much less of a struggle she was having dealing with the restrictions than she had expected. This also continued to be the case as she moved into the period of adding foods back into her diet. "I've really lost my taste for most of the sweets I used to binge on. I'm a much pickier eater now! But in a good way!"

Summary

Mindfulness-based interventions have much to offer individuals living with obesity. They take an "inside-out" approach to help people learn to attend to their own bodily signals and food-related thoughts and emotions when making eating decisions. This inner wisdom or ability to self-regulate is often lost when individuals participate in numerous diets that dictate how much, when, and what to eat without encouraging them to consider their own needs and preferences. Mindfulness practice cultivates greater awareness of and attention to thoughts, emotions, bodily sensations, and other stimuli. When attended to in a nonjudgmental, curious way, this can lead to greater understanding of how one makes decisions about eating. This provides information to more flexibly respond to eating cues in a manner that is sustainable, internalized, and consistent with goals and values. Mindfulness explicitly encourages acceptance and self-compassion, qualities that can help counter shame and feelings of futility about weight loss and improved health. MB-EAT, DBT, and ACT are all evidence-based interventions that explicitly incorporate the theoretical and practical aspects of mindfulness skills. Mindfulness practice is the predominant feature of MB-EAT, whereas ACT and DBT both include mindfulness as part of a larger package of clinical techniques that have been used with a variety of populations and presenting problems.

Key Points

- Mindfulness practice can help individuals living with obesity to change their relationship to food by gaining nonjudgmental awareness of food-related thoughts, feelings, and bodily sensations.
- MB-EAT was developed specifically to address eating concerns typical of individuals who are overweight/obese and the related disordered eating patterns, whereas DBT and ACT have been adapted for individuals with these concerns.
- The results of research conducted on these approaches show their effectiveness in improving binge eating, emotional eating, and weight loss.

References

1. R. J. Davidon and A. W. Kaszniak. Conceptual and methodological issues in research on mindfulness and meditation. *Am Psychol* 2015; **70**: 581–92.

2. J. L. Kristeller. Mindfulness. In S. Ayers, C. Llewellyn, C. McManus, et al., eds., *Cambridge Handbook of Psychology, Health and Medicine* (3rd edn). Cambridge: Cambridge University Press (in press).

3. G. A Marlatt and J. L Kristeller. Mindfulness and meditation. In W. D. Miller, ed., *Integrating Spirituality into Treatment: Resources for Practitioners.* Washington, DC: American Psychological Association, 1999: 67–84.

4. J. Kabat-Zinn. *Wherever You Go, There You Are: Mindfulness Meditation in Everyday Life.* New York, NY: Hyperion, 1994.

5. S. Jain, S. L. Shapiro, S. Swanick, et al. A randomized controlled trial of mindfulness meditation versus relaxation training: Effects on distress, positive states of mind, rumination, and distraction. *Ann Behav Med* 2007; **33**: 11–21.

6. P. Ekman, R. J. Davidson, M. Ricard, et al. Buddhist and psychological perspectives on emotions and well-being. *Curr Dir Psychol Sci* 2005; **14**: 59–63.

7. K. D. Neff. The science of self-compassion. In C. K. Germer and R. D. Siegel, eds., *Wisdom and Compassion in Psychotherapy: Deepening Mindfulness in Clinical Practice.* New York, NY: Guilford Press, 2012: 79–92.

8. S. Sauer and R. A. Baer. Mindfulness and decentering as mechanisms of change in mindfulness- and acceptance-based interventions. In R. A. Baer and R. A. Baer, eds., *Assessing Mindfulness and Acceptance Processes in Clients: Illuminating the Theory and Practice of Change.* Oakland, CA: Context Press/New Harbinger Publications, 2010: 25–50.

9. S. C. Hayes and K. G. Wilson. Mindfulness: Method and process. *Clin Psychol* 2003; **10**: 161–5.

10. J. Quaglia, S. Braun, S. Freeman, et al. Meta-analytic evidence for effects of mindfulness training on dimensions of self-reported dispositional mindfulness. *Psychol Assessment* 2016; **28**: 803–18.

11. J. Kabat-Zinn. An outpatient program in behavioral medicine for chronic pain patients based on the practice of mindfulness meditation: Theoretical considerations and preliminary results. *Gen Hosp Psychiatry* 1982; **4**: 33–47.

12. J. Kabat-Zinn. *Full Catastrophe Living: Using The Wisdom of Your Body and Mind to Face Stress, Pain, and Illness.* New York, NY: Delta Trade Paperbacks, 1990.

13. Z. V. Segal, J. M. G. Williams, and J. D. Teasdale. *Mindfulness-Based Cognitive Therapy for Depression: A New Approach to Preventing Relapse.* New York, NY: Guilford Press, 2002.

14. J. D. Teasdale, Z. V. Segal, J. M. G. Williams, et al. Prevention of relapse/recurrence in major depression by mindfulness-based cognitive therapy. *J Consult Clin Psych* 2000; **68**: 615–23.

15. J. Piet and E. Jougaard. The effect of mindfulness-based cognitive therapy for prevention of relapse in recurrent major depressive disorder: A systematic review and meta-analysis. *Clin Psychol Rev* 2011; **31**: 1032–40.

16. S. Bowen, N. Chawla, and G. A. Marlatt. *Mindfulness-Based Relapse Prevention for Addictive Behaviors: A Clinician's Guide.* New York, NY: Guilford Press, 2010.

17. J. Kristeller. *The Joy of Half a Cookie: Using Mindfulness to Lose Weight and End the Struggle with Food.* New York, NY: Penguin Books, 2015.

18. S. C. Hayes. Acceptance and commitment therapy, relationship frame theory, and the third way of behavioural and cognitive therapies. *Behav Ther* 2004; **35**: 639–65.

19. B. Wansink. *Mindless Eating: Why We Eat More Than We Think.* New York, NY: Bantam Books, 2010.

20. B. Wansink and J. Sobal. Mindless eating: The 200 daily food decisions we overlook. *Environ Behav* 2007; **39**: 106–23.

21. W. K. Simmons and D. C. DeVille. Interoceptive contributions to healthy

eating and obesity. *Curr Opin Psychol* 2017; **17**: 106–12.

22. R. E. Cole and T. Horacek. Effectiveness of the "My Body Knows When" intuitive-eating pilot program. *Am J Health Behav* 2010; **34**: 286–97.

23. E. Tribole and E. Resch. *Intuitive Eating: A Revolutionary Program That Works.* New York, NY: St. Martin's Griffin, 2003.

24. L. Bacon. *Health at Every Size: The Surprising Truth about Your Weight.* Dallas, TX: BanBella Books, 2010.

25. G. E. Schwartz. Biofeedback, self-regulation, and the patterning of physiological processes. *Am Sci* 1975; **63**: 314–24.

26. C. P. Herman and J. Polivy. A boundary model for the regulation of eating. *Psychiat Ann* 1983; **13**: 918–27.

27. J. Rodin. Current status of the internal-external hypothesis for obesity: What went wrong? *Am Psychol* 1981; **36**: 361–72.

28. S. Schachter and J. Rodin. *Obese Humans and Rats.* Oxford: Lawrence Erlbaum, 1974.

29. S. L. Shapiro and G. E. R. Schwartz. Intentional systemic mindfulness: An integrative model for self-regulation and health. *Adv Mind Body Med* 2000; **16**: 128–34.

30. S. S. Khalsa, D. Rudrauf, A. R. Damasio, et al. Interoceptive awareness in experienced meditators. *Psychophysiology* 2008; **45**: 671–7.

31. E. D. Capaldi. ed. *Why We Eat What We Eat: The Psychology of Eating.* Washington, DC: American Psychological Association, 1996.

32. J. Ogden. *The Psychology of Eating: From Healthy to disordered behavior* (2nd edn). New York, NY: Wiley-Blackwell, 2010.

33. C. S. Carver and M. F. Scheier. *On the Self-Regulation of Behavior.* New York, NY: Cambridge University Press, 1998.

34. J. L. Kristeller and E. Epel. Mindful eating and mindless eating. In A. Ie, C. Ngnoumen, and E. Langer, eds., *The Wiley Blackwell Handbook of*

Mindfulness. New York, NY: Wiley-Blackwell, 2014: 913–33.

35. J. Kristeller and R. Wolever. *Mindfulness-Based Eating Awareness Training (MB-EAT): A Treatment Manual.* New York, NY: Guilford Press (in press).

36. R. J. Sternberg. A balance theory of wisdom. *Rev Gen Psychol* 1998; **2**: 347–65.

37. P. B. Baltes and U. M. Staudinger. Wisdom: A metaheuristic (pragmatic) to orchestrate mind and virtue toward excellence. *Am Psychol* 2000; **55**: 122–36.

38. B. D. Ostafin and K. T. Kassman. Stepping out of history: Mindfulness improves insight problem solving. *Conscious And Cogn* 2012; **21**: 1031–6.

39. D. Goleman and R. J. Davidson. *Altered Traits: Science Reveals How Meditation Changes Your Mind, Brain, and Body.* New York, NY: Penguin Random House, 2017.

40. J. L. Kristeller. Mindfulness, wisdom, and eating: Applying a multi-domain model of meditation effects. *Construct Hum Sci* 2003; **8**: 107–18.

41. T. W. Meeks, B. R. Cahn, and D. V. Jeste. Neurobiological foundations of wisdom. In C. K. Germer and R. D. Siegel, eds., *Wisdom and Compassion in Psychotherapy: Deepening Mindfulness in Clinical Practice.* New York, NY: Guilford Press, 2012: 189–201.

42. L. Sobik, K. Hutchison, and L. Craighead. Cue-elicited craving for food: A fresh approach to the study of binge eating. *Appetite* 2005; **44**: 253–61.

43. G. S. Goldfield, K. B. Adamo, J. Rutherford, et al. Stress and the relative reinforcing value of food in female binge eaters. *Physiol Behav* 2008, **93**: 579–87.

44. J. L. Kristeller and J. Rodin. Identifying eating patterns in male and female undergraduates using cluster analysis. *Addict Behav* 1989; **14**: 631–42.

45. L. M. Bartoshuk. The psychophysics of taste. *Am J Clin Nutr* 1978; **31**: 1068–77.

46. L. M Bartoshuk and D. J. Snyder. The biology and psychology of taste. In K. D. Brownell and M. S. Gold, eds.,

Food and Addiction: A Comprehensive Handbook. New York, NY: Oxford University Press, 2012; 126–30.

47. A. Geliebter and S. A. Hashim. Gastric capacity in normal, obese, and bulimic women. *Physiol Behav* 2001; **74**: 743–6.

48. A. Geliebter, S. A. Hashim, and M. E. Gluck. Appetite-related gut peptides, ghrelin, PYY, and GLP-1 in obese women with and without binge eating disorder (BED). *Physiol Behav* 2008; **94**: 696–9.

49. R. Sysko, M. J. Devlin, B. T. Walsh, et al. Satiety and test meal intake among women with binge eating disorder. *Int J Eat Disorder* 2007; **40**: 554–61.

50. A. K. Remick, J. Polivy, and P. Pliner. Internal and external moderators of the effect of variety on food intake. *Psychol Bull* 2009; **135**: 434–51.

51. L. B. Sørensen, P. Møller, A. Flint, et al. Effect of sensory perception of foods on appetite and food intake: A review of studies on humans. *Int J Obesity* 2003; **27**: 1152–66.

52. H. A. Raynor and L. H. Epstein. Dietary variety, energy regulation, and obesity. *Psychol Bull* 2001; **127**: 325–41.

53. L. Brondel, M. Romer, V. Van Wymelbeke, et al. Sensory-specific satiety with simple foods in humans: No influence of BMI? *Int J Obesity* 2007; **31**: 987–95.

54. M. Grosshans, S. Loeber, and F. Kiefer. Implications from addiction research towards the understanding and treatment of obesity. *Addict Biol* 2011; **16**: 189–98.

55. A. Drewnowski. The behavioral phenotype in human obesity. In E. D. Capaldi and E. D. Capalidi, eds., *Why We Eat What We Eat: The Psychology of Eating*. Washington, DC: American Psychological Association, 1996: 291–308.

56. J. L. Kristeller and R. Q. Wolever. Mindfulness-based eating awareness training for treating binge eating disorder: The conceptual foundation. *Eat Disord* 2011; **19**: 49–61.

57. G. A. Marlatt and D. M. Donovan. *Relapse Prevention: Maintenance Strategies in the Treatment of Addictive Behaviors* (2nd edn). New York, NY: Guilford Press, 2005.

58. D. R. Vago and F. Zeidan. The brain on silent: Mind wandering, mindful awareness, and states of mental tranquility. *Ann NY Acad Sci* 2016; **1373**: 96–113.

59. D. M. Thomas, C. K. Martin, S. Lettieri, et al. Can a weight loss of one pound a week be achieved with a 3,500-kcal deficit? Commentary on a commonly accepted rule. *Int J Obesity* 2013; **37**: 1611–3.

60. J. L. Kristeller and C. B. Hallett. An exploratory study of a meditation-based intervention for binge eating disorder. *J Health Psychol* 1999; **4**: 357–63.

61. J. Gormally, S. Black, S. Daston, et al. The assessment of binge eating severity among obese persons. *Addict Behav* 1982; 7: 47–55.

62. J. L. Kristeller, R. Q. Wolever, and V. Sheets. Mindfulness-Based Eating Awareness Training (MB-EAT) for binge eating: A randomized clinical trial. *Mindfulness* 2014; **5**: 282–97.

63. A. J. Stunkard and S. Messick. The three-factor eating questionnaire to measure dietary restraint, disinhibition and hunger. *J Psychosom Res* 1985; **29**: 71–83.

64. J. L. Kristeller, K. Jordan, and K. Bolinskey. Mindfulness-Based Eating Awareness Training (MB-EAT) for weight loss: A randomized clinical trial (under review).

65. C. K. Miller, J. L. Kristeller, A. Headings, et al. Comparison of a mindful eating intervention to a diabetes self-management intervention among adults with type 2 diabetes: A randomized controlled trial. *Health Educ Behav* 2014; **41**: 145–54.

66. C. K Miller, J. L. Kristeller, A. Headings, et al. Comparative effectiveness of a mindful eating intervention to a diabetes self-management intervention among adults with type 2 diabetes: A pilot study. *J Acad Nutr Diet* 2012; **112**: 1835–42.

67. J. Daubenmier, P. J. Moran, J. Kristeller, et al. Effects of a mindfulness-based weight loss intervention in adults with obesity: A randomized clinical trial. *Obesity* 2016; **24**: 794–804.

68. V. A. Barnes, J. L. Kristeller, and M. H. Johnson. Impact of mindfulness-based eating awareness on diet and exercise habits in adolescents. *J Altern Complement Med* 2016; **3**: 70.

69. D. B. Sarwar, R. J. Dilks, and L. West-Smith. Dietary intake and eating behavior after bariatric surgery: Threats to weight loss maintenance and strategies for success. *Surg Obes Relat Dis* 2011; 7: 644–51.

70. J. Odom, K. C. Zalesin, T. L. Washington, et al. Behavioural predictors of weight regain after bariatric surgery. *Obes Surg* 2010; **20**: 349–56.

71. K. B. Grothe, P. M. Dubbert, and J. R. O'Jile. Psychological assessment and management of the weight loss surgery patient. *Am J Med Sci* 2006; **331**: 201–6.

72. M. Zimmerman, C. Francione-Witt, I. Chelminski, et al. Presurgical psychiatric evaluations of candidates for bariatric surgery, part 1: Reliability and reasons for and frequency of exclusion. *J Clin Psychiatry* 2007; **68**: 1557–62.

73. J. E. Mitchell, N. J. Christian, D. R. Flum, et al. Postoperative behavioral variables and weight change three years after bariatric surgery. *JAMA Surgery* 2016; **151**: 752–7.

74. M. A. Kalarchian, T. G. Wilson, R. E. Brolin, et al. Binge eating in bariatric surgery patients. *Int J Eat Disord* 1998; **23**: 89–92.

75. R. Saunders, L. Johnson, and J. Teschner. Prevalence of eating disorders among bariatric surgery patients. *Eat Disord* 1998; **6**: 309–17.

76. F. Stewart and A. Avenell. Behavioural interventions for severe obesity before and/or after bariatric surgery: A systematic review and meta-analysis. *Obes Surg* 2016; **26**: 1203–14.

77. T. M. Leahey, J. H. Crowther, and S. R. Irwin. A cognitive-behavioural mindfulness group therapy intervention for the treatment of binge eating in bariatric surgery patients. *Cogn Behav Pract* 2008; **15**: 364–75.

78. S. A. Chacko, G. Y. Yeh, R. B. Davis, et al. A mindfulness-based intervention to control weight after bariatric surgery: Preliminary results from a randomized controlled pilot trial. *Complement Ther Med* 2016; **28**: 13–21.

79. S. M. Wnuk, C. D. Du, J. Van Exan, et al. Mindfulness-based eating and awareness training for post-bariatric surgery patients: A feasibility pilot study. *Mindfulness* 2017, https://doi.org/10.1007/s12671-017-0834-7.

80. M. M. Linehan. *Cognitive-Behavioural Treatment of Borderline Personality Disorder*. New York, NY: Guilford Press, 1993.

81. T. F. Heatherton and R. F. Baumeister. Binge eating as escape from self-awareness. *Psychol Bull* 1991; **110**: 86–108.

82. J. Polivy and P. Herman. Etiology of binge eating: Psychological mechanisms. In C. G. Fairburn and G. T. Wilson, eds., *Binge Eating: Nature, Assessment, and Treatment*. New York, NY: Guilford Press, 1993: 173–205.

83. S. Wiser and C. F. Telch. Dialectical behaviour therapy for binge eating disorder. *J Clin Psychol* 1999; **55**: 755–68.

84. S. McMain, J. H. R. Sayrs, L. A. Dimeff, et al. Dialectical behavior therapy for individuals with borderline personality disorder and substance dependence. In L. A. Dimeff and K. Koerner, *Dialectical Behaviour Therapy in Clinical Practice*. New York, NY: Guilford Press, 2007: 145–73.

85. S. Bowen and A. Marlatt. Surfing the urge: Brief mindfulness-based intervention for college student smokers. *Psychol Addict Behav* 2009; **23**: 666–71.

86. L. Wisniewski, D. Safer, and E. Chen. Dialectical behaviour therapy and eating disorders. In L. A. Dimeff and K. Koerner, eds., *Dialectical Behaviour Therapy in Clinical Practice: Applications across Disorders and Settings*. New York, NY: Guilford Press, 2007: 174–221.

87. C. F. Telch. Skills training treatment for adaptive affect regulation in a woman with binge-eating disorder. *Int J Eat Disord* 1997; **22**: 7–81.

88. D. L. Safer, C. F. Telch, and W. S. Agras. Dialectical behaviour therapy for bulimia nervosa: A case study. *Int J Eat Disord* 2001; **30**: 101–6.

89. C. F. Telch, W. S. Agras, and M. M. Linehan. Dialectical behaviour therapy for binge eating disorder. *J Clin Psychol* 2001; **69**: 1061–5.

90. C. F. Telch, W. S. Agras, and M. M. Linehan. Group dialectical behaviour therapy for binge-eating disorder: A preliminary, uncontrolled trial. *Behav Ther* 2000; **31**: 569–82.

91. D. L. Safer, A. H. Robinson, and B. Jo. Outcome from a randomized controlled trial of group therapy for binge eating disorder: Comparing dialectical behaviour therapy adapted for binge eating to an active comparison group therapy. *Behav Ther* 2010; **41**: 106–20.

92. S. C. Hayes, K. D. Stroshal, and K. G. Wilson. *Acceptance and Commitment Therapy: The process and practice of Mindful Change* (1st edn). New York, NY: Guildford Press, 1999.

93. S. C. Hayes, K. D. Stroshal, and K. G. Wilson. *Acceptance and Commitment Therapy: The Process and Practice of Mindful Change* (2nd edn). New York, NY: Guildford Press, 2012.

94. S. C. Hayes. Acceptance and Commitment Therapy and the new behavior therapies: mindfulness, acceptance, and relationship. In S. C. Hayes, V. M. Follette, and M. Linehan, eds., *Mindfulness and Acceptance: Expanding the Cognitive-Behavioral Tradition*. New York, NY: Guilford Press, 2004.

95. S. C. Hayes, M. Levin, J. Vilardaga, et al. Acceptance and commitment therapy and contextual behavioral science: Examining the progress of a distinctive model of behavioral and cognitive therapy. *Behav Ther* 2013; **44**: 180–98.

96. K. G. Wilson and A. R. Murrell. Values work in Acceptance and Commitment

Therapy: Setting a course for behavioral treatment. In S. C. Hayes, V. M. Follette, and M. Linehan, eds., *Mindfulness and Acceptance: Expanding the Cognitive-Behavioral Tradition*. New York, NY: Guilford Press, 2004: 120–51.

97. S. C. Hayes, D. Barnes-Holmes, and B. Roche, eds. *Relational Frame Theory: A Post-Skinnerian Account of Human Language and Cognition*. New York, NY: Plenum Press, 2001.

98. R. M. Merwin and K. G. Wilson. Understanding and treating eating disorders: An ACT perspective. In J. T. Blackledge, J. Ciarrochi, and F. P. Deane, eds., *Acceptance and Commitment Therapy: Contemporary Theory Research and Practice*. Sydney: Australian Academic Press, 2009: 87–118.

99. S. C. Hayes, J. B. Luoma, F. W. Bond, et al. Acceptance and commitment therapy: Model, processes, and outcomes. *Behav Res Ther* 2006; **44**: 1–25.

100. A. Pearson, V. Follette, and S. Hayes. A pilot study of acceptance and commitment therapy as a workshop intervention for body dissatisfaction and disordered eating attitudes. *Cogn Behav Pract* 2012; **19**: 181–97.

101. M. L. Hill, A. Masuda, H. Melcher, et al. Acceptance and commitment therapy for women diagnosed with binge eating disorder: A case-series study. *Cogn Behav Pract* 2015; **22**: 367–78.

102. E. Forman, M. Butryn, K. Hoffman, et al. An open trial of an acceptance-based intervention for weight loss. *Cogn Behav Pract* 2009; **16**: 223–35.

103. S. Weineland, D. Arvidsson, T. Kakoulidis, et al. Acceptance and commitment therapy for bariatric surgery patients: A pilot RCT. *Obes Res Clin Pract* 2012; **6**: e21–30.

104. J. Lillis, S. Hayes, K. Bunting, et al. Teaching acceptance and mindfulness to improve the lives of the obese: A preliminary test of a theoretical model. *Ann Behav Med* 2009; **37**: 58–69.

105. H. M. Niemeier, T. Leahey, K. P. Reed, et al. An acceptance-based behavioral

intervention for weight loss: A pilot study. *Behav Ther* 2012; **43**: 427–35.

106. J. Kabat-Zinn. *Full Catastrophe Living: Using the Wisdom of Your Body and Mind to Face Stress, Pain, and Illness* (2nd edn). New York, NY: Random House, 2013.

107. R. S. Crane, S. Stanley, M. Rooney, et al. Disciplined improvisation: Characteristics of inquiry in mindfulness-based teaching. *Mindfulness* 2015; **6**: 1104–14.

108. A. Evans, R. Crane, L. Cooper, et al. A framework for supervision for mindfulness-based teachers: A space for embodied mutual inquiry. *Mindfulness* 2015; **6**: 572–81.

109. S. L. Woods. Training professionals in mindfulness: the heart of teaching. In F. Didonna, ed., *Clinical Handbook of Mindfulness*. New York, NY: Springer. 2010: 463–75.

110. S. L. Woods. Building a framework for mindful inquiry, 2013. Available at https://slwoods.com/wp-content/uplo ads/2016/02/aframeworkformindfulin quirydec2012.pdf (accessed November 27, 2017).

111. J. L. Kristeller and A. E. Lieberstein. Teaching individuals mindful eating. In D. R. D. McCown and M. S. Micozzi, eds., *Resources for Teaching Mindfulness: An International Handbook*. New York, NY: Springer, 2016: 359–79.

112. S. L. Woods, P. Rockman, and C. Evans. A contemplative dialogue: the inquiry process in mindfulness-based interventions, 2016. Available at www .mindfulnessstudies.com/wp-content/upl oads/2016/02/Woods-S.-L.-Rockman-P.- Collins-E.-2016-A-Complentative- Dialogue.pdf (accessed November 27, 2017).

113. Z. V. Segal, J. M. G. Williams, and J. D. Teasdale. *Mindfulness-Based Cognitive Therapy for Depression: A New Approach to Preventing Relapse* (2nd edn). New York, NY: Guilford Press, 2013.

Chapter 11

Compassion-Focused Therapy in Severe Obesity

Jacqueline C. Carter, Kerri Bojman, and Allison C. Kelly

Case Vignette

Sarah is a 41-year-old single woman who lives alone and is employed as a nurse at a general hospital. She is currently on sick leave related to her struggles with depression. She has never been married and does not have children. At the first appointment she stated, "I spend a lot of time alone." Her main concerns are described as overeating and difficulty controlling her weight. Her body mass index (BMI) is 43 kg/m². On a typical day, her eating is quite controlled while at work, but after work she experiences intense urges to overeat and usually stops for large quantities of takeout food on the way home. She states, "I feel like sometimes I have no control over my eating or my weight, and this makes me feel horrible about myself." Sarah also speaks of difficulties with assertiveness, particularly at work, and with social anxiety. She has been feeling bullied by an outspoken coworker but feels unable to stand up for herself. "It's like I have a huge lump in my throat, and I can't speak." Growing up, her mother was passive and quiet, and her father was described as a judgmental, critical, and unpredictable man who struggled with alcohol abuse. Her mother's weight had always been in the normal range, whereas her father was always overweight. As a child and adolescent, Sarah was terrified to speak around her father because he would criticize her, calling her "stupid" and telling her to "keep her mouth shut." She first began to overeat in secret as a child, and by the time she reached adolescence, she was significantly overweight and was teased by her peers about her weight in school. Sarah has continued to gain weight since then and reports that feelings of shame about her weight have caused her to isolate herself over the years. Fear of judgment and rejection has led her to avoid social situations and to avoid expressing her views at work. Currently, Sarah binge eats nearly every night on large quantities of fast food that she uses to "stuff down [her] feelings" and to fill a void inside herself. Afterwards, she experiences intense feelings of guilt and shame and increased worries about her weight. She says that she never feels full or satisfied after binges. She reports intense self-criticism after overeating and feels disgusted by her body size and shape. She frequently calls herself "fat" and blames herself for her loss of control over eating and her weight problems.

Introduction

In this chapter, we present an overview of compassion-focused therapy (CFT) and discuss the relevance of this approach for patients with severe obesity. Next, we describe a number of CFT strategies and exercises that may be useful for healthcare practitioners working with individuals to manage severe obesity [1–3]. These include CFT case formulation, psychoeducation, breathing meditations, thought records aimed at fostering more compassionate thinking, compassionate letter writing, and compassionate visualization. Finally, relevant research supporting the usefulness of CFT interventions for patients with obesity is reviewed. Throughout the chapter, we present examples of implementing the various CFT strategies based on the Case Vignette.

Compassion-Focused Therapy

Compassion-focused therapy (CFT) is a transdiagnostic and integrative therapeutic approach that was developed to help individuals who suffer from high levels of self-criticism, shame, and self-directed hostility [4]. The approach was designed to help shame-prone individuals increase access to affiliative feelings such as warmth and reassurance by helping them to increase their capacities for receiving compassion from others and having compassion both for self and others [1,5]. *Compassion*, which is defined as both a sensitivity to the suffering of self and others and a motivation to help alleviate or prevent it, is thought to promote the feelings of reassurance and warmth that are necessary to lower self-criticism and shame, facilitate healthy emotion regulation, and promote adaptive behavior change [1,4]. Gilbert observed that our evolved brains make it possible for us to relate to ourselves in the same type of caring and compassionate manner that others might relate to us during difficult times [6]. Of note, CFT is not meant to be a stand-alone treatment but rather is designed to be integrated into disorder-specific interventions such as cognitive-behavior therapy (CBT; see Chapters 8 and 9). The idea is that all psychotherapeutic tasks are approached from a compassionate mind-set, and only through this mind-set can these tasks provide more lasting relief from shame, self-criticism, and the symptoms they under-pin such as depression or overeating [6].

Drawing on evolutionary psychology, neuroscience research, attachment theory, and CBT, CFT posits that humans have evolved to have three distinct yet interacting emotion regulation systems: the threat system, the drive system, and the soothing system [7]. The threat system is oriented toward signs of danger in the environment. In response to a real or perceived threat, this system generates feelings such as fear, anger, and/or shame and promotes defensive behaviors such as withdrawal or aggression. It is thought that real or imagined criticism from others, as well as self-criticism, activates this system. Therefore, in the case of obesity, weight stigma or negative body image thoughts may activate this system. The drive system motivates individuals to acquire evolutionarily important resources, including status and respect from others. In response to experiences of success, this system produces feelings of excitement and pride and promotes continued striving [8]. Importantly, imagining oneself as successful in others' eyes and/or praising oneself stimulates these same responses. Therefore, successful weight loss or food restriction may activate this system. Finally, the soothing system is activated by signs that one is safe, and also in response to signals of compassion and caring from others. This system is also activated in response to images and memories of others as compassionate, as well as self-generated care and compassion. When the soothing system is active, it promotes feelings of safeness, soothing, calmness, and contentedness, as well as behaviors aimed at social connection and trust [8]. Of note, some individuals might come to rely on food and eating to temporarily activate their soothing systems, but unlike affiliation and compassion, these methods of self-soothing can result in self-criticism and shame, which can make those individuals vulnerable to more overeating [2]. Individuals who struggle with shame and self-criticism are thought to have an overactive threat system and an underactive soothing system due to early negative experiences such as criticism, neglect, or abuse and/or the absence of warmth and affection. From a CFT perspective, in order for these individuals to overcome their difficulties, they must learn to access feelings of safeness and connectedness as a primary way of regulating feelings of distress and shame [9]. It is through developing their capacities for compassion that this becomes possible. This is the rationale for CFT strategies.

Gilbert developed CFT specifically to help shame-prone individuals access the soothing, affiliative emotions that are viewed as necessary for shame and self-criticism to abate and for healthy affect regulation to develop [1,8]. The main goal of CFT is therefore to cultivate a more compassionate and caring way of relating to oneself and others and to become more receptive to compassion and caring from other people. Various compassionate mind training exercises are used to help self-critical and shame-prone patients pay attention, think, feel, and behave in a way that promotes compassionate relationships with others and with themselves.

Shame and Obesity

Gilbert defines *shame* as a painful self-conscious emotion triggered and perpetuated by perceiving oneself as flawed (internal shame) and believing that others share this view (external shame) [1]. Studies suggest that individuals with obesity struggle with high levels of shame [10,11]. This may be due to the influence of Western culture on beauty standards, since it is filled with messages of idealized images of how we should look, making it inevitable for people to internalize this thin ideal and subsequently feel like they do not measure up. Pressures to diet and lose weight are pervasive, while at the same time environmental factors actually promote a high level of food consumption and a sedentary lifestyle.

Weight-based stigma refers to negative attitudes or behaviors toward people based on their body weight or shape [12–15] (see Chapter 3). Individuals with obesity commonly experience weight-based stigma, including negative stereotypes and attributions of blame, which tend to be internalized as weight-related self-criticism, body shame, and negative social comparisons contributing to feelings of inferiority and inadequacy [10,11,16]. Shame and self-criticism have been linked to a wide variety of mental health problems [6]. Further, growing evidence suggests that self-criticism and shame predict worse weight management outcomes. In a recent cross-sectional study, Duarte and colleagues found that higher levels of weight-focused shame, self-criticism, and feelings of inferiority were all significantly associated with greater difficulties controlling eating behavior as well as poorer weight loss outcomes in a sample of individuals with obesity attending a community-based behavioral weight loss program [16]. The relationship between shame and loss of control over eating was mediated by weight-related negative affect. Further, higher self-reassurance and favorable social comparisons predicted better weight loss outcomes. These findings suggest that self-criticism, shame, and feelings of inferiority may make long-term weight control more difficult by making it more challenging for patients to stick to weight management plans.

Weight-based stigma and weight-related self-criticism can trigger depressed feelings and social withdrawal, thereby making people more vulnerable to engaging in further maladaptive behaviors like overeating [17]. Evidence for the negative impact of self-criticism on weight loss outcome was uncovered in a qualitative study of men and women taking part in weight loss treatment [18]. The results suggested that when setbacks were met with self-criticism rather than self-caring, poorer weight loss outcomes were observed. Further evidence of the negative impact of shame on weight loss outcomes emerged in a recent longitudinal study of individuals with obesity [19]. In this study, shame appeared to fuel weight loss behaviors in the short term by motivating individuals to be seen less critically by self and others. However, over time, this pressured form of motivation appeared to undermine rather than sustain the continued effort needed to maintain weight loss because the strength of the shame–weight loss relationship decreased over time. Thus successful weight loss may initially provide feelings of pride that may temporarily reduce and/or distract from underlying feelings of shame, but the relief may be brief. Shame is unlikely to provide sustained motivation for weight loss.

Recognizing that weight-based stigma can contribute to shame and self-criticism in individuals with obesity and adversely affect health outcomes, a CFT approach appears to be highly relevant to the management of severe obesity. In support of this idea, Hilbert and colleagues found that self-compassion partially mediated the relationship between self-criticism and poor mental and physical health in a sample of individuals with obesity, suggesting that increasing the capacity for self-compassion in these individuals may improve health-related quality of life [20].

Compassion-Focused Treatment Strategies

In this section, we describe a number of key CFT strategies that may be useful for healthcare practitioners working with individuals to manage severe obesity. These exercises include CFT case formulation, psychoeducation, breathing meditations, thought records aimed at fostering more compassionate thinking, compassionate letter writing, and compassionate visualization [1,17].

Patients who feel overwhelmed by threat, such as those high in self-criticism, tend to have limited access to soothing or supportive memories. Not surprisingly, this interferes with their ability to self-soothe [4]. CFT uses interventions that focus on deepening the capacity to self-soothe and to feel compassion toward oneself and others. For this to occur, it is necessary for patients to feel compassion on an experiential level [3]. Given that CFT is meant to be integrated into empirically supported treatments for a given disorder, key CBT principles and interventions are still essential when using CFT strategies with patients who struggle to control their eating or weight [21,22] (see Chapters 8 and 9). Integrating CFT involves an explicit focus on approaching all interventions with a compassionate mind-set and with the aim of activating patients' soothing system.

Compassion-Focused Case Formulation

Drawing on Goss and Allan's adaptation of CFT for eating disorders, the CFT therapist helps the patient to develop a functional analysis of his or her weight problem through the lens of the tripartite model of affect regulation [17]. The therapist works collaboratively with the patient to identify the origins and functions of the patient's self-criticism, shame, and associated symptoms (e.g., overeating) with the goal of helping him or her recognize the initially adaptive nature of these patterns so as to replace self-blame with self-compassion [1]. For example, in the case of Sarah, her comfort eating began as a child to help her cope with the fear and shame she felt when her father was hostile toward her. Through her psychotherapy, she became aware of how her childhood experiences made her hypervigilant to threat and led her to develop a highly activated threat system, which, in turn, contributed to increased self-criticism and shame. Sarah came to understand how she was caught in a vicious cycle of self-criticism and shame that triggered overeating to comfort herself but which perpetuated further self-deprecation and shame. Thus self-criticism and shame both triggered and maintained her binge eating episodes. Sarah also came to understand how social isolation and depression fueled this cycle. Feelings of shame about her weight led her to avoid social situations, and food became a way to comfort herself and fill the void caused by isolation and loneliness. Through this type of functional analysis, patients come to recognize how self-criticism is actually maintaining their weight problem and how increasing their access to affiliation and social connection could help to interrupt the cycle. In Sarah's case, she came to realize the link between her tendency to be self-critical and her reliance on binge eating to cope with the feelings of shame produced by her self-criticism. In CFT, patients also come to understand how associated symptoms (e.g., non-assertiveness) are related to activation of the threat system, associated safety behaviors (e.g., avoidance), and unintended consequences (e.g., isolation). The patient is helped to see that for most people, care, support, and encouragement are more motivating than scorn and criticism.

CFT therapists also work to increase the patient's motivation to become more self-compassionate and to experience compassion from and for other people, to guide the patient through compassionate mind training interventions designed to increase capacities for compassion, and to identify, normalize, and reduce any fears of compassion that commonly arise (e.g., worries that one is undeserving of compassion, fears that becoming self-compassionate will lead to a drop in personal standards) [23]. This latter part of CFT is a key part of the therapy, given that individuals high in self-criticism are more likely to be afraid of compassion [24]. For example, Sarah was worried that becoming more self-compassionate would cause her to indulge more frequently in comfort foods. However, during the course of treatment, she found that by being kinder to herself and less socially avoidant, she actually felt less driven to overeat.

Psychoeducation

Drawing on the CFT psychoeducation outlined by Goss [2], the CFT therapist emphasizes that humans evolved to eat for energy conservation and weight gain in the context of food scarcity. Humans also evolved to share food and eat together as a way of social affiliation. Therefore, eating tends to be related to feeling cared for or caring for others. Eating is typically experienced as soothing. Patients are taught that these evolved responses may be problematic if eating is the only way that patients know how to self-soothe. In addition, in Sarah's case, her father had always been overweight, and therefore, she likely had a genetic predisposition to obesity.

The CFT therapist also explains the tripartite affect regulation system. Eating is one way to regulate emotions. However, relying solely on eating for affect regulation, as in Sarah's case, can lead to using certain mind-sets and safety strategies (e.g., binge eating) to temporarily reduce negative affect (e.g., shame), but this can lead to unintended negative consequences (e.g., further guilt and shame, further weight gain). Importantly, the CFT therapist stresses that the patient's mind-set and strategies are not his or her fault but are the consequences of many different factors, including his or her biology, evolution, learning history, social and cultural contexts, and current environment. Although patients did not cause their own problems, only they can take responsibility for making changes.

Breathing Meditations and Attention Training

In CFT, mindfulness practices are routinely used to help patients become more aware of their self-critical thoughts, view their thoughts more objectively, and reflect on their own mental states and those of others. *Mindfulness* refers to paying attention to the present moment on purpose in a nonjudgmental way [25] (see Chapter 10). Over time, patients learn to become better able to direct their attention to the present moment – and away from self-critical and ruminative thoughts [1,3]. Patients learn that it is possible to experience emotions and thoughts in a nonshaming, nonjudgmental way and to approach these experiences in a curious and compassionate manner, making them more manageable and helpful [3].

A common breathing meditation in CFT refers to engaging in a soothing-rhythm breathing (SRB). Patients are instructed to breathe a little deeper than normal and to look for a rhythm in their breathing, resulting in feeling like they are slowing down [1]. By slowing down the breath, the parasympathetic nervous system is activated, and the intensity of threat emotions decreases [3]. Patients who encounter tension during this exercise are taught that CFT views tension as part of the threat protection system. Patients are instructed to release their tension with gratitude because while tension is not necessary, it developed as a way to protect and prepare them for action [1]. By becoming more aware of the link between bodily feelings and breathing [1,3], patients are better able to use their breath to help activate their soothing system and decrease threat-based emotions.

Aside from SRB, a number of other breathing meditations are used in CFT. Mindful breathing is used to teach patients to notice their breath and return to their breath when their attention wanders. During mindful breathing, patients are instructed to sit in an upright, comfortable position and breathe at a comfortable rate. Patients are asked to focus their attention on wherever they feel their breath most easily in their body. When attention wanders, patients are encouraged to gently bring their attention back to their breath. After the practice is complete, patients are encouraged to explore and reflect on their experience using the CFT framework [3].

Compassionate Imagery

Imagery is a skill that facilitates experiential work [3]. This occurs because internal stimuli can operate like external stimuli; that is, memories, images, and thoughts can have a physiologic effect on the brain and body [1]. In compassionate imagery work, images are used to stimulate the affiliative and soothing system and create mental experiences for patients that enhance feelings of safeness, reassurance, and well-being [1,2]. Common imagery practices in CFT focus on trying to create the experience of receiving or giving compassion [3]. They are broadly focused on five different domains [1], including

1. **Developing the Inner Compassionate Self.** This exercise is focused on creating a sense of a compassionate self. Patients are asked to pay attention to their body and engage in behaviors including slowing down their breathing, maintaining a relaxed but alert state and posture, relaxing their face, and comfortably curving their mouth. Patients are then invited to imagine themselves as their ideal compassionate self – confident, wise, calm, kind, assertive, warm, and helpful [1].

2. **Compassion Flowing into the Self.** This exercise is focused on opening up to the kindness of others. Patients may be asked to focus on memories or past events where

others were kind to them or imagine an ideal compassionate being and relating to that being [1].

3. **Compassion Flowing Out from the Self to Others.** This exercise is focused on wishing happiness and freedom of suffering to others. Patients are encouraged to direct compassionate feelings toward a chosen person or animal [1,3]. This exercise is designed to stimulate the affiliative and soothing system by creating the experience of giving compassion.

4. **Compassion for Self.** This exercise is focused on developing feelings, thoughts, and experiences that are directed toward developing compassion for the self [1]. Patients are encouraged to imagine seeing themselves in a compassionate way, wishing themselves happiness and freedom from suffering [1]. Patients can imagine a future compassionate self and are encouraged to provide details of their future self, such as what being happy would look like or how being happy would feel [1].

5. **Compassionate Images at Work.** This exercise involves developing compassionate images to promote engaging with and tolerating different emotions and behaviors and then courageously changing the emotion and/or behavior [1]. Patients are asked to imagine their compassionate self and then to focus their attention on another aspect of the self that causes distress (e.g., the critical self). Patients are asked to imagine having compassion for their critical self and to imagine what they would like to say to or how they would like to help that part of the self [1].

When starting compassionate imagery work with patients, a useful first step is to help them "create a safe place" [1]. In this exercise, patients are asked to imagine themselves in a place that is associated with feeling safe, calm, and peaceful. They are asked to describe details about their sensory experience in their safe place [3]. Compassion-focused therapy focuses on the affiliative component of the imagery, and the therapist may add instructions to the imagery, including, "If there are other people in your safe place, imagine that they welcome you and are happy to see you" [3: 143]. For patients who have difficulty imagining a safe place, it can be helpful for therapists to provide sensory anchors, such as asking patients to imagine certain soothing aspects of their place (e.g., "Imagine what the warm breeze would feel like on your face") [3: 146]. The following two imagery exercises were adapted from Gilbert's work [1] for use in the CFT intervention in the study by Kelly and Carter [26]:

Imagery 1. When you are ready, try to engage in some deep, slow breathing. Once you find a comfortable rhythm, take a few moments to recall a time when you felt someone was being warm, caring, understanding, and nonjudgmental with you. Close your eyes or look down as you try to recall this memory. Really try to bring it to mind as vividly as you can.

Imagery 2. When you are ready, try to engage in some deep, slow breathing. Once you find a comfortable rhythm, take a few moments to recall a time when you felt warm, *caring, understanding,* and *nonjudgmental* toward another person (adult or child) or toward an animal that has some distress. Close your eyes or look down as you try to recall this memory. Really try to bring it to mind as vividly as you can.

Next, the therapist may ask some of the following questions or make the following statements:

- What was happening in the situation?
- If you can see yourself, how did you look?

- What were you feeling?
- What do you notice happens in your body as you recall this time you were being compassionate?
- Try to sit with these feelings and sensations.
- Notice the warmth, understanding, and kindness you can feel toward another person (or animal).
- Notice your genuine care for his or her well-being.

Another common imagery intervention in CFT is called the *perfect nurturer practice* [27]. In this practice, patients are helped to imagine qualities of an ideal figure (be it a person or otherwise) who unquestionably meets their needs [27]. The perfect nurturer understands the patient; has compassion for him or her; is kind, supportive, and encouraging; and is never critical or judgmental [3]. Patients are asked to imagine the emotional and physical qualities of the perfect nurturer and the orientation that the perfect nurturer has toward them. The rationale is that repeated practice of the perfect nurturer image helps to activate self-soothing emotions and build new sensory-based memories in the neural network, enhancing the likelihood that this soothing memory will be activated again in the future [27].

Compassionate Letter Writing

In compassionate letter writing, patients are encouraged to think about a personally relevant and difficult event in their lives and write themselves a letter about the event from a compassionate point of view [1,28]. The purpose of writing the letter is not just to focus on difficult feelings but to help patients empathically connect with their thoughts and feelings and work with them in compassionate and balanced ways [1]. The letter may be written in a variety of ways. Patients may be instructed to imagine the voice of a compassionate person talking to them and write down their words. Patients may also write from a compassionate mode, or imagine a friend writing to them, or imagine what they would say to a friend. The letter can be written in or out of session. Once the letter is written, the therapist can invite the patient to read the letter in session [1]. In order for the letter to be compassionate, it is important for the letter to (1) express concern and caring, (2) be sensitive to the patient's needs and distress, (3) be helpful in facing and becoming more tolerant of emotions, (4) be helpful in becoming more understanding of emotions and difficulties, (5) be nonjudgmental and noncondemning, (6) be warm, understanding, and caring, and (7) be helpful in determining what the patient needs to do to move forward [3]. The patient is encouraged to write a letter that is compassionate, warm, and supportive.

For example, in one compassionate letter writing exercise, Sarah chose to write a letter to herself from her grandmother, who she remembered as the only person who was warm and kind toward her when she was growing up. The letter was about Sarah's experience of being criticized and silenced by her father as a child and adolescent. In the letter, her grandmother expressed warmth and caring toward Sarah, reassuring her that her father's behavior toward her was not her fault, encouraging her to be kind to herself, and empathizing with how hard it is to change.

For individuals with severe obesity, compassionate letter writing may focus on empathy about how hard it is to change deeply ingrained eating habits and to maintain those changes in the longer term, wisdom into knowing what is best, strength to cope with setbacks, nonjudgment in the face of setbacks, warmth in the way they relate to themselves, and compassionate encouragement [26]. For example, the letter may look something like, "Dear Sarah, You are having a tough time with this food plan, and no wonder – it is so hard to try and change eating patterns that you've had since you were a kid. Anyone would find this process to be really hard. You've made a lot of difficult changes lately and are showing courage by trying out the strategies learned in therapy. Tomorrow, try your best to care for yourself by sticking to your meal plan as much as possible. Remind yourself that it is understandable that this is hard and uncomfortable and that, over time, it will become easier. Be patient with yourself, and focus on the courage you are showing in caring for yourself through this new way of eating."

Compassionate Self-Talk

Compassionate self-talk has been used in CFT interventions for people with binge eating disorder (BED) [26]. During compassionate self-talk exercises, patients are encouraged to think of themselves as a child they have a strong desire to take care of. Patients are encouraged to (1) reassure themselves with care, strength, wisdom, and warmth to engage in the behaviors that will help to prevent overeating (e.g., developing and sticking to a meal plan) yet still (2) understand and empathize with their struggle to make changes, and (3) forgive themselves if they do overeat [26]. For example, a patient who engaged in an overeating episode may tell himself or herself, "So you overate. Although in some ways that's not what you wanted to do, it's hard to change habits you've been doing since you were a kid. You had a hard day at work, and overeating is how you've always dealt with hard days. Think of all the times you didn't overeat, all the urges you have resisted, and try to focus on what's most important – the fact that you're trying to help yourself. Don't beat yourself up over this – see it as a great opportunity to learn something. You're only human – think about what you can do to help yourself feel better tomorrow."

Compassionate Thought Balancing

CFT therapists may benefit from using thought records with patients. The form resembles what would be used in standard cognitive therapy, with columns in which to identify triggering events, feelings, and thoughts (see Chapter 8). However, there is a focus on identifying self-critical, shame-based thoughts in particular and to recognize thoughts that reflect internal shame (e.g., "I am disgusting") and external shame (e.g., "People think I'm a fat pig. People are grossed out by me"). Then, when the patient lists alternatives to his or her negative thoughts, he or she is asked to focus on shifting to a compassionate mind-set and respond to those self-critical thoughts from this perspective. For example, patients may be encouraged to write down what they would tell a friend in the same situation, such as: "It's *so* hard to have these kinds of thoughts in your head and to go out in the world every day. No wonder you'd prefer to be at home by yourself" and "Try to remind yourself of times when people have been caring and compassionate with you." The focus is less on challenging the content of the thoughts with evidence than instead trying to dissolve the shame underlying the thoughts with compassion. Finally, the patient is asked to write down any subsequent changes in his or her feelings. As in standard cognitive therapy, the therapist uses guided discovery and Socratic questioning during this exercise [4].

Addressing Fears of Self-Compassion

Often patients have mixed feelings about overcoming self-criticism and being more self-compassionate. This ambivalence frequently relates to beliefs around the benefits of self-criticism. For example, Sarah believed that being harsh and self-critical about her body image would motivate her to lose weight. In fact, the opposite seemed to be true – self-criticism and shame actually seemed to make her vulnerable to overeating. To help patients overcome fears of self-compassion, it can be helpful to explore nonjudgmentally the perceived function served by the self-criticism [3]. This is illustrated in the following dialogue.

CLINICIAN: You often criticize and attack yourself for being overweight, and you have observed that this tends to make you feel ashamed of your body and more depressed. How would you feel about working on relating to yourself in a kinder, more compassionate way when you notice yourself struggling rather than criticizing yourself?

SARAH: [*Pauses*] Well, to be honest, I think I might find that hard.

CLINICIAN: It sounds like maybe there are some mixed feelings about letting that harsh inner critic go?

SARAH: Yes, I think there are . . .

CLINICIAN: What are you afraid might happen?

SARAH: Well, since I was a child, I have always tried to motivate myself to lose weight by calling myself fat and disgusting. I know we've figured out that calling myself fat makes me feel bad, but I guess I'm just afraid that if I stop being so hard on myself, I'll give up and gain even more weight.

CLINICIAN: It's understandable that you're afraid of gaining weight. So you use self-criticism to motivate yourself to lose weight, and you're afraid that you would give up trying if that self-critical voice eased off?

SARAH: Yes, I'm afraid I'd just give up and lose control completely.

CLINICIAN: So, it sounds like if we are going to try to work on lowering that self-critical voice, we need to find some other, more helpful ways to motivate you? Would you be willing to explore whether developing self-compassion might actually help to motivate you to stay on track with your eating and exercise plan?

SARAH: Yes, I'd be willing to try it out.

Sometimes it can be helpful to clarify with patients that being more self-compassionate does not mean being permissive with oneself, for example, telling oneself to go ahead and overeat because that's what one feels like doing in the moment. Instead, self-compassion involves warmly and patiently directing oneself to do what is *best for one's well-being in the longer term* while acknowledging how hard and painful it can be to do that.

Another common obstacle to working on developing self-compassion is feeling undeserving of self-compassion. This feeling often relates to having grown up in an emotionally neglectful or abusive environment. In such cases, it can be helpful to use the strategy of *decentering*, that is, asking the patient to take a moment to imagine saying similar harsh critical things to a friend or family member who was struggling with similar issues, discussing what the likely effect would be on how that person would think or feel about themselves, and then relating it back to the patient's own situation. Typically, patients describe feeling very uncomfortable even imagining saying such harsh and disapproving things to someone else. Similarly, it can be helpful to ask the patient what he or she would say to a friend who was struggling to control his or her weight or eating and what the rationale would be. It can be helpful to discuss whether the patient would try to motivate his or her friend through harsh criticism or by warmness and kindness and why. Decentering has the effect of allowing patients to step outside themselves and see the negative effects of self-criticism and the benefits of compassion. Psychoeducation may also be helpful. For example, one study found that among people prone to overeating, being told that everyone overeats from time to time and that it's okay to do so actually made them less likely to overeat when given the chance [29]. Therefore, in some ways, thinking about eating struggles from a compassionate frame of mind might actually help to overcome them.

Empirical Evidence for the Effectiveness of CFT for Obesity

Research on the effectiveness of CFT interventions for the management of obesity is at an early stage. Kelly and Carter found evidence for the usefulness of CFT for individuals with BED [26]. Binge eating disorder is characterized by recurrent episodes of binge eating in the absence of extreme compensatory behaviors [30]. Most people with BED are overweight or obese. In this pilot randomized, controlled trial (RCT), a CFT-inspired intervention was compared with a CBT-inspired intervention that focused on behavioral strategies. Forty-one individuals with BED were randomly assigned to one of these two interventions, administered via the Internet, or to a wait list control group. In both treatment conditions, participants were asked to monitor and plan their eating on a daily basis for three weeks and were educated about basic CBT principles regarding the importance of regular, flexible eating throughout the day. Participants in the CFT group were then taught about the importance of self-compassion during the process of trying to change their eating and were asked to respond to urges to binge and to actual binge episodes with a compassionate inner dialogue. Compassionate imagery and letter-writing exercises were taught as a way to help access these compassionate feelings. Participants in the behavioral strategies group were taught about the importance of distracting themselves with binge-incompatible activities to avoid acting on urges to binge. They were asked to develop a list of alternate activities they could perform during these moments and to select one or more activities during the urges. No CFT-based strategies were taught in the behavioral strategies group. The results indicate that both active interventions reduced binge eating more than the control condition. However, only the CFT-based intervention was more effective than the control condition at improving self-compassion, concerns about overeating, concerns about weight, and overall eating pathology. These findings suggest that integrating CFT-based exercises into CBT treatments for individuals with binge eating may yield benefits not only in terms of reductions in behavioral symptoms but also in terms of psychological vulnerability factors that may interfere with the management of obesity, such as low self-compassion.

Two other recent studies also provided preliminary evidence for the applicability of CFT to the management of obesity. The first study examined a 12-week group intervention that integrated CFT strategies with mindfulness as well as acceptance and commitment therapy (ACT) [31]. Thirty-six women with BED who were overweight or obese experienced improvements in binge eating, acceptance of internal experiences related to body image, and other indicators of better psychological functioning following the group treatment, whereas a wait list control group did not show these improvements [31]. In a second study of the same group treatment, the group intervention resulted in significantly greater improvements in health-related quality of life, increases in physical activity, and decreases in weight-related self-stigma compared with treatment as usual in 73 women who were overweight or obese [32].

Taken together the results of these studies provide preliminary evidence that integrating CFT interventions into the management of severe obesity may be beneficial, although the specific contribution of CFT to the treatment is not yet known and warrants further research.

Case Vignette Revisited

With the support and guidance of her therapist, Sarah became more aware of her self-critical thoughts and their impact on her emotions and behavior. She realized that rather than helping her to achieve her goals of gaining control of her eating and weight, self-criticism and shame were both triggering and perpetuating maladaptive behaviors such as binge eating. While she was skeptical at first, she was willing to practice compassionate imagery and letter-writing exercises and gradually strengthened her self-compassionate voice and learned to be kinder to herself when she was struggling. These exercises helped her to become more motivated to follow her meal planning and find other ways of soothing herself besides comfort eating. Sarah also significantly increased her physical activity by reminding herself how much better she felt after exercising and by finding a social form of exercise that she enjoyed. The way she went about increasing her exercise was care based rather than control based, and this approach helped her sustain her efforts.

Summary

In this chapter, we have described the theoretical model on which CFT is based and provided an overview of key CFT strategies. We have provided a case vignette to illustrate the integration of CFT and CFT-based exercises in working with shame-prone patients with severe obesity. In addition, we have discussed the likelihood that self-critical individuals will have strong fears of self-compassion and have provided examples of how clinicians might help their patients understand and work through these fears. Finally, relevant research supporting the usefulness of CFT interventions with patients with obesity was reviewed.

Key Points

- Individuals with obesity are prone to shame and self-criticism.
- Compassion-focused therapy was developed specifically to help individuals who struggle with shame and self-criticism; thus its theoretical model can be a helpful framework for clinicians working with individuals with severe obesity who struggle with these issues.
- Various CFT-based interventions can be used to help patients develop greater capacities for self-compassion, both from self and from others. These exercises not only may

reduce patients' shame and self-criticism but also may help them to take and sustain efforts to manage their eating and weight.

- Clinicians should expect that their patients will be fearful of developing more compassion for themselves and devote time to exploring and validating these fears while encouraging patients to experiment with this new care-based approach to behavior change.

References

1. P. Gilbert. *Compassion-Focused Therapy: Distinctive Features*. Hove: Routledge, 2010.

2. K. Goss. *The Compassionate-Mind Guide to Ending Overeating: Using Compassion-Focused Therapy to Overcome Bingeing and Disordered Eating*. Oakland, CA: New Harbinger Publications, 2011.

3. R. L. Kolts. *CFT Made Simple: A Clinician's Guide to Practicing Compassion-Focused Therapy*. Oakland, CA: New Harbinger Publications, 2016.

4. P. Gilbert and C. Irons. Focused therapies and compassionate mind training for shame and self-attacking. In P. Gilbert, ed., *Compassion: Conceptualisations, Research and Use in Psychotherapy*. Hove: Routledge, 2005: 263–325.

5. P. Gilbert. *Using the Power of Mindfulness and Compassion to Transform Our Lives*. London: Constable & Robinson, 2013.

6. P. Gilbert. The origins and nature of compassion focused therapy. *Br J Clin Psychol* 2014; **53**: 6–41.

7. P. Gilbert. Introducing compassion-focused therapy. *Adv Psychiatr Treat* 2009; **15**: 199–208.

8. R. A. Depue and J. V. Morrone-Strupinsky. A neurobehavioural model of affiliative bonding: Implications for conceptualizing a human trait of affiliation. *Behav Brain Sci* 2005; **28**: 313–49.

9. C. Irons, P. Gilbert, M. W. Baldwin, et al. Parental recall, attachment relating and self-attacking/self-reassurance: Their relationship with depression. *Br J Clin Psychol* 2006; **45**: 297–308.

10. J. D. Latner, L. E. Durso, and J. M. Mond. Health and health-related quality of life among treatment-seeking overweight and obese adults: Associations with internalized weight bias. *J Eat Disord* 2013; **1**: 3.

11. J. Lillis, J. B. Luoma, M. E. Levin, et al. Measuring weight self-stigma: The weight self-stigma questionnaire. *Obesity* 2010; **18**: 971–6.

12. S. E. Cassin and A. Friedman. Weight-based stigma and body image in severe obesity. In S. Sockalingam and R. Hawa, eds., *Psychiatric Care in Severe Obesity: An Interdisciplinary Guide to Integrated Care*. Toronto, Springer International, 2017: 93–105.

13. J. D. Latner, K. S., O'Brien, L. E. Durso, et al. Weighing obesity stigma: The relative strength of different forms of bias. *Int J Obes* 2008; **32**: 1145–52.

14. R. Puhl and K. D. Brownell. Bias, discrimination, and obesity. *Obes Res* 2001; **9**: 788–805.

15. M. H. Schafer and K. F. Ferraro. The stigma of obesity: Does perceived weight discrimination affect identity and physical health? *Soc Psychol Q* 2011; **74**: 76–97.

16. C. Duarte, M. Matos, R. J. Stubbs, et al. The impact of shame, self-criticism and social rank on eating behaviours in overweight and obese women participating in a weight management programme. *PLoS One* 2017; **12**: 1–14.

17. K. Goss and S. Allan. The development and application of compassion-focused therapy for eating disorders (CFT-E). *Br J Clin Psychol* 2014; **53**: 62–77.

18. J. Gilbert, R. J. Stubbs, C. Gale, et al. A qualitative study of the understanding and use of "compassion focused coping strategies" in people who suffer from serious weight difficulties. *J Compassionate Health Care* 2014; **1**: 9.

19. K. Bojman, J. C. Carter, A. C. Kelly, et al. Weight regain in obesity: The role of shame and self-compassion. Manuscript in preparation, Memorial University of Newfoundland, 2017.

20. A. Hilbert, E. Braehler, R. Schmidt, et al. Self-compassion as a resource in the self-stigma process of overweight and obese individuals. *Obes Facts* 2015; **8**: 293–301.

21. S. E. Cassin, S. Sockalingam, S. Wnuk, et al. Cognitive behavioural therapy for bariatric surgery patients: Preliminary evidence for feasibility, acceptability, and effectiveness. *Cogn Behav Pract* 2013; **20**: 529–43.

22. Z. Cooper, C. G. Fairburn, and D. M. Hawker. *Cognitive-Behavioural Treatment of Obesity: A Clinician's Guide.* New York, NY: Guilford Press, 2003.

23. C. Gale, P. Gilbert, N. Read, et al. An evaluation of the impact of introducing compassion focused therapy to a standard treatment programme for people with eating disorders. *Clin Psychol Psychother* 2014; **21**: 1–12.

24. P. Gilbert, K. McEwan, L. Gibbons, et al. Fears of compassion and happiness in relation to alexithymia, mindfulness, and self-criticism. *Psychol Psychother T* 2012; **85**: 374–90.

25. J. Kabat-Zinn. *Full Catastrophe Living: Using the Wisdom of your Body and Mind to Face Stress, Pain, and Illness* (15th anniversary edn). New York, NY: Delta Trade Paperback/Bantam Dell, 2005.

26. A. C. Kelly and J. C. Carter. Self-compassion training for binge eating disorder: A pilot randomized controlled trial. *Psychol Psychother Theor Res Pract* 2015; **88**: 285–303.

27. D. A. Lee. The perfect nurturer: A model to develop a compassionate mind within the context of cognitive therapy. In P. Gilbert, ed., *Compassion: Conceptualisations, Research and Use in Psychotherapy.* New York, NY: Routledge, 2005: 326–51.

28. M. R. Leary, E. B. Tate, C. E. Adams, et al. Self-compassion and reactions to unpleasant self-relevant events: The implications of treating oneself kindly. *J Pers Soc Psychol* 2007; **92**: 887–904.

29. C. E. Adams and M. R. Leary. Promoting self-compassionate attitudes toward eating among restrictive and guilty eaters. *J Soc Clin Psychol* 2007; **26**: 1120–44.

30. American Psychiatric Association. *Diagnostic and Statistical Manual of Mental Disorders* (5th edn). Arlington, VA: American Psychiatric Publishing, 2013.

31. J. Pinto-Gouveia, S. A. Carvalho, L. Palmeira, et al. BEfree: A new psychological program for binge eating that integrates psychoeducation, mindfulness, and compassion. *Clin Psychol Psychother* 2017; **24**: 1090–8.

32. L. Palmeira, J. Pinto-Gouveia, and M. Cunha. Exploring the efficacy of an acceptance, mindfulness and compassionate-based group intervention for women struggling with their weight (Kg-free): A randomized, controlled trial. *Appetite* 2017; **112**: 107–16.

Chapter

Family-Focused Interventions in Severe Obesity

Anna Wallwork and Annie Basterfield

Case Vignette

Sam is a 44-year-old man who has been struggling with weight gain and poor health over the past few years. He has been married for 23 years and lives at home with his wife and their 22-year-old daughter and 18-year-old son with special needs. He asked his family doctor to refer him for bariatric surgery. When he met with the social worker for an initial psychosocial surgical assessment, he indicated that he has been off work for two years subsequent to a major fall that resulted in surgery on both of his knees, which left him unable to resume his role as an independent landscaper. Though he has finally been cleared to return to work, he has been advised that he will not be able to resume work as a landscaper due to his vulnerable knees. As such, Sam stated that he is interested in pursuing bariatric surgery because he does not believe he can achieve optimal health on his own, and he would like to return to his landscaping business.

In speaking about his weight gain over the past few years, Sam informed the social worker that since being off work and unable to support his family financially, he has felt depressed, unmotivated, and socially withdrawn and has maintained a mostly sedentary lifestyle. He reported that his wife does not want him to have bariatric surgery at this time, believing it to be extreme and unnecessary. She also feels that it will require him to continue being off work, whereas if he goes back to work in another field, she feels that he will lose weight and feel better about himself because he will become more active and contribute financially again. Sam stated that the financial strain on the family has been a major stressor in his relationship with his wife, who is feeling burdened with being the only breadwinner in the family. In addition, his children have been asked to contribute more financially given the high costs of their academic pursuits.

When the social worker assessed Sam's readiness and motivation to make dietary and lifestyle changes, he provided various reasons as to why he has not been able to do so up to this time, including being enrolled in additional career-building courses in order to expand his occupational options, helping his son build his résumé and driving him around in his pursuit of a part-time job, not wanting to burden others in the home with any changes to the dietary status quo they all maintain, as well as stating confidently that once he has the surgery, he will be 100 percent committed to the lifestyle changes needed. When exploring the role of family and other social supports in his life in order to maximize his outcomes before and after surgery, Sam noted that other than his wife, who would ultimately be available to care for his instrumental needs if he did have surgery, he has not told anyone about his intentions for surgery, including his adult children. He stated that he feels somewhat ashamed to admit to others that he is "resorting to surgical means as an answer to weight issues."

Introduction

This chapter discusses the role of family-focused interventions in the treatment of individuals with severe obesity and those pursuing bariatric surgery. The rationale and empirical support for family-focused interventions in obesity care are reviewed, as well as the theoretical frameworks and common treatment modalities for approaching this work. The majority of this chapter presents common challenging clinical presentations where family-focused interventions are warranted. Strategies and practical tips for working with patients and their family members are also provided. The chapter concludes with the integration of the information presented in the resolution of the Case Vignette (see Case Vignette Revisited).

The Role of Family-Focused Interventions in Severe Obesity Care

Evidence is emerging that supports the inclusion of family-focused interventions in the treatment of individuals with severe obesity. Family-based approaches have already been established as the "gold standard" in pediatric obesity treatment [1]. In addition, clinical practice guidelines for the treatment of preadolescents and adolescents with obesity have emphasized the importance of parent/family inclusion in order to optimize family competency and support for the patient, family knowledge and understanding of the process, and commitment to long-term lifestyle changes [2]. A review of meta-analyses of randomized, controlled trials (RCTs) of family-based interventions in healthcare supports the effectiveness of family-based care over usual medical care for patients' physical and mental health, particularly in the case of cardiovascular disease, with emergent focus on cancer, arthritis, and diabetes care [3]. At this time, empirical evidence for the efficacy of family-focused interventions in the treatment of adult obesity is limited, but given that obesity has strong intergenerational effects and that health risk factors cluster within families who reside in shared environments [4–6], addressing obesity through a family-based lens should be considered an important intervention for clinicians in the field.

Clinically speaking, family-focused interventions can be considered to be any treatment or intervention that includes the patient and one additional family member, but a standard definition of *family* or *family member* is no longer relevant; therefore, clinicians must account for the diversity of single, blended, and multigenerational families and respect sources of family support as best defined by patients themselves [1].

Family Systems Theory

Adopting a family-based perspective can be a helpful framework for professionals involved in the treatment of severe obesity. Family systems theory proposes that families are complex systems in which multiple reciprocal interactions occur simultaneously, and each family member's thoughts and behaviors are shaped by other members' thoughts and behaviors [7]. This perspective encourages an exploration of family processes and functions and suggests that a person can only be understood within the context of his or her whole family. This theory does not seek to explain *why* families engage in particular behaviors but rather provides a lens through which to view families as an "open, ongoing, goal-seeking, self-regulating social system" [8]. A large body of research has demonstrated that family unit dynamics have a strong influence on one's lifestyle and health behaviors and that these dynamics can be developed, maintained, or changed over time and therefore encourage or preclude the successful adoption of healthy lifestyle behaviors in patients with obesity [4,9]. As such, recent studies have argued for the importance of approaching adults with obesity, including bariatric surgery patients, with a family-focused lens [10–13]. Clinically speaking, when patients and their families mutually ascribe the patient's health threat as equally important to the group as a whole, the greater is the likelihood of health behavior modification as a family through a communal coping approach to the challenges generated by surgery [14]. Families presenting in this way provide an ideal foundation for which to work collaboratively with patients and family members in the treatment of severe obesity and health optimization.

Modalities of Family-Focused Interventions

Various forms of family-focused interventions can be provided when working with patients with severe obesity. These include psychoeducational interventions, relationship-focused interventions, behavioral interventions, support groups, and family therapy.

Psychoeducational Interventions. Psychoeducational interventions are quite common and are largely directed at increasing knowledge of weight loss management and healthy lifestyles to cope better collectively with changes brought about by treatment. They may also address family responses to challenges encountered, ineffective coping styles, and expansion of the patient's/family's social support network [15]. Treatment can include educating patients and their family members about medical conditions, lifestyle and dietary changes necessary for weight loss management and optimal health, and the ways in which the patient and family may be affected by the processes of change or lack thereof if nonadherent. Particularly in relation to those pursuing bariatric surgery, patients and families should be encouraged to broaden their knowledge of what a healthy lifestyle means and to identify health improvement goals in many forms rather than solely focusing on weight loss as the desirable outcome.

Relationship-Focused Interventions. Relationship-focused interventions direct attention to the emotional and supportive aspects of the patient's care, as well as building the skills needed to enhance family/relationship cohesion while living with the demands of obesity care and weight loss management. Treatment can include addressing skill-building elements in problem solving, family communication, and conflict management [3]. Particularly in the case of bariatric surgery, family units are often so acutely affected by the patient's significant lifestyle changes that they will be challenged to either best use their resources in order to reorganize as a whole or dissolve altogether [10]. Often a multimodal combination of both of these types of interventions can be applied to maximize patient and family outcomes when it comes to adherence to clinical weight loss advice and improved health overall.

Behavioral Interventions. Behavioral interventions are a prevailing approach used in obesity management, and they can often go hand-in-hand when working with families in this capacity. For example, patients and their family members can be educated on self-monitoring techniques, goal setting, problem solving, behavioral contracting, and relapse-prevention strategies (see Chapters 8 and 9) [5]. Supportive family members can also be advised on how to best provide positive reinforcement regarding a patient's desirable behavior without criticism of the patient's weight or progress in behavioral change.

Support Groups. Facilitated patient and family support groups can be an excellent avenue for families to learn from similar others' lived experiences within their own families in terms of lifestyle transitions throughout obesity or bariatric surgical treatment. Support groups are often welcome sources of informational, practical, and emotional support for patients embarking on their own weight loss journey as well as their family members [4]. These groups do not include direct assessment of family dynamics by a clinician or address problem-solving or coping skills for specific individuals. However, often these areas can be addressed by peers within the group, and professional facilitators can amend shared information from other patients/families that may be inaccurate or misguided.

Family Therapy. A family therapy approach typically identifies any problems with family adjustment to changes brought about by treatment recommendations as being a result of preexisting dysfunctional family dynamics. Treatment focus often involves working with members to reduce familial stressors, optimize family resources, and address emotional needs and concerns to shift relational climates at home as best as possible [4,5]. When the psychosocial clinician involved in obesity care is not able to provide this level of therapy directly, patients and their family members may be referred externally to couple or family counseling prior to continuing with or alongside their obesity treatment.

Clinical Presentations That Warrant Family-Focused Interventions

When assessing a patient pursuing bariatric surgery or other treatment for severe obesity, an examination of the perceived support a patient feels and the quality of his or her family life and important relationships is paramount to deciding how best to apply family-focused treatment. Eliciting family behavioral change requires a thorough understanding of family function, competence, roles, and normative day-to-day processes in order to best target identified needs. This section outlines some examples of challenging clinical presentations that clinicians may encounter in the context of treating severe obesity that may warrant a family-focused intervention. Table 12.1 provides a quick reference guide to the clinical challenges and possible interventions addressed in this section.

Table 12.1 Common Clinical Presentations and Possible Family-Focused Interventions

Presentation	Possible interventions
Stigmatizing attitudes toward obesity and/or bariatric surgery	• Inviting family members to attend all appointments • Providing psychoeducation • Facilitating nonjudgmental dialogue with patients and families • Recommending patient/family support groups
Family members engaging in unhealthy eating behaviors	• Facilitating a family support meeting to problem solve, strategize, and set goals • Identifying health behaviors that family members can engage in together
Family members sabotaging the patient's progress	• Assessing the negative impact of weight loss on patient's relationships • Assessing for relationships that may revolve around food and cautioning about potential for interpersonal strain

Table 12.1 (cont.)

Presentation	Possible interventions
	• Engaging saboteur in all stages of the treatment process and providing an opportunity for him or her to process the experience • Exploring strategies for coping • Psychoeducation regarding potential positive impact of healthy changes on the family system • Recommending patient/family support groups
Patient's perspective that diet/lifestyle changes should not apply to the rest of the family	• Assessing patient confidence and assertiveness in asking for support • Identifying problematic behaviors that patients want their family members to change • Coaching patients to ask for support (using techniques such as role playing) • Advocating for patient needs within family support meetings and aiding in problem solving and solution generation
Other familial stressors that can challenge the patient's pursuit of and adherence to obesity treatment	• Assessing the nature and intensity of familial stressors, as well as coping skills • Providing recommendations and referrals to appropriate resources to enhance coping with different familial stressors • Encouraging patients to reflect on timing of treatment and whether they can manage multiple stressors • Respect patient's autonomy for decision making in his or her own care
Identifying optimal support people for different support functions	• Encouraging the patient to identify different support needs and family members from whom the patient can receive support
Cultural considerations with regard to family diet and nutritional behaviors	• Exploring culturally based dietary and nutrition practices • Working with patients and families to make culturally sensitive treatment recommendations while also prioritizing obesity treatment

Stigma Related to Bariatric Surgery

When patients explore the option of surgical interventions for obesity and inform their family members of their intentions for surgery, family members can often express judgments about surgery being an acceptable option [16]. Clinical presentation of this issue is demonstrated in the following vignette.

Vanessa is considering bariatric surgery as an option for treating her obesity. She also has type 2 diabetes and obstructive sleep apnea, and her family doctor strongly recommended bariatric surgery as an option for treating her comorbidities. Her support people, including her partner and her siblings, have said that they think surgery is too extreme. They have made comments such as, "Why can't you just eat better?" and "If you just go to the gym regularly, you will lose the weight." These comments are leaving Vanessa feeling unsupported by her family and ashamed that she has not been able to lose the weight on her own.

In addition to the well-documented stigma toward obesity (see Chapter 3), there are likely many factors that influence stigmatization associated with bariatric surgery. For example, bariatric surgery is perceived as an "easy way out" or a "quick fix" to weight loss [16–18]. Research has shown that surgical interventions for weight loss are viewed more negatively than other weight loss interventions and that individuals who pursue surgical interventions are perceived as lazier, less responsible for their weight loss, and less attractive than those who lose weight through diet and exercise alone [19,20]. In addition, family members often express their concern over the risk of medical complications and fatality associated with surgical interventions, which can cause family members to be unsupportive of bariatric surgery. Media and popular culture likely play an important role in shaping common perceptions of and attitudes about bariatric surgery – a study analyzing representations of bariatric surgery in American mainstream magazines found that surgery is often portrayed as medically risky and costly [17].

It is possible that the stigma expressed by family members could be due to misunderstanding and lack of education about bariatric surgery. Therefore, clinicians should encourage inclusion of family members in the assessment process, where psychoeducation about bariatric surgery is provided in detail. In addition, assessments should include an opportunity for patients and family members to discuss their perceptions and concerns about bariatric surgery. Specifically, this could include inviting family members to attend specific preoperative appointments with patients. Clinicians can provide psychoeducation to patients and their family members about the eligibility criteria for bariatric surgery (including age, body mass index [BMI], weight-related comorbidities) and the potential weight loss and health benefits that can be expected with bariatric surgery. Perhaps most important, clinicians can provide further psychoeducation to patients and family members about the serious commitment to diet and lifestyle changes that is required to do well after bariatric surgery and reinforce the message that the focus should not be on weight but rather on improving overall general health. Although surgery is often perceived as an "easy way out," this is certainly not the case: patients must understand the lifelong changes to diet and lifestyle that are required in order to be successful with weight loss and maintenance of improved overall health following bariatric surgery.

Clinicians conducting psychosocial assessments with bariatric surgery patients should inquire with patients and their family members directly about their perceptions and potential concerns regarding bariatric surgery. Clinicians can ask patients, "What response have you received from your family members when you have shared your intentions to have bariatric surgery?" They can also ask family members, "What are your thoughts about [the patient] having bariatric surgery?" If patients or their family members express stigmatizing perceptions and/or concerns, clinicians can create a nonjudgmental environment for open conversation by acknowledging that these particular perceptions and concerns are quite common, considering the messages that we receive about bariatric surgery in our environments and in the media. When family members are particularly concerned about the medical risks associated with surgery, it is important to validate the importance of seriously considering the risks and potential complications of bariatric surgery. Beyond acknowledging and validating family members' perceptions and concerns, it is important to focus on strengthening support for the patient's intentions for surgery by advocating on behalf of patients. Focusing on the potential health benefits associated with bariatric surgery is a way that clinicians can help families to identify the ways in which bariatric surgery could be beneficial rather than focusing on stigmatizing attitudes. In addition, clinicians should ask patients to share with their families why it is important to them to pursue bariatric surgery and similarly create a space for family members to ask questions. Recommending support groups as an intervention can be particularly helpful because this forum provides patients and family members with an opportunity to hear the perspectives of other families who are going through bariatric surgery. By giving patients and family members the opportunity to discuss their concerns and providing accurate health-focused psychoeducational information, myths about bariatric surgery can be debunked, and patients can experience increased support from their family members.

The Maintenance of Negative Health Behaviors by Family Members

It is not unusual for patients to discuss how their loved ones support their pursuit of obesity treatment, but they also continue to engage in negative health habits that make it challenging for patients to be successful. This is highlighted in the following vignette.

Louisa is meeting with the social worker for psychosocial treatment at a medical weight loss program for severe obesity. When discussing the role of social supports in her life, Louisa states that her family members continue to bring unhealthy foods into the home in spite of her best efforts to refrain from doing so. She also notes that at times her husband will indulge in treats right in front of her and even offer her some, saying things like, "A little bit won't hurt you!" Moreover, Louisa complains that despite numerous requests for help and accommodation from her family members, meals are still being prepared in a way that does not support the dietary recommendations she is trying to follow. Louisa states to the social worker that she is greatly concerned about her home life affecting her ability to be successful. The social worker suggests that they brainstorm solutions to manage the frequent challenges she encounters at home and discuss how best to implement such solutions in a way that encourages positive family interactions.

In situations similar to Louisa's, patients may defend their loved ones, indicating that their family members' intentions do not appear ill-willed but merely show ignorance or forgetfulness around the patient's efforts to make changes. Certainly, if the patient identified these patterns as being a barrier to implementing lifestyle changes, then his or her primary support persons in the home would be invited and strongly encouraged to attend an appointment with the patient so that collaborative problem solving, strategizing, and common goal setting could occur with the help of professional facilitation for this process. Often it is the case that the loved ones do not possess a similar readiness to embark on such a lifestyle change (i.e., they are not at the same stage of change as the patient [21]). Spouses/parents who disagree on basic health tenants and behaviors for their family are also unlikely to be successful in treatment [1]. Although different family member perspectives on making healthy changes can be a challenge, it should not necessarily be viewed as a barrier to the patient's success, particularly when family members do demonstrate emotional support toward the patient's efforts. Generally, problem solving around family roles and patterns in a way that maximizes the patient's control over most aspects of his or her diet (e.g., grocery shopping, meal preparation for the family or at least for himself or herself, determining hidden locations for storage of tempting foods in the home) and finding compromises for other family members to maintain some or most of their preferred habits (e.g., continuing to have their treats but doing so while at work, away from the patient, in another area of the home, or when the patient is not around or only bringing home indulgent foods that the patient may not be interested in, e.g., agreeing not to bring in the patient's favorite treats or bringing less desirable flavors of items the patient might otherwise be tempted by) can be win-wins for all members in the home.

Educating all members of the family about the potential for improved health benefits to all when they embark on a "joint journey" or as "joint collaborators" in the weight loss treatment process can be planting a seed for family members in terms of their own readiness to make changes [12,22]. Furthermore, finding any common goal among family members can also go a long way toward establishing more joint patterns as a family. For example, a spouse may not be motivated to engage in physical activity but may show an interest in spending more quality time with his or her partner and/or family. Brainstorming solutions that may meet all of their needs – such as joining a recreation league of a commonly enjoyed activity or taking evening or weekend walks outside the home as a couple or to a local park as a family – may be common ground at which family members are able to meet.

Intentional Sabotage by Family Members

Preexisting marital or familial strain within the home, often manifested in emotional distress, conflict, or dysfunction, is likely to have a negative impact on a family member's engagement and participation in obesity treatment. In the psychosocial treatment of severe obesity, it can be helpful for clinicians to ask their patients, "Might you anticipate a significant weight loss negatively affecting any of your important relationships?" Initially, most patients may not identify this as a concern for them, but when family or social relations are explored in more detail, the patient may be able to identify relationships that occur and flourish predominantly around enjoyment of food (e.g., destressing with a particular colleague over a daily coffee and snack break, always meeting a particular friend at a favorite restaurant) and/or through socialization where unhealthy habits may be common (e.g., frequent pub nights where decadent fare and alcoholic beverages are consumed, cottage weekends where binge drinking and frequent snacking are common). In order to avoid temptation and relapses, the patient may make the conscious decision not to engage in these social endeavors with his or her loved ones while pursuing obesity treatment; as such, this may contribute to interpersonal strain within those relationships and/or lead to feelings of jealously, neglect, or ill-will in the patient's loved ones. When viewed through a family systems lens, when a family member feels that the status quo or equilibrium at home has been threatened or disturbed by lifestyle changes instigated by the patient, that family member may feel that his or her attachment or position of power is weakened or lost, resulting in resistance to such change by trying to sabotage it [23]. Family members who experience such negative emotions toward the patient's pursuit of obesity treatment may identify with a limited readiness to change, jealousy that the patient is ready and able to make such a commitment, a lack of confidence in being able to be successful with such treatment themselves, or not having qualified or having met the criteria for the same treatment as the patient and therefore not having the same professional support. As such, family members may engage in intentional sabotage toward the patient in an effort to keep him or her from losing weight. This scenario may look similar to Louisa's case example described earlier, but it occurs more deliberately and with negative intent, which can pose a major challenge for patients and care teams. Often the patient struggles with the dilemma either to continue in his or her pursuit of change and accept that some of his or her close relationships may be jeopardized or to give up on the changes to protect and preserve the familial status quo [23].

As a clinician, dismissing the challenge of family saboteurs and focusing only on the patient will likely end in limited success or relapse back into old habits for the patient. At all opportunities, the identified challenging family member should be overtly included at any stage of the treatment process – that is, be present at all clinical assessments and follow-up visits, educational sessions, and support group sessions or programs. Given the known impact of obesity treatment including bariatric surgery on family members' lives, it is imperative that a specific forum is provided to explore and process their personal experiences as well. This forum may be particularly important for spouses or close family members who also struggle with their weight and health. At each encounter, benefits and stressors to the relationship throughout all treatment interventions can be explored, and strategies to cope with any identified stressors can be collaboratively negotiated [23]. In addition, directly targeting the challenging family member's well-being and worries about the future may be important in reducing strain in his or her relationship with the patient and in garnering that family member's ongoing support [24].

The provision of psychoeducation to both patients and family members (through group or one-on-one sessions or in written form) related to the potential positive health outcomes for all individuals and the family unit as a whole can enhance family members' understanding of the treatment process, manage their expectations, and provide guidance for navigating transitional challenges along the weight loss journey [13]. Moreover, patient and family support groups provide an opportunity for family members to learn more about the treatment process from the patient/family member perspective. They also offer a safe forum for communicating concerns and provide an opportunity to learn strategies for best managing their emotional distress when it comes to the patient's changes. Over time, challenging family members may show a shift in their support for the patient, and they may also have enhanced personal motivation toward behavioral change.

"It's Not Fair for My Family to Make the Same Sacrifices!"

The dietary and lifestyle changes that are essential in treating severe obesity undoubtedly have an impact on family systems. The significant changes that a patient makes to his or her diet (e.g., making nutritious food choices, eating smaller portions, eating regular meals and snacks, eating more slowly) and lifestyle (e.g., exercising regularly and consuming less alcohol) take place within the patient's familial environment. These changes can have a positive impact on families, in that healthy behaviors can be adopted by other family members when they are flexibly responsive to change, or they can create challenges for family members who are resistant to change [13,25].

A family-focused clinical issue that can arise in the context of treatment for severe obesity is that patients may believe that the necessary lifestyle changes should only apply to themselves and that their family members should be immune to such changes. Given that it is their personal choice to target their weight and health, their perspective may be that it is unfair to impose dietary and lifestyle changes on their family members. For example, patients who have young children may say that it is not possible to keep "treats" out of the house because otherwise they would be depriving their children.

The clinician should further explore this perspective with the patient by asking why it is important for the patient to maintain the status quo for his or her family members. In some cases, patients would ideally prefer for their family members to adapt to their dietary and lifestyle changes, but they lack the confidence or assertiveness to ask for support. The clinician can offer support by coaching the patient to reach out to his or her family members using role-playing techniques. The clinician should work with the patient to clearly identify what specific behaviors he or she would like family members to change. For example, a patient may request that his or her family reduce the number of takeout and/or fast-food meals they consume during the week.

It may be important to invite the patient's loved ones in for a family support meeting, particularly if patients continue to experience difficulty requesting support assertively. During a family support meeting, the clinician can assist by advocating for the patient and giving volume to his or her voice. In some cases, it may be more influential for families to hear recommendations from a healthcare professional than from the patients themselves. As such, clinicians can help patients and their families to identify areas for support and specific strategies that can be used to help the patient, as well as problem solve and create solutions with the family.

Finding the "Right Time" for Surgery

A number of stressors can present a challenge to obesity treatment, including timely familial stressors (e.g., financial/employment concerns, major life events such as pregnancy, separation, moving) or personal stressors (e.g., caring for an ill loved one, mental health concerns, academic pressures, taking on a new job or a promotion). In the Case Vignette involving Sam presented at the beginning of this chapter, although Sam is motivated to pursue weight loss surgery, his wife's priority is for him to return to work because she is more concerned with the financial burden placed on the family with Sam being unemployed. Some patients may find it challenging to manage their family stressors and undergo obesity treatment at the same time and must account for these interacting stressors when making decisions to pursue treatment [1]. Additionally, one member pursuing intensive obesity treatment or bariatric surgery can often exacerbate the burden on a family due to the frequent clinic visits and tests needed, the tracking of behaviors in order to demonstrate adherence, and any associated costs [1].

The clinician should assess the nature and intensity of the patient's family stressors, as well as the patient's coping skills and confidence in his or her ability to take on obesity treatment alongside potential stressors. If patients have stressors such as mental health concerns or financial/employment concerns and are not accessing resources (e.g., psychosocial treatment, income support, employment counseling), clinicians can help direct and connect patients to appropriate resources in order to address the stressors that may adversely affect their obesity treatment. If the patient's family stressors are significant and appear to be poorly managed by the patient at home, it is important for clinicians to have patients consider whether it is the optimal time to pursue obesity treatment. Clinicians may encourage patients to take some time to contemplate their stressors and discuss plans for treatment in the context of the family system with their family members. In an adult treatment program, clinicians must inform patients that obesity treatment can often be experienced as an additional strain that can add pressure to other life stressors but also must respect the patient's autonomy to make decisions about their health and coping abilities [26]. Clinicians should always follow up with patients who take time to make a decision about treatment in order to discuss patients' decisions and future treatment options.

Patient's Support Person Is Not the "Best Fit"

Patients pursuing obesity treatment often default to their partner or closest family member as their primary support person. However, this person may not be best suited for the role if he or she has not adopted a communal coping approach alongside the patient [14]. While it is important to have the support of partners and close family members, it is equally important for patients to consider the different kinds of support they may require while they pursue obesity treatment. There are many different recognized functions of social support, including companionship and emotional, informational, and instrumental support [27]. In order to help patients make their support functions more robust, clinicians can assist patients in identifying how they would best receive these different kinds of support and from whom they would receive it.

Patients can access support from other family members (actual and chosen) in order to make their support system well rounded. For example, family members who have also experienced difficulties with obesity may be able to offer a unique type of support because they can relate to and empathize with the patient's journey. Further, a family member who has undergone the particular obesity treatment that the patient is considering can offer a specific perspective, support, and guidance on how to navigate treatment.

There is evidence to suggest that individuals can be more successful at weight loss and improved health maintenance when they have a support person who is also motivated to get healthy alongside them [28]. Furthermore, when patients are guided and encouraged to consider broader health improvement goals, as opposed to weight loss alone, their path to long-term success will be more likely. Therefore, clinicians may encourage patients to identify a family member who is interested in making positive lifestyle changes as well. Patients may ask the family member to enroll in treatment with them or at least engage in some of the dietary and behavioral changes with them. This kind of support can improve treatment adherence [28].

The following case vignette demonstrates the benefit of identifying different support functions from different family members in order to strengthen the support system for the patient.

Lisa is undergoing a dietary and lifestyle intensive treatment program. She lives with her husband and her 23-year-old son, both of whom are supportive of her treatment and her weight loss pursuits. Lisa's husband has been providing her with encouragement and reassurance when she experiences challenges with behavior changes. Lisa's son also struggles with his weight and has decided to support his mom by making changes to promote better health along with his mother. Lisa and her son cook, eat, and exercise together, which is very helpful because Lisa's husband travels for work and is not always available. In addition, Lisa's cousin went through the same program three years ago and has been successful in maintaining the weight loss and health improvements. Lisa's cousin has offered a great deal of support, providing information, encouragement, and mentorship. Both Lisa's son and cousin have attended clinical appointments with Lisa throughout her treatment.

Culturally Diverse Family Norms

Inquiry into the specific needs and responses of culturally diverse families cannot be overlooked in the management of severe obesity. Families demonstrate different dynamics within different cultures, and therefore, family-based interventions should consider the unique role of culture – specifically how it influences dietary patterns and nutrition in terms of food choices and portioning, celebration, and religious fasting and diet. For example, when it comes to treatment recommendations around self-regulation and measuring portions, challenges may be faced within cultures that have food beliefs around set meals and predetermined quantities of food [29]. Furthermore, there are various cultural family norms/routines regarding who occupies the roles in the home related to food purchasing and preparation and authoritative hierarchies and/or cultural traditions that may demand certain foods/dishes be available in the home. Certainly, from a family systems perspective, when stable cultural family norms and rituals are disrupted by one member's drastic lifestyle changes, family-adopted behavioral change is challenged and therefore should be regularly reevaluated by clinicians throughout the treatment process [1]. Specific cultural components need to be explored in detail and addressed in order to optimize patient and family success in obesity management. It is critical that the treatment team, patient, and family members establish mutually agreed on goals through ongoing open dialogue. There are racial, ethnic, and cultural differences in the perception of obesity that may influence other family members' motivation for adopting changes. In addition, in some cases, it may be necessary for clinicians to modify dietary recommendations to account for specific cultural fare. Approaching cultural diversity among family units often requires cultural curiosity and culturally sensitive perspectives and tools in order to effect behavior change [29].

Case Vignette Revisited

The bariatric assessment team made recommendations to Sam based on his current circumstances. The social worker invited Sam back for another appointment and strongly encouraged him to bring his wife and children. Sam attended the appointment with his wife and his son. The purpose of the social work follow-up appointment was to create a nonjudgmental environment for Sam and his loved ones to openly discuss his intentions for surgery and how this particular treatment may affect the entire family. The social worker first invited Sam's wife and son to share their concerns about surgery and validated these concerns. Psychoeducation was then provided about the potential health and lifestyle benefits that can occur after bariatric surgery. By the same token, the social worker emphasized the necessary hard work involved with making changes to diet and lifestyle in order to be successful with maintenance of improved health after bariatric surgery. Sam's family and the social worker explored different diet and lifestyle behaviors that occur in the home that could potentially be problematic for Sam afterwards. Under the hypothetical scenario that Sam is to proceed with surgery, strategies were discussed for how Sam's family could support him, for example, by not bringing tempting foods into the home, meal planning and grocery shopping together, and engaging in some regular physical activity together. Additionally, the social worker collaborated with the family to problem solve around decreasing some of the other familial stressors in the home (e.g., advising on employment support services for Sam's son, balancing roles at home to allow Sam more dedicated time to focus on the dietary recommendations). To Sam's surprise, his wife and son were receptive to making changes as a family to support him. The social worker made it clear that surgery is a serious decision and, while providing many health benefits, can be a major stressor for patients and their family. Given all the stressors considered, including Sam's depression, unemployment, and supporting his son's needs, the social worker encouraged Sam and his family to take some time to reflect on whether or not this is the right time to pursue surgery. Before the end of the session, the social worker provided Sam with some psychotherapy referrals and encouraged the family to attend the bariatric program's support group for patients and families. The social worker also made herself available to Sam and his family for any follow-up discussions or in-person meetings as required.

Sam and his family took a few months to consider the decision of whether or not he should pursue bariatric surgery. During this time, Sam's wife encouraged him to pursue the psychotherapy referral for treatment of his depression and to see his family doctor. With medication and psychotherapy, Sam found that his mood improved, and he was motivated to start making some diet and lifestyle changes. Even though he lost minimal weight with the diet and lifestyle changes alone, he felt greatly encouraged by other health improvements he was experiencing, and his family gained valuable practice in providing practical support to assist Sam with his weight loss. Sam also reached out to his sister for support, who had gone through bariatric surgery five years ago. His sister answered some of Sam's questions and invited his whole family to meet with her partner and children to offer some insight into what life might be like for the family after surgery. Moreover, Sam and his wife attended the support group a few times, and hearing the stories of bariatric patients and the experience of family members helped Sam's wife to understand further his motivations for the surgery and the reasons why going back to work immediately may not be the solution to Sam's health issues. However, Sam's family was still under financial stress with him being out of work, and this would be an ongoing stressor until he is able to return to work.

The social worker followed up a few months later in order to discuss Sam's decision regarding the pursuit of bariatric surgery. Sam had come to the decision that he would not like to pursue bariatric surgery at this time but planned to do so in the future. With the strengthened support of his family through openly discussing how they could support his lifestyle changes, he and his family were starting to collectively modify aspects of their lifestyle. Although he felt that he now had more support from his wife, they had decided that the financial stressor and subsequent relationship strain were barriers to him being successful with surgery at this time. He had set a goal to find employment in a new career and become more financially stable before pursuing surgery. The social worker supported Sam in this decision and provided resources for employment counseling. The social worker also encouraged Sam and his family to continue with the changes they had made so far and invited Sam back to be reassessed for surgery when he felt ready.

Summary

Family-focused interventions in the area of severe obesity management and bariatric care are becoming more prominent in research and should be encouraged in clinical practice. Family systems theory informs the perspective that family dynamics have a strong influence on lifestyle and health behaviors. In family-based treatment, all members of the family should be collectively viewed as the "patient" and encouraged to share accountability and work together toward the common goal of improved health behaviors [1,9]. In the treatment of severe obesity, where changes to diet and lifestyle are crucial, clinicians can integrate family-focused treatment modalities including psychoeducation, relationship-focused interventions, behavioral interventions, support programs/groups, and family therapy to address familial issues in order to enhance patients' environments for optimizing health. In comparison with patient-focused approaches, family-focused interventions have been shown to be advantageous in terms of long-term sustainability of behavioral change. Addressing family members' concerns throughout the treatment process may also protect against erosion of their support for the patient [30]. Application of family-focused interventions should be tailored to each family's unique relations, patterns, competencies, resiliencies, and vulnerabilities. Some of the ineffectiveness of such treatments may be the result of a weak understanding of the familial dynamics that underlie many health behaviors prior to implementation [4].

Key Points

- Family-focused interventions include the patient and at least one additional "family member" as identified by the patient.
- Family unit dynamics have a strong influence on one's lifestyle and health behaviors and can encourage or preclude successful long-term change in patients with obesity.
- Addressing family members' concerns throughout the treatment process may protect against erosion of their support for the patient.
- Family-focused interventions should be uniquely tailored to each collective "patient."
- Ineffective family-focused interventions may be due to poor understanding of family dynamics that underlie health behaviors and patterns.

References

1. J. A. Skelton, C. Buehler, M. B. Irby, et al. Where are family theories in family-based obesity treatment? Conceptualizing the study of families in pediatric weight management. *Int J Obes* 2012; **36**: 891–900.

2. V. A. Shrewsbury, K. S. Steinbeck, S. Torvaldsen, et al. The role of parents in pre-adolescent and adolescent overweight and obesity treatment: A systematic review of clinical recommendations. *Obes Rev* 2011; **12**: 231–53.

3. C. A. Chesla. Do family interventions improve health? *J Fam Nurs* 2010; **16**: 355–77.

4. T. L. Campbell and J. M. Patterson. The effectiveness of family interventions in the treatment of physical illness. *J Marital Fam Ther* 1995; **21**: 545–83.

5. P. Sung-Chan, T. W. Sung, X. Zhai, et al. Family-based models for childhood-obesity interventions: A systematic review of randomized controlled trials. *Obes Rev* 2013; **14**: 265–78.

6. D. C. Vidot, G. Prado, N. De La Cruz-Munoz, et al. Review of family-based approaches to improve postoperative outcomes among bariatric surgery patients. *Surg Obes Relat Dis* 2011; **11**: 451–8.

7. S. Minuchin. *Family and Family Therapy.* Cambridge, MA: Harvard University Press, 1974.

8. B. Broderick. *Understanding Family Process: Basics of Family Systems Theory*. Thousand Oaks, CA: SAGE Publications, 1993.

9. K. J. Pratt, E. Holowacz, and N. L. Walton. Marriage and family therapists' perspectives on treating overweight clients and their weight-related behaviors. *Am J Fam Ther* 2014; **42**: 364–85.

10. A. Byland, E. Benzein, and C. Persson. Creating a new sense of we-ness: Family functioning in relation to gastric bypass surgery. *Bariatr Surg Pract Patient Care* 2013; **8**: 152–60.

11. M. R. Lent, L. Bailey-Davis, B. A. Irving, et al. Bariatric surgery patients and their families: Healthy, physical activity, and social support. *Obes Surg* 2016; **26**: 2981–8.

12. M. L. Pories, J. Hodgson, M. A. Rose, et al. Following bariatric surgery: An exploration of the couples' experience. *Obes Surg* 2016; **26**: 54–60.

13. A. Wallwork, L. Tremblay, M. Chi, et al. Exploring partners' experiences in living with patients who undergo bariatric surgery. *Obes Surg* 2017; **27**: 1973–81.

14. M. A. Lewis, C. M. McBride, K. I. Pollak, et al. Understanding health behaviour change among couples: An interdependence and communal coping approach. *Soc Sci Med* 2006; **62**: 1369–80.

15. W. R. McFarlane. Psychoeducation: A potential model for intervention in family practice. In R. Sawa, ed., *Family Health Care*. Thousand Oaks, CA: SAGE Publications, 1992: 200–12.

16. L. R. Vartarian and J. Fardouly. Reducing the stigma of bariatric surgery: Benefits of providing information about necessary lifestyle changes. *Obesity* 2014; **22**: 1233–7.

17. P. Drew. "But then I learned . . . ": Weight loss surgery patients negotiate surgery discourses. *Soc Sci Med* 2011; **73**: 1230–7.

18. K. S. Groven. "They think surgery is just a quick fix." *Int J Qual Stud Health Well-Being* 2014; **9**: 1–14.

19. B. A. Mattingly, M. A. Stambush, and A. E. Hill. Shedding the pounds but not the stigma: Negative attributions as a function of a target's method of weight loss. *J Appl Biobehav Res* 2009; **14**: 128–44.

20. L. R. Vartarian and J. Fardouly. The stigma of obesity surgery: Negative evaluations based on weight loss history. *Obes Surg* 2013; **23**: 1545–50.

21. J. O. Prochaska and C. C. DiClemente. Stages and processes of self-change of smoking: Toward an integrative model of change. *J Consult Clin Psychol* 1983; **51**: 390–5.

22. J. P. Ogle, J. Park, M. L. Damhorst, et al. Social support for women who have undergone bariatric surgery. *Qual Health Res* 2016; **26**: 176–93.

23. G. Andrews. Intimate saboteurs. *Obes Surg* 1997; **75**: 445–8.

24. L. M. Martire, R. Schulz, V. S. Helgeson, et al. Review and meta-analysis of couple-oriented interventions for chronic illness. *Ann Behav Med* 2010; **40**: 325–42.

25. S. Garbers, C. McDonnell, S. C. Fogel, et al. Aging, weight, and health among adult lesbian and bisexual women: A metasynthesis of the multisite "health weight initiative" focus groups. *LGBT Health* 2015; **2**: 176–87.

26. S. I. Saarni, H. Anttila, S. E. Saarni, et al. Ethical issues of obesity surgery: A health technology assessment. *Obes Surg* 2011; **21**: 1469–76.

27. A. Wallwork and L. Tremblay. The role of social support in weight loss management for morbidly obese individuals. In S. Sockalingam and R. Hawa, eds., *Psychiatric Care in Severe Obesity: An Interdisciplinary Guide to Integrated Care*. New York, NY: Springer International, 2017: 207–19.

28. A. Gorin, S. Phelan, D. Tate, et al. Involving support partners in obesity treatment. *J Consult Clin Psychol* 2005; **73**: 341–3.

29. S. Caprio, S. R. Daniels, A. Drewnowski, et al. Influence of race, ethnicity, and culture on childhood obesity: Implications for prevention and treatment. *Obesity* 2008; **16**: 2566–77.

30. L. M. Martire and R. Schulz. Involving family in psychosocial interventions for chronic illness. *Curr Dir Psychol Sci* 2007; **16**: 90–4.

Chapter 13

Support Groups for Severe Obesity

Susan Wnuk, Lorraine Gougeon, and Annie Basterfield

Case Vignette

Horizons Medical Weight Management Center is an outpatient program located in a medium-sized city in North America. The multidisciplinary clinical team is composed of family physicians, nurses, dietitians, social workers, an internist, and a kinesiologist. Other medical specialists including an endocrinologist, psychologist, and psychiatrist are available to provide consultations or time-limited treatment on an as-needed basis. Treatment options include medication, nutrition counseling and follow-up, brief behavior therapy, exercise counseling, and a time-limited liquid meal replacement. To be eligible for treatment, patients must have a body mass index (BMI) of 27 kg/m^2 or higher and obesity-related comorbidities. Patients are expected to attend appointments one to three times per month. The typical patient at Horizons attends regular appointments for one to two years with the goal of achieving a weight loss of at least 10 to 20 percent excess body weight. Patients are predominantly female, Caucasian, between the ages of 40 and 60 years, and working to middle class. Horizons also refers patients to a bariatric surgery clinic if indicated.

During a monthly business meeting at Horizons, a social worker raised the idea of starting a patient support group. She explained that over the past few months, several different patients had inquired about local support groups as a way to meet others experiencing similar problems and to share ideas about local resources and strategies for healthy living. The team discussed the logistical concerns related to starting a support group, including identifying the facilitator(s), the frequency and scheduling of the group, and the physical space for the group. They decided that they would start by hosting a monthly 60-minute meeting during a weekday evening that would be facilitated by the social worker and a dietitian. They set the date of the first meeting in three months to provide enough time to advertise the meeting to patients. They advertised by posting flyers in the clinic's waiting room and on the clinic's website.

The social worker and dietitian facilitating the group met approximately one month prior to the first session to discuss their hopes for the group and the content and structure of the first session. They identified several possible goals for the group, ranging from promoting and supporting weight loss through diet and exercise, to discussing relationship issues, to identifying strategies for healthy food preparation and eating. Since they were not sure how best to make decisions about these issues, they decided to ask their patients via a needs assessment that they would distribute over the next two weeks. In addition, the dietitian raised concerns about group members seeking individual nutrition advice from her during sessions. The social worker suggested that family members and friends be allowed to accompany patients. Based on these concerns, they established group guidelines they would announce to patients at the beginning of the first session. They planned to have members sign in at each session and to add new members as requested.

Introduction

Good social support is critical in helping individuals make and sustain health-related behavioral changes. Support groups can be an effective means for providing this support, particularly when it is not available in other ways. The modern support and self-help group movement began in the twentieth century, with participation in these groups increasing beginning in the 1960s [1]. Individuals reporting less support and more conflict in their existing personal social networks were more likely to participate in self-help groups compared with those with more supportive personal networks. In a 2002 report based on survey findings, self-help organizations and other consumer-run services for individuals with mental health problems greatly outnumbered traditional mental health organizations [2].

For a variety of mental and physical health conditions, there is strong evidence to suggest that a social structure, such as self-help and support groups centered on a specific topic or problem, encourages the expression of associated emotions and buffers people from stress [3]. Support groups can provide a sense of community for individuals struggling with health problems, can be an important mediating factor in dealing with stressful health issues such as obesity, and can even improve health outcomes [3–5].

The aim of this chapter is to describe the conceptual and practical considerations related to beginning and maintaining a support group for adults with obesity and associated health conditions. The chapter is divided into sections, beginning with a brief review of theories, principles, and research on support groups, followed by practical recommendations for translating these findings into practice, and concluding with a discussion of factors to consider when facilitating support groups for specific populations.

Psychotherapy, Self-Help, and Support Groups

While support groups, self-help groups, and psychotherapy groups have many features in common, for the purposes of this chapter, support groups are differentiated from psychotherapy and self-help groups with the understanding that the latter two types of groups have the explicit aim of creating change in the members [6]. Support groups, on the other hand, meet for the purposes of providing emotional support and information to individuals with a common problem [6].

Self-Help Groups

Self-help groups are not usually led by professionally trained facilitators and do not charge members a fee for participating. Anyone who is interested in attending can typically do so. The member intake and attendance format is open so that individuals are free to attend sessions when they wish. These groups may have a national or international organizational structure but are not usually dependent on local organizations that host the group. For example, while meetings may take place in a community center, if needed, the group can move to another location without affecting its mission. Self-help groups usually follow some type of program, such as a workbook or steps. The most well-known and prototypical group in this category is Alcoholics Anonymous, which has led to offshoots including Overeaters Anonymous.

Psychotherapy Groups

Psychotherapy groups are usually led by a mental health professional trained in a psychotherapeutic approach who directs the group in accordance with a particular structural and/or theoretical understanding and agenda. This agenda is in service of specific psychological or behavioral goals such as treating binge eating disorder. The session plan often includes exercises or interventions at certain points in a session. For example, in a typical cognitive-behavioral group, homework is reviewed, followed by instruction and discussion about thought and behavior monitoring. Psychotherapy groups are also driven by a theoretical understanding of the meaning of member behaviors, thoughts, and emotions, and this understanding informs interventions. For example, in a relational process group, the group facilitator may explicitly comment on group member behaviors that interfere with maintaining stable relationships. In psychotherapy groups, members are usually charged a fee and are asked to commit to attending a certain number of sessions, and groups are usually hosted in a healthcare or mental healthcare facility. Potential members are interviewed and screened to ensure that they meet criteria for the group and may be discharged from the group if they miss a certain number of sessions or repeatedly exhibit disruptive behavior.

Support Groups

Like psychotherapy groups, support groups are also led by a facilitator, but this person's role is usually more administrative and organizational. The facilitator may make arrangements for the physical space of the group, communicate with members to remind them of meeting times, make announcements, and start and end each session. These tasks may be shared between more than one person, and roles may rotate over time. The leader is not looked to as the definitive source of knowledge and wisdom. Instead, knowledge and wisdom are understood to reside within each member, who contributes from his or her own perspective and life experience. The content of each session is not usually highly structured or agenda driven and instead flexibly accommodates the needs and wishes of the group. Because support groups are facilitated by professionals who are usually linked to a healthcare organization or community agency, members will likely be required to be registered or otherwise affiliated with the hosting organization. Like self-help groups, support groups tend to have an open admission and attendance policy so that members can attend sessions when they wish. While change may be desired and may occur in members, change goals are subordinate to those of emotional support and information sharing. In this way, support groups are an adjunct to active treatment, not active treatment in and of themselves.

Therapeutic Factors in Support Groups

Yalom's *therapeutic factors* are intended to answer the question of how group therapy works. They were first published in the original 1970 text, *Theory and Practice of Group Psychotherapy*, which is now in its fifth edition [7]. The 11 therapeutic factors were created to identify the mechanisms of change in group psychotherapy, and although they are identified separately, it is understood that they overlap and are interdependent. Due to individual differences, participants in the same group might benefit from different factors or groups of factors. Research has shown that many of these factors are relevant in support groups for a variety of health conditions, including bariatric surgery patients. They have also been found to be helpful in a support group for improving self-esteem and general coping skills for women [8–10]. The 11 factors and how they may affect support groups for obesity are summarized next.

Instillation of Hope

This factor is crucial in any form of individual or group psychotherapy. Support groups offer a unique advantage, however, in that members will be at various stages of development in addressing their shared problem or aspects of the problem. Members can be inspired and encouraged by others who have overcome or are successfully managing the problems with which they are still struggling.

Universality

Individuals often seek support because they feel alone in their struggles and "flawed" for having these struggles. Meeting other group members who share similar experiences and feelings can provide a profound sense of relief. Importantly, in relation to this factor, obesity is a highly stigmatized condition [11] (see Chapter 3). Individuals with obesity may internalize societal messages that they are failing or out of control; thus, meeting others who understand the damaging effects of these messages can relieve shame and feelings of isolation. The authenticity of this shared firsthand experience lends credence to group members' suggestions. Universality has been found to be relevant in research on support groups for patients with cancer and bariatric surgery patients [9,12].

Imparting Information

Information can be conveyed by group members or facilitators. In groups for individuals with obesity, the variety of topics can range widely and will depend on the focus of the group. For example, information might be provided about diabetes management, mental health concerns, or exercise that is gentle on joints. Ideally, the spirit from which information is shared is one of collaboration.

Altruism

Although most individuals do not join a support group with the conscious intention of helping others, over time this factor tends to emerge as members gain experience with the group and with managing their own concerns. Altruism naturally occurs as a result of imparting information. The experience of being able to give something to another member, such as information about one's own struggles with a similar difficult experience, can boost the member's self-esteem, confidence, and interpersonal skills.

Corrective Recapitulation of the Primary Family Experience

This factor is not usually explicitly named and discussed in support groups. However, individuals with obesity come from diverse backgrounds that might include childhood and adult trauma, neglect, or other emotionally painful experiences. They will carry their expectations of others, whether for good or for ill, into the group, and this may be expressed in their behavior. In well-functioning support groups, members will feel safe to express themselves, seek information and support, and encourage each other. These experiences can implicitly provide a corrective experience to dysfunctional early relationships. Problematic interpersonal behaviors such as monopolizing the group through excessive talking or advice giving can be seen as learned behaviors arising from past difficult experiences.

Development of Socializing Techniques

The group setting ideally provides a safe and supportive environment for members to take risks by extending their repertoire of interpersonal behavior and improving their social skills. This factor is not usually explicitly addressed in support groups, especially those that focus on a shared condition such as obesity. However, as group members become more comfortable with each other, they may become more willing to share vulnerable feelings, and the response from the group can provide useful feedback.

Imitative Behavior

Group members learn from watching and hearing how they each tackle various problems. Imitative behavior may be more important in the early stages of a group and each individual member's first few sessions attending a group, when the other group members and facilitators are looked to as role models for how to behave. Through this process, members learn how to express personal feelings, show concern, and support others.

Interpersonal Learning

This factor is based on three aspects: the importance of interpersonal relationships to human beings as a species, corrective emotional experiences (members having a meaningful emotional experience in the group that disconfirms problematic beliefs usually learned early in life, for example, that others will hurt or abandon them), and the group as a social microcosm (i.e., over time, group members will feel comfortable and safe and will display the interpersonal style they default to in other parts of their lives). Interpersonal learning is not typically explicitly addressed in support groups but will operate implicitly. Understanding this factor can be helpful for group facilitators in addressing group member behaviors.

Group Cohesiveness

A cohesive group is one in which all members feel a sense of belonging, acceptance, and validation. This factor is akin to the therapeutic relationship in individual psychotherapy, and just as a positive therapeutic relationship is needed for individual therapy to be effective, group cohesiveness is necessary for the other therapeutic factors to operate in a group. Cohesiveness encompasses the relationship of each member with every group member as well as with the facilitators. Cohesiveness is not static but rather fluctuates during the course of the group. In the case of support groups, cohesiveness will vary each session because different members will be present.

Catharsis

Catharsis is the experience of relief from emotional distress through the free and uninhibited expression of emotion. When group members tell their stories to a supportive audience, they can find relief from chronic feelings of shame and guilt. Importantly, the intensity of emotional expression must be appreciated from the perspective of the member, not the facilitator. Catharsis does not always involve crying, a raised voice, or other clearly visible signs of emotion. A seemingly unemotional expression might feel very important and vulnerable to the person making the expression.

Existential Factors

This factor is composed of five items: the recognition that life is unfair and unjust at times, that there is no escape from some of life's pain or death, that ultimately one must face life alone, the importance of facing the basic issues of life and death and thus living life more honestly and less caught up by trivialities, and learning to take ultimate responsibility for the way one lives their life, regardless of advice and support from others. This factor is particularly relevant to individuals who are seriously medically ill, including individuals with medical comorbidities related to obesity.

Practical Considerations in Planning a Support Group

Before beginning a support group, decisions should be made about several practical or structural aspects. These decisions can change over time in response to facilitator experience, group member feedback, and the natural evolution of the group.

Goals and Purpose of the Group

The goals and purpose of the group will depend on the nature of the patient population. There are many subpopulations within the general condition of obesity; for example, individuals with type 2 diabetes, those who struggle with binge eating disorder (BED), young adults, and bariatric surgery patients. Depending on the setting, the treatment and perspective of the hosting organization will vary and will be reflected in the mission of the group. In a medically supervised weight loss clinic, for instance, it would follow that the purpose of the group would be to support weight loss and weight loss maintenance. In a BED treatment clinic, the goal of the group might be to normalize eating behaviors and discuss strategies for preventing binges, while weight loss would be secondary. To clarify the purpose and goals further, it can be helpful to conduct a needs assessment of potential group members. The needs assessment should include questions about practical concerns such as the timing and frequency of the group as well discussion topics.

In order for support groups to be optimally productive and helpful to members, group guidelines or rules that are in keeping with the group's purpose should be developed. Group guidelines should be reviewed at the start of each session to familiarize new members with the expectations and to emphasize their importance for returning members. Guidelines to consider include arriving on time and staying for the duration of the group, keeping other group members' private information and identities confidential, avoiding providing direct advice and instead speaking from personal experience, not interrupting others when they are speaking, being aware of how frequently and for how long one speaks so as to provide others the chance to contribute, and muting and putting away cell phones.

Support Group Facilitators

A stance of openness, genuineness, caring, and empathy is the foundation for effective group facilitation [7]. Clinicians who wish to facilitate support groups should have training in basic group facilitation skills. An understanding of group dynamics, types of groups, typical member roles, stages of group development, and interventions is very useful in successfully running a group. This may mean that a clinician interested in running a support group who does not possess this background experience will partner with a colleague who does.

Wasserman and Danforth propose a useful set of goals for support group facilitators: (1) information exchange, (2) an atmosphere of mutual support, (3) group cohesion, (4) increased coping and self-efficacy, (5) reduction in social isolation, (6) stress reduction, (7) an atmosphere of safety, and (8) reinforcement of members' positive activity in and outside the group [13]. To accomplish these general goals, support group facilitators do not rely on interpretation of behavior, as would be typical in psychotherapy groups, and do not emphasize a particular approach, as in self-help groups. Instead, the facilitator will open and close the group, make announcements about community resources, refocus the group's communication or propose a discussion topic, and review the group guidelines and intervene when these are being infringed upon.

Ideally, two facilitators run a group. This allows for the sharing of facilitation duties and less disruption within sessions when an individual member requires assistance outside the session. There may be times when a facilitator is not able to attend a session or may discontinue his or her facilitation role altogether and a new facilitator joins. These changes need to be communicated to the group in advance whenever possible because members become accustomed to interacting with particular individual facilitators and may require time to adjust.

Composition of the Group

In terms of membership, groups will naturally be composed of patients from the healthcare organization where the facilitators work, and facilitators should consider their knowledge of patients' needs and expectations. For example, is the support group appropriate for all patients or just those who are at a particular stage in treatment? If patients vary widely in age, should the group be subdivided based on age? These and similar questions should be considered to anticipate potential challenges. Decisions about whether to permit group members' family and friends will depend on the nature of the treatment of the hosting organization. For example, it may be appropriate for nonpatients to attend diabetes management support groups or bariatric surgery support groups to learn how they can best support the patient. These decisions should be made based on the facilitators' and group members' comfort and preferences. Based on the authors' experience, groups with more than 20 members become difficult to manage. If attendance repeatedly exceeds this number, the group may need to be divided into two smaller groups.

Group Member Intake and Attendance

Regarding group member intake and attendance, open groups continuously admit new members and allow members to attend sessions when they are available. These groups are usually ongoing and do not have a defined end date. Advantages are that a greater number of individuals can be supported, and the changing composition of the group from session to session leads to greater diversity of discussion. The main disadvantage is that group cohesion may be a challenge because members do not have as much contact with each other. In a closed group, members are asked to commit to attending each session as scheduled, and these groups often end after a certain number of sessions. Advantages of this format are the greater degree of cohesion among individuals and greater feelings of emotional safety over time as members come to know each other more intimately.

Meeting Frequency, Schedule, and Location

Meeting frequency, schedule, and location will depend on facilitator and organizational limits combined with the needs of the greatest number of potential members. Evening meetings are usually best for accommodating members' work schedules. The location is typically in the setting that houses the health organization, such as hospitals or other clinical settings. Care should be taken to ensure that appropriately sized chairs are available in the group room. In settings where patients have limited physical mobility or require assistive devices, the space should be accessible.

Meeting Structure and Agenda

Support group sessions are not agenda driven to the same extent as psychotherapy and self-help groups. In early sessions while the group is forming, it can be helpful to have a sequence of activities planned. When beginning support group sessions, especially in open-format groups, facilitator and patient introductions and check-ins are helpful in guiding the session's discussion. Facilitators should introduce themselves and their professional role within the treatment program and then invite members to introduce themselves. In addition to stating their first names, it can be helpful for members to briefly describe their stage in the treatment process as well as any topics they would like to discuss during the session. As these introductions and check-ins are taking place, the facilitator should take note of discussion topics raised by members. If time and group size permit, icebreaker questions can be a helpful tool to use during introductions in order to initiate group discussion and help group members feel more at ease [14]. Sample icebreaker topics are favorite television shows and favorite holiday locations. In closed support groups, early sessions may begin with introductions and check-ins similar to open groups. However, as members become more familiar with each other, it may be more useful for sessions to begin with check-ins related to the obesity treatment. For example, facilitators may ask patients to update the group on their treatment progress since the last session and whether there have been any positive experiences and/or challenges. In both open and closed groups, a check-out can be helpful for members to reflect on what they learned from the session and to provide feedback. Table 13.1 lists suggested topics for obesity support groups.

Self-help and psychotherapy group interventions and techniques, such as readings and goal setting, can be incorporated into support groups. The intention should remain consistent with the overall purpose of the particular group. For example, if the purpose of the group is to support members with weight loss goals, interventions focused on effective goal setting may be particularly useful. Similarly, short activities and exercises such as brief mindfulness exercises can be helpful. Facilitators should ensure that activities do not take too much time away from the general purpose of the support group model, which focuses on the provision of information and support. If members are required to complete homework or report back on behavioral change, the group will evolve into a therapy group, and another set of considerations and decisions will be required of the facilitators. These skill-building opportunities are more suited to closed and/or time-limited support groups because the group will be composed of the same members from session to session, and therefore, all attendees will be familiar with the readings or information discussed from session to session.

Table 13.1 Suggested Topics for Obesity Support Group Meetings

Category	Suggested topics
Nutrition	• Specific nutrition concerns (e.g., fiber intake, vitamins) • Protein sources • Recipe exchange • Healthy snack ideas • Methods for tracking food intake • Tips for eating at restaurants • Planning and organizing meal plans • Grocery shopping and cooking • Weight plateaus
Exercise	• Types of exercise • Starting an exercise program • Exercising with mobility challenges and pain • Hiring a fitness professional • Lack of familiarity with exercise facilities
Social	• Enlisting the support of family and friends • Managing reactions to lifestyle changes and weight loss • Dating, healthy eating, and weight loss • Impact of lifestyle changes on work and workplace relationships • Sexual health and lifestyle changes
Psychological	• Binge eating • Food cravings • Grazing • Emotional eating • Body image • Depression, anxiety, and other mental health problems • Professional mental health treatment
Medical	• Gastrointestinal issues (e.g., irritable bowel syndrome, constipation) • Fertility concerns and weight • Excess loose skin following weight loss • Joint problems • Diabetes • Medications and weight

Support Group Creation and Maintenance Cycle

Taken from a wider perspective, creating and maintaining a successful, productive support group involves many identifiable and interconnected steps that are outlined below. Steps 7 and 8 can be repeated as often as needed.

1. **Suggest the Purpose of the Group and Membership.** The first step in creating a support group is to identify the purpose of the group and who the group is meant to serve.
2. **Conduct a Needs Assessment.** Once the general purpose and member composition of the group have been identified, a needs assessment of prospective group members should be conducted. This assessment is most easily accomplished via a brief self-report

questionnaire and should include questions to solicit information from potential group members about their hopes and expectations for the group.

3. **Establish Group Purpose and Membership.** Based on the results of the needs assessment, the purpose of the group and membership can be clarified and established.

4. **Develop a Session Plan and Schedule.** The session plan can be brief and should include a description of group activities.

5. **Advertise.** Means for notifying potential group members should be identified. This can include posting notices in the physical space of the clinic, online on obesity-related websites or forums, and by email. Sufficient time for advertising should be provided prior to the first session. Advertisements should include the name of the support group, location and dates of the meetings, and contact information for the group facilitator(s).

6. **Facilitate Sessions.** With the above-mentioned preparation completed, meetings can be facilitated as planned.

7. **Solicit Group Member Feedback.** Group member feedback is important for making the group relevant to the largest number of patients. When the facilitators ask for feedback, they communicate that they take members' needs seriously and intend to collaborate with members to improve the group. Before asking for group member feedback, it is important for the facilitators or hosting organization to clarify the type of information that would be helpful as well as the purpose of the information. Some examples include querying the overall helpfulness of the group, members' experience of the group dynamics and/or facilitators, and asking for suggestions for discussion topics. This information can be collected for program evaluation or for a formal research project.

Feedback can be collected through questionnaires administered following each session or at monthly or quarterly intervals. Several self-report questionnaires that measure various aspects of group functioning have been developed and used in research and can be considered for this purpose. Brief measures include the Group Sessions Rating Scale [15], which contains four items to measure group members' feelings of being respected by the leader and group, their sense that the group is relevant, and the extent to which they discussed relevant topics. The Group Climate Questionnaire Short Form [16] is composed of 12 items that assess group members' perception of their engagement in the group, sense of responsibility for group work, and conflict between members. Longer and more comprehensive measures include the Therapeutic Factors Inventory Short Form [17], which includes 19 items to assess Yalom's therapeutic factors. The original long form of this measure contained 99 items [18]. The Group Questionnaire [19] contains 40 items to measure group members' sense of belonging to the group, ability of the group to work effectively on shared goals, and trust between members and leaders. Finally, the Working Alliance Inventory [20] assesses the therapeutic alliance between the group leaders and members and has 36 items that measure the extent of the emotional bonding between group therapist and members and their agreement on tasks and goals of therapy.

8. **Implement Changes.** Changes based on the group member feedback should be implemented if feasible. Facilitators should review feedback to identify themes and common requests. After taking into account the facilitators' abilities and practical and institutional limits, changes suggested by group members can be implemented as a way of enhancing group cohesion and better meeting the needs of the group.

Challenges in Facilitating Support Groups

While support groups offer many benefits to patients and can be rewarding for facilitators, challenges will occur. Facilitators should reflect on potential challenges, become aware of their boundaries, and consider responses that are empathic yet firm. Challenges in groups are usually interpersonal in nature and thus are often difficult to navigate emotionally. Facilitators should also keep in mind the power imbalance between themselves and the members and approach these situations with sensitivity. Although support group leaders do not explicitly take on an expert role, members will nonetheless cast them in that role to some extent based on their professional identity and leadership of the group. Some challenges relate to group member nonadherence to group guidelines, while others relate to factors such as personal boundaries and mental health concerns. Below are several examples of common group challenges and suggested facilitator responses.

The Monopolizing Group Member

Depending on personality and interpersonal style, some members may be so eager to discuss certain topics that they monopolize group discussions. One of the tasks of the facilitator is to monitor the discussion and to shape group members' behavior so that everyone has an opportunity to speak [7]. This can be done in reference to group guidelines to reinforce that facilitator corrections are not arbitrary.

> FACILITATOR: [*Interrupting a group member during a session*] I appreciate you have a lot you want to share with us, but for the sake of time and to let others contribute, I need to stop you there. One of our group guidelines is to be mindful about how much airtime each person takes in the group.

On occasion, there may be a member who is consistently nonadherent to the group guideline of sharing speaking opportunities. Facilitators should meet with the group member individually to explain the purpose of this guideline and to problem solve. This private discussion may be enough, or the member may need more support or reminders from the facilitator during sessions. If after an individual meeting a group member is still unable to change his or her behavior, the facilitator may offer other forms of support or ask the member to leave the group.

> FACILITATOR: [*Speaking with a member privately after a session*] I notice that you've been struggling with sticking to the group guideline of limiting how much airtime you take. An important goal for the group is for everyone to have a chance to contribute. I'm wondering what would help you remember this guideline?
>
> GROUP MEMBER: Sometimes I get carried away when talking about things that are important to me, especially when I get upset about family stuff. I don't know what would help me stop. I have a hard time controlling myself, and besides, lots of the people in the group are really quiet and don't talk much, so I might as well talk.
>
> FACILITATOR: I think we have a couple of options. If you'd like to keep working on this in the group, I could signal you once you've taken up an appropriate amount of time. If that's

not something that seems doable right now, the other option would be for you to do some individual therapy so that you can address those family issues in more depth than we can in the group; then you could return to the group later. What do you think?

Conflict between Group Members

Repeated nonadherence to group guidelines, emphasis on personal struggles without apparent efforts to change behavior, and interpersonal differences can lead to conflict between group members. Conflict often manifests as more subtle cues that can easily go unnoticed by facilitators. For example, if one member is monopolizing the discussion, other group members may express their frustration by rolling their eyes, whispering, or even turning their backs away from the offending group member. Although it can be difficult to notice these subtle body language expressions and identify the reason for them, facilitators should be aware of the potential for these expressions.

If the facilitator notices a group member expressing conflict through body language, it is best to meet with that member individually to identify the nature of the conflict and discuss steps for more effectively managing it. Signs of conflict should be addressed sooner rather than later; otherwise, the conflict can escalate and members could leave permanently. The following dialogue is a suggested way of responding to such a situation.

FACILITATOR: [*To a group member, speaking privately after the session*] I noticed that through-out today's group, you seemed to be turning your back to one particular group member every time he spoke, and you made loud sighs that seemed to distract other group members. I'm wondering what was going on?

GROUP MEMBER: Oh, I just can't stand that person! I find him very annoying!

FACILITATOR: That does sound really frustrating. Is there anything specific that has happened between the two of you to cause conflict?

GROUP MEMBER: Well, not specifically – but he just irritates me. Every time he talks, I can't help but roll my eyes and sigh because I'm so annoyed.

FACILITATOR: I understand. It's unlikely that everyone will get along in a group when you are all coming from different backgrounds. However, I need to remind you of the group guideline that we accept each group member as they are and try to avoid judgments. While it's not expected that everyone will like everyone in the group, it is expected that we show everyone respect, which includes body language. Even if you feel annoyed, I hope that you're willing to stop the sighing, eye rolling, and turning away?

Finally, group members may at times come into conflict with the facilitators or institution about policies or guidelines. For example, members may object to a guideline about not eating during support group sessions. In these situations, the facilitators should allow the members to voice their concerns and then validate those concerns and explain the rationale for that particular guideline. It may not always be possible to accommodate individual members' preferences, and this may lead to member frustration, but as much as possible the needs of the group as a whole must be balanced with institutional/facilitator limits and policies.

Responding to Personal Questions

Group members naturally become curious about the group facilitators' personal lives. In the case of support groups for individuals living with obesity, members may be interested in the facilitators' own experiences with weight and their eating practices. While most group members will be aware of appropriate interpersonal boundaries in clinician-patient relationships, some members will ask direct questions. Self-disclosure in therapeutic contexts is a controversial topic, and recommendations vary greatly depending on psychotherapy philosophy and modality [21]. It is beyond the scope of this chapter to review these different perspectives, but for the purposes of support group facilitation, it is important to be aware of one's own personal limits around self-disclosure and to formulate possible responses to personal questions.

> GROUP MEMBER: [*Turning to facilitators*] You're both thin and look like you've never had to watch what you eat. Have either of you ever been overweight or on a diet?
>
> FACILITATOR: [*Option 1*] I appreciate you wanting to know more about me, but this group is about you, and my weight isn't something I talk about with patients.
>
> FACILITATOR: [*Option 2*] Yes, I've struggled with my weight for most of my life and have been maintaining a healthy weight with the help of a dietitian I see regularly. I've also had psychotherapy to work on emotional eating.
>
> FACILITATOR: [*Option 3*] I don't talk about my weight with patients, but I can assure you that I've also struggled with different things in my life.

Significant Mental Health Issues

While the purpose of support groups for obesity is unlikely to be focused specifically on mental health concerns, discussion of topics related to obesity, such as body image, eating behaviors, and psychological processes related to eating can result in members becoming more aware of their mental health. Further, discussion of these topics may result in some members feeling distressed. In addition, members who have already self-identified that they are experiencing challenges with their mental health may use the support group as an opportunity to seek help and/or reach out for more support. In rare cases, members may also express suicidal ideation within the support group setting.

Whenever possible, a facilitator who is a trained mental health clinician should be present at support group sessions to intervene in crisis situations. If this is not possible, a plan for addressing these situations should be developed. If mental health concerns are identified for a specific group member that do not require crisis intervention, facilitators should make a serious effort to connect with that group member after the session to offer support and suggest additional resources if needed. If time and resources do not allow for more individualized follow-up after the support group session, facilitators may consider creating a list of resources that can be distributed to members.

Special Populations and Settings

Individuals attending obesity support groups may have little else in common besides their weight status. Two individuals medically classified as obese may be of different genders, ages, physical abilities, medical conditions, and educational and socioeconomic classes, to name but a few characteristics that contribute to one's lived experience. These characteristics should be taken into account because they may have a significant impact on group members' experience and may require sensitive and appropriate facilitator responses. In this section we discuss the needs of women and men, minority groups, young adults, bariatric surgery patients, and Internet-based support groups.

With regard to gender, the bulk of the research on obesity support groups has focused on men and women as identified groups. The authors recognize that the focus on men and women in this section does not include other gender identities, expressions, and experiences and that the considerations for individuals of nonbinary gender identities, expressions, and experiences may be different from what is recommended in this chapter.

Women

Women experience a number of unique medical risks associated with obesity, including difficulties with reproductive health and risks during pregnancy, including polycystic ovarian syndrome [22,23]. Research has suggested that women experience more body dissatisfaction than men [24,25], and therefore, body image may be a primary focus for women living with obesity. When working with women in obesity support groups, facilitators should consider that these particular concerns can be important for some women to discuss.

Research has focused on the importance of social support for women during weight loss treatments, including lifestyle-focused interventions and bariatric surgery. In a lifestyle and online weight loss intervention for veterans, it was found that in the online forum component, women participated more in social support than men [26]. Other qualitative studies have demonstrated the self-identified importance of social support within the weight loss program by women [27–29]. While support from family members and friends is very important, support from "like others" (others who are also going through weight loss treatment) has been highlighted as particularly important for women because these individuals can provide empathetic understanding and unique feedback [29]. When designing support groups for women, facilitators should consider the importance of the social support component and allow group members time and opportunities to engage in this form of support.

Men

Men are typically more reluctant to seek help when dealing with health-related issues [30]. Davies and colleagues conducted focus groups of male college students to determine what health concerns the students had, what barriers prevented them from seeking help, and what recommendations could be adopted to help men lead healthier lifestyles [31]. The most common health concerns focused on alcohol use, followed by personal fitness and physical appearance, including maintaining desired weight and healthy eating habits. The most cited barriers to seeking health services were the desire to conceal vulnerability and to demonstrate independence. The focus groups provided strategies for improving services to male students. Free services such as health classes, a call-in telephone line, and information workshops that included some incentive to attend were suggested. It was felt that peer presenters would decrease feelings of vulnerability, and a small-group setting would improve comfort levels of men seeking help.

Health of Men (HoM) is a weight management program started in 1997 to develop health services for men in Bradford and Airedale, United Kingdom [32]. Goals of the program include establishing weight management groups in community settings and workplace locations, providing the groups with support information and advice, and eventually enabling the men to run their own groups. Eight groups were established, and all completed a free six-week course of one-hour meetings during work time. They also had the support of a dietitian and an exercise specialist who provided direct expert information. Although some of the groups dissolved at the end of the six weeks, the majority continued to meet regularly for weight monitoring and group support. Aspects of the groups that the participants valued were confidentiality, the friendly environment, and the provision of skill-building tools.

A systematic review by Robertson and colleagues sought to determine what strategies could be used to increase the use of health services by men in the United Kingdom [33]. They found some evidence that men respond better to healthcare interventions that offer tests, facts, and figures (e.g., cholesterol testing), those that are offered in workplace settings, and those that also target men's partners. Overall, they were unable to determine from this review whether programs specifically targeting men are warranted.

Many men perceive dieting and weight loss as female concerns to the detriment of their own health, as shown by rising obesity rates and health conditions associated with obesity, such as diabetes, coronary heart disease, hypertension, and arthritis. Support groups may be beneficial to men with severe obesity if they are offered in familiar settings, target health goals, have input from healthcare professionals, and are peer led.

Minority Groups

When designing support groups, facilitators need to be sensitive to the fact that group members may come from diverse backgrounds, including ethnic/cultural minorities, socio-economic backgrounds, sexual identities, gender identities, and various physical and non-physical abilities. In addition, there may be barriers that prevent group members from attending support groups, including language barriers, lack of transportation and accessibility, lack of child care, and timing of groups [34–36]. The needs of diverse group members may vary within the support group, and therefore, facilitators should make an effort to make support groups as inclusive as possible for their diverse group members. This could include implementing considerations such as using inclusive language, ensuring the availability of accessible facilities, providing transportation reimbursement, providing child care, holding support groups in community settings, and integrating guidelines around respecting and celebrating the diversity of group members.

In settings where there is a high concentration of individuals from a particular background, it can be worth considering designing a support group specifically targeted to those individuals. Within the context of obesity, culture can play a very significant role in the understanding of food and eating practices, body image, and physical activity [37]. Brown and colleagues designed a culturally competent intervention for diabetes management among Mexican Americans, in which the following cultural considerations were implemented: preferred language, integration of cultural dietary preferences, focus on social activities and family involvement, and opportunity for discussion about culturally based health beliefs and practices [38]. Similarly, a study examining the perceived barriers and treatment preferences for obesity among urban postpartum African-American women determined that interventions need to address cultural factors, including affordability and cultural perceptions of body image [36]. When facilitators are designing a support group for individuals from a particular cultural background, it is important that facilitators demonstrate culturally competent interventions and become as culturally aware and grounded as possible in order to understand and serve the unique needs of the population.

Young Adults

Consideration of young adults within the scope of treatment for adulthood obesity is very important. In addition to young adulthood being a unique transitional stage in one's life, some young adults may transition between pediatric and adult obesity treatment programs [39]. Therefore, it is important to recognize that the treatment of obesity in young adults will need to address factors associated with this transitional period, including the balance between emerging independence and self-identity and shifting roles of the family in the lives of young adults [39].

Young adulthood is a crucial time for promoting health and disease prevention [39]. In a qualitative study with college students, a number of factors were identified as contributing to weight, diet, and physical activity, including availability of food on campus, snacking and late-night eating, alcohol consumption, and negative experiences using campus recreation facilities [40]. Researchers have suggested that postsecondary campuses are important sites for obesity-related interventions with young adults, considering the number of contributing factors toward weight problems that can be present in this setting [39,40]. Support groups for obesity could also be considered in this setting, focusing on the particular weight-related issues that young adults attending postsecondary institutions encounter.

Bariatric Surgery Patients

The success of bariatric surgery requires lifelong lifestyle changes that include dietary modifications, increased physical activity, and commitment to adhering to vitamin and mineral supplement recommendations. Other factors such as patient education and social support may also contribute to weight loss and improved health. Attendance and participation in bariatric support groups can make aftercare easier and more efficient for patients. Ideally, the group process will generate alternate behaviors and coping strategies to assist patients in the development of choices that will lead to improved health functioning [3].

Face-to-face groups, as well as online forums and chat rooms, offer pre- and postoperative bariatric surgery patients information and support. Beck and colleagues reviewed the evidence regarding the effect of psychotherapeutic interventions, such as individual therapy, group therapy, and support groups, on weight loss after bariatric surgery [41]. They found in three of four studies that attendance at support groups was significantly associated with increased weight loss up to 36 months after surgery. In two studies, a *dose effect* was found. Patients who attended five or more support group meetings lost more weight than those who attended five or fewer meetings in the first year after surgery.

A self-report survey of 274 gastric bypass patients was conducted to determine what variables are associated with successful weight loss one year after bariatric surgery [42]. Their results supported previous research that regular attendance at support group meetings improved weight loss. Additionally, participants rated their adherence to dietary recommendations on a scale from 0 to 9. Participants who reported low to moderate adherence (3 out of 9) had significant postoperative success only if they attended support group meetings. This study recommended that support group attendance (online or in person) should be highly encouraged because it provides social support, information sharing, and accountability and promotes adherence, especially for those in a low to moderate adherence group.

Given the positive relationship between support group attendance and weight loss after surgery, it is important to look at barriers to attending group meetings. Varied or flexible meeting times, structured agendas, innovative topics, and expert speakers may contribute to better attendance.

Support groups led by healthcare providers can provide the bariatric surgery patient with consistent psychological, nutritional, and health information. Madan and colleagues found that patients often did not remember advice that was given to them before surgery, so support groups can provide ongoing education in addition to providing coping strategies for the recurrence of old habits and problematic eating behaviors, such as grazing or binge eating [43].

Although there is no standard model for establishing a support group for bariatric surgery patients, some common themes are expected to be addressed, such as nutrition and physical activity recommendations, surgery-related concerns, body image issues, relapse prevention, and learning from peers. A systematic review by Livhits and colleagues found four studies that provided suggestions for topics of discussion for support groups [44]. Nutrition-related topics included protein, recipe ideas, portion control long term, replacing the coping aspect of eating, dealing with weight loss plateaus, and managing various postoperative diet phases. Exercise, plastic surgery, and dealing with anxiety and depression also were common topics.

Little is known about the efficacy of patient-led bariatric surgery support groups. Bariatric surgery patients are increasingly turning to online patient forums for support. Barriers such as distance, transportation, mobility, and fear of healthcare provider stigmatization were found to limit attendance at face-to-face support group meetings [45,46]. Atwood and colleagues analyzed the frequency of various types of social support exchanged on pre- and postoperative online discussion forums [47]. Most messages exchanged in the preoperative forum provided emotional (49 percent) or informational (39 percent) support. In the postoperative forum, most messages provided informational (52 percent) or emotional (39 percent) support. Other types of support included network support, esteem support, and tangible support. Emotional support included online posts of encouragement, sympathy/empathy, and validation. Informational support included suggestions and advice, such as adhering to dietary guidelines and educating about the requirements for surgical approval. This advice is similar to that which is offered at support groups at bariatric centers. The authors concluded that online bariatric surgery discussion forums may provide valuable support that is otherwise difficult to access, particularly for individuals who do not live in close proximity to the settings offering face-to-face support groups.

Case Vignette Revisited

At a business meeting six months after holding monthly support group meetings, the group facilitators reported back about positive as well as challenging experiences. One of the positive developments was the increase in participation from six patients in the first three sessions to 12 to 15 patients per session in the past two months. They also found that the discussion lagged somewhat for the first two months, with long silences that left some group members appearing visibly uncomfortable. To remedy this, the facilitators developed a list of discussion topics that they brought to each session and would suggest a topic when long silences occurred. This restarted the discussion. They found this to no longer be an issue as many of the original group members attended regularly and became more comfortable with each other. Both facilitators received feedback from various members about how much they valued and enjoyed the group. One member in particular said the group inspired her to continue walking regularly because it improved her blood sugar control even though she hadn't lost weight.

In terms of challenges, many members felt that 60 minutes was not long enough and requested that sessions be extended to 90 minutes. The facilitators likewise found that they usually had to interrupt productive conversations near the end of the allotted session time. They identified a regular group member who tended to dominate sessions, leaving little time for others to speak. Other members appeared visibly frustrated, and they noticed that a few members had stopped attending. There was also a member who frequently complained about her physical and mental health and marriage but rejected suggestions. They noticed that some group members rolled their eyes in annoyance when this particular member spoke. Just as she had feared prior to the first session, the dietitian frequently stayed late to answer pressing nutrition questions posed by members. Finally, one group member brought her 10-year-old son to a session because she was unable to find childcare. The facilitators felt reluctant to confront her and allowed her son to sit in, though other members appeared uncomfortable, and the discussion that night seemed stilted.

After presenting this information, the team discussed ways to improve the group and address challenges. Importantly, the facilitators realized that they were not able to answer some of the questions posed by their colleagues, such as the average age of the members, members' medical concerns, or members' ideas and hopes for the group. Therefore, they decided to distribute a group feedback questionnaire. They considered the option of engaging the group in a discussion to solicit their feedback in the next session but decided against going this route because it would not have permitted enough time for other important topics to be discussed. In addition, some members might not feel comfortable offering criticisms about the group directly to the facilitators. To address the problematic behavior of some individual members, the team suggested speaking with those individuals privately at the end of a session when that behavior occurred to gently point out the problematic behavior and suggest concrete ways to improve. Regarding group members who sought the dietitian's advice after sessions were over, the team decided to add a group guideline, that members who required individualized advice would be directed to make an appointment. Likewise, to prevent inappropriate guests from attending, they added a group guideline that guests must be over the age of 18.

Summary

Support groups can be a valuable resource for individuals living with obesity. The overall purpose of an obesity support group is to provide a forum for the facilitators and members to provide information and emotional support and not to deliver a treatment intervention per se. Support groups nonetheless can be a powerful means for inspiring members to take action to improve their health and wellness. Support groups also provide a venue for clinicians to better understand their patients' experiences and challenges and therefore to provide more effective patient-centered care.

Key Points

- Support groups can be an effective means for providing social support, particularly for patients who lack support in their personal networks.
- Before beginning a support group, facilitators should consider the setting, the needs of potential group members, the purpose of the group, and their own group facilitation skills.
- Individuals with obesity come from varied backgrounds and life experiences, and the needs of special populations within the patient group should be accommodated.
- Support group facilitators should regularly seek feedback from members and implement changes where possible and clinically appropriate.

References

1. R. C. Kessler, K. D. Mickelson, and S. Zhao. Patterns and correlates of self-help group members in the United States. *Soc Policy* 1997; **27**: 27–46.

2. I. D. Goldstrom, J. Campbell, J. A. Rogers, et al. National estimates for mental health mutual support groups, self-help organizations, and consumer-operated services. *Admin Pol Ment Health* 2006; **33**: 92–103.

3. J. D. Marcus and G. R. Elkins. Development of a model for a structured support group for patients following bariatric surgery. *Obes Surg* 2004; **14**: 103–6.

4. D. Spiegel, J. R. Bloom, and E. Gottheil. Effect of psychosocial treatment on survival of patients with metastatic breast cancer. *Lancet* 1989; **334**: 888–91.

5. D. Spiegel. Social support: How friends, family, and groups can help. In D. Goleman and J. Gurin, eds., *Mind Body Medicine*. Yonkers, NY: Consumer Report Books, 1993.

6. L. F. Kurtz. *Self-Help and Support Groups: A Handbook for Practitioners*. Thousand Oaks, CA: SAGE Publications, 1997.

7. I. Yalom and M. Leszcz. *The Theory and Practice of Group Psychotherapy* (5th edn). New York, NY: Basic Books, 2005.

8. L. Ferreira Santos, L. M. de Almeida Cavalcante Oliveira, D. Bouttelet Munari, et al. Therapeutic factors in group support from the perspective of the coordinators and group members. *Acta Paul Enferm* 2012; **25**: 122–7.

9. S. E. Hildebrandt. Effects of participation in bariatric support group after Roux-en-Y gastric bypass. *Obes Surg* 1998; **8**: 535–42.

10. V. Blackmon, C. Cassell, C. G. McElderry, et al. A qualitative impact evaluation of the First Love Yourself (FLY) women's support group. *IJPHS* 2016; **5**: 123–8.

11. R. M. Puhl and C. A. Heuer. Obesity stigma: Important considerations for public health. *Am J Public Health* 2010; **100**: 1019–28.

12. J. Ussher, L. Kirsten, P. Butow, et al. What do cancer support groups provide which other supportive relationships do not? The experience of peer support groups for people with cancer. *Soc Sci Med* 2006; **62**: 2565–76.

13. H. Wasserman and H. E. Danforth. *The Human Bond: Support Groups and Mutual Aid*. New York, NY: Springer, 1988.

14. L. D. DeSilets. Using icebreakers to open communication. *J Contin Educ Nurs* 2008; **39**: 292–3.

15. B. L. Duncan and S. D. Miller. *The Group Session Rating Scale*. Jensen Beach, FL: Authors, 2007.

16. K. R. MacKenzie. The clinical application of a group measure. In R. R. Dies and K. R. MacKenzie, eds., *Advances in Group Psychotherapy: Integrating Research and Practice*. New York, NY: International Universities Press, 1983.

17. A. S. Joyce, R. MacNair-Semands, G. A. Tasca, et al. Factor structure and validity of the Therapeutic Factors Inventory–Short Form. *Group Dyn* 2011; **15**: 201–19.

18. K. P. Lese and R. R. MacNair-Semands. The Therapeutic Factors Inventory: The development of a scale. *Group* 2000; **24**: 303–17.

19. J. Krogel, G. Burlingame, C. Chapman, et al. The Group Questionnaire: A clinical and empirically derived measure of group relationship. *Psychother Res* 2013; **23**: 344–54.

20. A. O. Horvath and L. S. Greenberg. Development and validation of the Working Alliance Inventory. *J Couns Psychol* 1989; **36**: 223–33.

21. B. A. Farber. *Self-disclosure in psychotherapy*. New York, The Guilford Press, 2006.

22. M. J. Legato. Gender-specific aspects of obesity. *Int J Fertil Womens Med* 1997; **42**: 184–97.

23. D. Ryan. Obesity in women: a life cycle of medical risks. *Int J Obes* 2007; **31**: 53–7.

24. T. F. Cash and K. F. Hicks. Being fat versus thinking fat: relationships with body image, eating behaviours, and well-being. *Cognit Ther Res* 1990; **14**: 327–41.

25. M. B. Schwartz and K. D. Brownell. Obesity and body image. *Body Image* 2004; **1**: 43–56.

26. B. Holtz, S. L. Krein, D. R. Bentley, et al. Comparison of veteran experiences of low-cost, home-based diet and exercise interventions. *J Rehabil Res Dev* 2014; **51**: 149–60.

27. L. M. Hayward, C. Nixon, M. P. Jasper, et al. The process of restructuring and the treatment of obesity in women. *Health Care Women Int* 2000; **21**: 615–30.

28. J. H. Cho, S. Y. Jae, I. L. Han Choo, et al. Health-promoting behaviour among women with abdominal obesity: A conceptual link to social support and perceived stress. *J Adv Nurs* 2014; **70**: 1381–90.

29. J. P. Ogle, J. Park, M. L. Damhorst, et al. Social support for women who have undergone bariatric surgery. *Qual Health Res* 2016; **26**: 176–93.

30. A. E. Addis and J. R. Mahalik. Men, masculinity, and the contexts of seeking help. *Am Psychol* 2003; **58**: 5–14.

31. J. Davies, B. P. McCrae, J. Frank, et al. Identifying male college students' perceived health needs, barriers to seeking help, and recommendations to help men adopt healthier lifestyles. *J Am Coll Health* 2000; **48**: 259–67.

32. A. Harrison. Health of men: Weight management partnership. *Commun Pract* 2007; **80**: 31–4.

33. L. M. Robertson, F. Douglas, A. Ludbrook, et al. What works with men? A systematic review of health promoting interventions targeting men. *BMC Health Serv Res* 2008; **8**: 141.

34. E. A. Jacobs, D. S. Shepard, J. A. Suaya, et al. Overcoming language barriers in health care: Costs and benefits of interpreter services. *Am J Public Health* 2004; **94**: 866–9.

35. B. A. Careyva, M. B. Johson, K. Shaak, et al. Patient-reported barriers and limitations to attending diabetes group visits. *J Prim Care Commun Health* 2015; **6**: 279–81.

36. R. Setse, R. Grogan, L. A. Cooper, et al. Weight loss for urban-based, postpartum African American women: Perceived barriers and preferred components. *Matern Child Health J* 2008; **12**: 19–27.

37. S. Caprio, S. R. Daniels, A. Drewnowski, et al. Influence of race, ethnicity, and culture on childhood obesity: Implications for prevention and treatment. *Obesity* 2008; **16**: 2566–77.

38. S. A. Brown, S. A. Blozis, K. Kouzekanani, et al. Dosage effects of diabetes self-management education in Mexican Americans. *Diabetes Care* 2008; **28**: 527–32.

39. M. C. Nelson, M. Story, M. I. Larson, et al. Emerging adulthood and college-aged youth: An overlooked age for weight-related behaviour change. *Obesity* 2008; **16**: 2205–11.

40. M. C. Nelson, R. Kocos, L. A. Lytle, et al. Understanding the perceived determinants of weight-related behaviours in late adolescence: A qualitative analysis among college youth. *J Nutr Educ Behav* 2009; **41**: 287–92.

41. N. N. Beck, M. Johannsen, R. K. Stoving, et al. Do postoperative psychotherapeutic interventions and support groups influence weight loss following bariatric surgery? A systematic review and meta-analysis of randomized and nonrandomized trials. *Obes Surg* 2012; **22**: 1790–7.

42. A. H. Robinson, S. Adler, H. B. Stevens, et al. What variables are associated with successful weight loss outcomes for bariatric surgery after one year? *Surg Obes Relat Dis* 2014; **10**: 697–704.

43. A. K. Madan, D. S. Tchansky, and R. J. Taddeucci. Postoperative laparoscopic bariatric surgery patients do not remember potential complications. *Obes Surg* 2007; **17**: 885–8.

44. M. Livhits, C. Mercado, I. Yermilov, et al. Is social support associated with greater weight loss after bariatric surgery? A systematic review. *Obes Rev* 2011; **12**: 142–8.

45. I. Peytremann-Brideaux and B. Santos-Eggimann. Health correlates of overweight and obesity in adults aged 50 years old and over: Results from the survey of health, ageing and retirement in Europe (SHARE). *Swiss Med Wkly* 2008; **138**: 261–6.

46. D. A. Anderson and T. A. Wadden. Bariatric surgery patients' views of their physicians' weight-related attitudes and practices. *Obesity* 2004; **12**: 1587–95.

47. M. E. Atwood, A. Friedman, B. A. Meisner, et al. The exchange of social support on online bariatric surgery discussion forums: A mixed-methods content analysis. *Health Commun* 2018; **33**: 628–635.

Chapter 14

Telephone-Based Psychological Interventions in Severe Obesity

Stephanie E. Cassin, Adrienne Mehak, and Sanjeev Sockalingam

Clinical Vignette

Mrs. Edwards is a 32-year-old recently divorced woman. She and her ex-husband have a fairly amicable relationship and share custody of their children, ages four and six. She previously worked as an administrative assistant, but she has been on disability for the past 18 months due to mobility issues and chronic back and knee pain secondary to obesity (body mass index [BMI] = 59 kg/m^2). She also has type 2 diabetes, as well as social anxiety and recurrent major depressive episodes with occasional suicidal ideation. Since being off work, her eating habits have become quite chaotic during the day, and her weight has been increasing.

Mrs. Edwards' physician strongly encouraged her to enroll in a behavioral weight loss program and to consider being referred to a bariatric surgery program as well. She is receptive to the idea of being referred to a hospital-based obesity program, but she resides in a rural community, and the nearest specialized program is in a major city 125 kilometers away. Mrs. Edwards owns a vehicle but finds it difficult to drive for extended periods due to her chronic pain. Moreover, it would be challenging for her to visit the obesity program regularly because she has to transport her children to and from school on most days, and the fuel and parking costs associated with driving to the obesity program are problematic given her limited income. Her depression and social anxiety are fairly well controlled at the moment, but she does occasionally have days when she finds it challenging to leave the house.

After much contemplation, Mrs. Edwards decides to request a referral to the obesity program so that she can at least attend a consultation and learn more about the program. The barriers to attend appointments are significant, but after trying to lose weight on her own for so many years without much long-term success, she feels that it may be necessary to have the support of an obesity program.

Introduction

In this chapter, we provide an overview of the various types of telephone-based psychological interventions that have been used in the management of severe obesity. We discuss the benefits of telephone-based interventions, as well as the limitations, and provide recommendations to address these limitations. We also describe some important ethical considerations in delivering psychological interventions by telephone. We review the empirical evidence supporting the effectiveness of telephone-based interventions in patients with severe obesity throughout the chapter. Finally, we provide some recommendations for delivering telephone-based interventions in reference to the Case Vignette.

Telephone-Based Psychological Interventions in Severe Obesity

Telehealth (also known as *telemedicine*) refers to the use of telecommunications and information technologies to provide clinical care at a distance in order to expand access, exchange information, or deliver care in alternate formats [1]. These technologies may include telephone, mobile devices, short message services (text messages), videoconferencing, email, and interactive websites and apps, among others [2]. These forms of communication may be synchronous (e.g., a telephone conversation between a healthcare provider and patient in real time) or asynchronous (e.g., a text message sent by a healthcare provider and received by a patient at a later time) [2]. This chapter focuses primarily on the use of telephone-based psychological interventions in the management of severe obesity, either as a stand-alone psychological intervention or to supplement traditional face-to-face interventions.

Types of Telephone-Based Psychological Interventions for Severe Obesity

Cognitive-Behavioral Telephone Interventions

Formal telephone-based cognitive-behavioral therapy (tele-CBT) interventions consist of CBT principles and strategies for severe obesity (see Chapters 8 and 9) delivered by a therapist via telephone. Often tele-CBT uses handouts provided in advance or intersession via email to reinforce tele-CBT session activities and homework. The efficacy of tele-CBT has been established in a range of medical patient populations, such as those with chronic pain [3], postnatal concerns [4], traumatic brain injury [5], and depression [6,7]. Although relatively little research to date has examined tele-CBT specifically for individuals with severe obesity, tele-CBT is increasingly being used as a result of the encouraging results in other medical populations.

Although group and individual face-to-face CBT has been shown to be effective in treating binge eating disorder (BED) and emotional eating symptoms in bariatric surgery candidates [8,9], the long travel distances required for patients to attend CBT sessions limits access and adherence to CBT interventions. In response to this need, a tele-CBT intervention was developed and piloted in patients to determine the feasibility and acceptability of this intervention [10]. This tele-CBT intervention was developed after reviewing the literature and consulting with experts in the field, including bariatric psychosocial clinicians. The result was a six-session tele-CBT intervention offered weekly that focused on the following clinical domains:

- Session 1: Socializing to the CBT model of obesity
- Session 2: Self-monitoring food intake and weight
- Session 3: Planning pleasurable activities and engaging in self-care activities
- Session 4: Identifying triggers for maladaptive eating
- Session 5: Reducing vulnerability to triggers for maladaptive eating by solving problems and challenging maladaptive thoughts (cognitive distortions)
- Session 6: Preparing for bariatric surgery (preoperative) *or* keeping on track after bariatric surgery (postoperative)

Empirical Evidence for Cognitive-Behavioral Telephone Interventions. Several studies have examined the efficacy of this six-session tele-CBT intervention in bariatric surgery patient populations before and after surgery. An initial pilot study demonstrated the feasibility, acceptability, and preliminary effectiveness of this tele-CBT intervention in eight patients [10]. Patients reported improvements in binge eating, emotional eating, and depressive symptoms following the intervention. The authors expanded this initial study and conducted a randomized, controlled trial (RCT) involving 47 patients randomized either to this tele-CBT intervention preoperatively or a wait list control group [11]. The tele-CBT group demonstrated significant improvements in binge eating, emotional eating, depressive symptoms, and anxiety symptoms, with large effect sizes. A total of 70 percent of patients completed tele-CBT in this study, and patients who discontinued treatment cited time constraints and lack of privacy for phone call sessions as the most common reasons for discontinuation.

In a follow-up study, the tele-CBT protocol was examined in postoperative bariatric surgery patients. In this open-trial study, a total of 19 patients received the tele-CBT intervention six months after bariatric surgery and reported significant improvements in binge eating, emotional eating, depressive symptoms, and anxiety symptoms after treatment [12]. The treatment effect sizes were larger than in the study examining preoperative tele-CBT, and the retention rate of 74 percent was comparable with other tele-CBT trials [13]. Additional studies suggest that postoperative psychosocial interventions may offer the greatest benefit to patients in terms of sustained weight loss and reinforce the need for further long-term studies on the effectiveness of tele-CBT after bariatric surgery [14]. In summary, these studies provide evidence for the efficacy of tele-CBT in treating obesity-related eating psychopathology and offer an accessible alternative to face-to-face CBT in obesity care.

Health-Coaching Telephone Interventions

In addition to tele-CBT, several other "telehealth" interventions have been applied with the goal of weight management and improving behaviors relevant to the treatment of severe obesity. The most extensively studied telephone-based approach to treating obesity and related behaviors is health coaching. *Health coaching*, also known as *wellness coaching, life coaching*, or simply *coaching*, refers to a category of interventions aimed at increasing health-promoting behaviors [15]. Coaching interventions include a range of patient-centered treatments that are based on an interpersonal relationship between the patient and the coach. Typically, coaches provide assistance with goal setting and achievement, as well as increased accountability and self-awareness in the process of working toward those goals [16]. Coaching has become a popular form of intervention for many chronic conditions [15], including overweight and obesity [16], and, in part due to its flexibility, appears well suited to application via telemedicine [17].

Unlike telephone-delivered CBT, telecoaching is not standardized or manualized and therefore has been implemented in different formats with varying treatment outcomes. In the context of weight management, it has been applied as a stand-alone intervention [8,19], as one aspect of a multicomponent treatment [20], and as a follow-up component of another style of intervention [21,22]. Interventions involving telecoaching have targeted many goals relevant to the treatment of severe obesity, such as reducing body weight and/or body fat percentage, reducing caloric intake, increasing overall physical activity and moderate/vigorous physical activity, and modifying various health-promoting lifestyle-related factors (e.g., increasing fruit and vegetable consumption, decreasing sedentary time) [23–28].

Despite differing end goals, some recurring elements have been applied across telecoaching interventions. Often, coaching has been implemented as a brief, relatively low-intensity treatment, with the typical number of phone sessions ranging from 10 to 14 [23,26], although some have been as brief as four sessions [29] and others have included as many as 78 follow-up sessions [30]. The phone sessions themselves are also relatively brief, lasting on average between 10 and 20 minutes [18,20]. These sessions usually occur at regular intervals (weekly or biweekly) and are almost always delivered by healthcare professionals with training in areas relevant to the intervention's goal.

In addition to these logistical considerations, several common treatment ingredients have been shared by telecoaching interventions related to the treatment of severe obesity. Most interventions include a didactic or psychoeducational component, and it is not uncommon to supplement coaching with psychoeducational resources (e.g., a handbook) [31]. Many telecoaching interventions have also included elements of self-monitoring (e.g., food logging), goal setting, and identification of barriers to success in the program, as well as problem solving to overcome those obstacles. Although it is not always explicitly mentioned as an aspect of the intervention, the provision of encouragement and reinforcement by the coach appears to be a significant component of telecoaching [20,32].

Empirical Evidence for Health Coaching Telephone Interventions. Findings from the coaching literature are inconsistent, likely reflecting the fact that coaching is unstandardized and therefore not consistently implemented across interventions. Despite these inconsistencies, telecoaching research suggests that it may be an appropriate, nonsurgical treatment for severe obesity, with promising results in weight management and health-promoting behaviors.

Studies examining telecoaching in individuals with severe obesity have demonstrated that participants receiving telecoaching experience greater reductions in BMI than control participants after six months of treatment [33], as well as decreased overall body weight, waist circumference, and body fat percentage [19,23,33]. Improvements in weight-related outcomes have been maintained for up to 24 months [27]. Notably, in one intervention, individuals with inadequate weight loss or weight regain following bariatric surgery demonstrated significant weight loss following telecoaching and maintained the weight loss 12 months after treatment [24]. Other studies examining individuals who are overweight or obese have demonstrated similar findings [18,19,34,35], as have interventions among children and adolescents who are overweight or obese [20–22]. It is important to note, however, that some interventions have not resulted in weight loss [e.g., 32]. In addition, although initial weight loss appears to be the norm, maintenance of weight loss is less consistently reported [23,27,35].

Telecoaching has led to improvement in other behaviors of interest. A number of dietary improvements were noted in a sample including individuals with severe obesity, such as increased consumption of fruits and vegetables and decreased consumption of takeaway meals and sweetened drinks [33]. Other telecoaching interventions have lead to dietary improvements [34], with increased consumption of fruits and vegetables most frequently reported [25,31]. Telecoaching appears well suited to increasing physical activity, both generally [18,26,30,33,36] and specifically, among those who are overweight or obese [32]. Finally, telecoaching has led to improvements in various psychological outcomes, such as anxiety, depression, quality of life, perceived social support, and self-efficacy [26,29,31,32,37].

Telecoaching interventions have numerous benefits. It is delivered from a distance, making it ideal for participants with barriers to attending traditional face-to-face treatments, such as those living in rural areas [18,19,22,23,27,34,37]. These interventions have repeatedly been noted for their wide reach, allowing for the simultaneous treatment of several hundreds of individuals over a short time period [23,27,30,33]. Telecoaching has also consistently been noted as a relatively low-cost intervention [18,25,31,34].

Additionally, patients are generally satisfied with telecoaching interventions. With some exceptions [33], most interventions have retained a large majority of participants [18,19,24,36]. When satisfaction ratings have been explicitly solicited from patients, they have usually been high [36], with telecoaching components being noted as particularly useful [20,26], One hundred percent of participants in one study reported that they were satisfied with the coaching they received and would recommend it to others [31]. This is an important finding given that those with greater treatment adherence generally achieve greater success across multiple outcomes [18,27,30]. Presumably, higher satisfaction should improve treatment adherence, which may, in turn, improve outcomes. Other benefits of telecoaching interventions include increased comfort in sharing personal or sensitive information [22] and the potential for successful outcomes when the intervention is delivered by paraprofessionals [32].

Perhaps the most significant limitation of coaching is the lack of standardization across different interventions, which makes it difficult to interpret research findings [17]. It is difficult to isolate which elements improve or worsen outcomes, and further research is required to clarify key ingredients and establish best-practice guidelines (e.g., optimal number of calls or duration of the intervention) [37]. Despite many of the positive outcomes reported following telecoaching interventions, it is currently difficult to establish telecoaching as an evidence-based treatment for severe obesity given the large variability across telecoaching interventions and the level of detail describing the interventions [38].

Motivational Interviewing Telephone Interventions

Another common telephone-delivered treatment for severe obesity is motivational interviewing (MI), a method of counseling first developed to treat alcohol abuse that has since been applied to a wide range of health-related behaviors, including obesity [39,40] (see Chapters 5, 6, and 7). Motivational interviewing is appropriate for conditions in which ambivalence toward change is common and behavior change can improve clinical outcomes. It aims to elicit patients' intrinsic motivation to initiate behavior change and increase treatment adherence [40].

As with telecoaching, MI has been applied as both the core component of an intervention [41–44] and as one aspect of a multicomponent intervention [45–47]. The central therapeutic skills used in telephone-delivered MI are reflective listening, asking open-ended questions, and providing patients with direct support and affirmation [46–53]. The elicitation of *change talk* (e.g., comments that signify that the patient is considering change or taking steps toward change) is often noted in these interventions. Elicitation of change talk may include exploring patients' motivation for behavior change, examining the pros and cons of altering the target behavior, and contrasting patients' current behaviors with their values and goals [44–47,53,54]. Other recurring elements in MI interventions relevant to severe obesity include health-related psychoeducation and psychoeducational resources (e.g., pamphlets, cookbooks), behavior-modification skills, barrier identification and problem solving, and self-monitoring components (e.g., step counting, food logging) [41–48,54,56].

Most interventions have included one face-to-face MI session prior to a series of telephone-delivered sessions [48,49,52], but some interventions have been successful with telephone contact alone [41,44,47,56]. The MI sessions themselves are brief, typically ranging from 10 [42] to 30 minutes [49]. These are generally low- to moderate-intensity interventions, with the average number of sessions ranging from three [48] to eight [41], although some more extensive interventions have included up to 18 sessions [52]. Typically sessions are delivered more frequently initially (i.e., weekly) and then taper off toward the end of the intervention [44,50,56], an approach noted to be successful in weight-related lifestyle interventions [57]. In interventions relevant to obesity, MI has almost exclusively been delivered by professionals with additional specific training in MI.

Empirical Evidence for Motivational Interviewing Telephone Interventions. Investigations of telephone-delivered MI have typically not targeted weight loss as a primary outcome, but studies that did assess that outcome reported reductions in body weight and BMI [43,45]. Interventions featuring MI as the central component have led to reductions in waist circumference and maintenance of current weight compared with an increase in weight among control group participants [42], as well as improvement in important lifestyle behaviors among individuals with obesity (e.g., physical activity, diet) [41,42,52]. Much of the MI research has focused on these lifestyle behaviors, with improvements found in overall and moderate/vigorous physical activity, sedentary or screen time, total calorie intake, fruit and vegetable consumption, fat consumption, sodium intake, and processed food consumption [41,42,45,48,55].

Importantly, where follow-up research has been conducted, improvements in diet and physical activity have been maintained for periods of up to 24 months after intervention [42,49,56,58], with one study finding continued postintervention improvement in physical activity [44]. MI interventions have also led to improved psychosocial outcomes among those who are overweight or obese, including overall psychological health, depression, quality of life, and self-efficacy [45,48,49,52]. Recent research suggests that MI may also be efficacious when delivered via the Internet for weight loss among individuals who are overweight or obese [59], although not all studies support this finding [54].

Where it has been examined, patient satisfaction with MI is high [41]. Moreover, patients who receive MI as an adjunctive treatment have consistently provided higher satisfaction ratings than those who only received the other component [45,47]. Further, treatment adherence for telephone-delivered MI is usually high, with the proportion of completed call sessions frequently reaching 90 percent or greater [43,46,48].

Given that it can be conducted from a distance, telephone-delivered MI addresses common barriers to face-to-face counseling such as geographic distance, time constraints, and transportation issues [49]. Further, telephone delivery of MI circumvents obstacles to attending treatment such as disability and stigma [49]. Finally, telephone-delivered MI allows for some level of continued follow-up contact, which may be necessary for maintenance of gains [52,58].

As mentioned earlier, telephone-delivered MI improves health-related lifestyle behaviors when delivered as a brief intervention, making it suitable for use in general practice [42]. This efficiency in combination with the low intensity of treatment required to achieve significant outcomes posits MI as a cost-effective treatment option [49]. Although higher-cost treatment approaches (e.g., combining MI with other approaches) yield greater treatment outcomes, improvements are still evident with the lower-cost approach of providing MI alone [43,50]. Motivational interviewing increases treatment adherence when employed with other treatment methods [51] and is well suited for incorporation into other interventions; for example, a combination of MI and telecoaching led to significant improvements in weight and related lifestyle behaviors that were maintained one year postintervention [31,60]. It is notable that MI in general has been found to be effective for weight loss and weight management [39], and there does appear to be ample support for the efficacy of telephone-delivered MI in lifestyle behaviors relevant to the treatment of severe obesity.

Other Telephone Interventions

Other telephone-based interventions relevant to the treatment of severe obesity are not subsumed under the categories previously described (i.e., CBT, telecoaching, MI) and are not yet widespread enough to be considered a category of their own. One novel approach is the use of automated interactive voice messages designed to provide continual support in promoting health-related lifestyle changes. This method has resulted in weight loss, as well as improved health literacy and health behaviors [61]. The use of mobile phones to promote health-related lifestyle changes is predicted to be increasingly relevant in the future [62], and has been found to be a useful component of weight loss interventions to assist individuals with obesity in self-monitoring health behaviors (e.g., food logging) [63]. Additionally, text messaging has been used to promote healthier lifestyle choices: for example, when used as one aspect of a face-to-face group behavioral lifestyle intervention [64], participants with obesity responded favorably to the text-message component itself [65]. Further, the use of text messages to encourage increased physical activity appears promising, but little research has been conducted to date [66].

Benefits of Telephone-Based Interventions for Severe Obesity

Telephone-based psychological interventions offer many benefits, the greatest of which is likely treatment accessibility. Patients limited by geographic location (e.g., rural communities), medical condition (e.g., severe obesity, mobility challenges, severe pain), psychiatric diagnosis (e.g., severe depression, social anxiety, agoraphobia), financial constraint, or other barriers may gain access to high-quality psychological services via telehealth. Many patients reside great distances from specialized obesity programs, and travel distance has an adverse impact on attendance at appointments, which, in turn, has negative implications for long-term weight loss and maintenance [67]. With telephone-based interventions, there is no need to travel to appointments, thereby reducing or eliminating the need to take time off from work or make childcare arrangements in order to participate in treatment. In addition, there may be greater flexibility to schedule sessions outside of traditional office hours, such as during evenings or on weekends. Given that patients can receive services from the comfort of their own home, telephone-based interventions can also be delivered by treatment providers whose offices are not entirely accessible and barrier free.

Weight-based stigma and discrimination are well documented among individuals with severe obesity [68] (see Chapter 3), and telephone-based interventions may be a helpful modality in reaching out to patients who have had negative healthcare experiences and feel conflicted about seeking services in person for fear of encountering further weight-based stigma or discrimination at the hands of healthcare professionals or the public. In addition to weight-based stigma and discrimination specifically, the stigma concerning treatment seeking that is particularly prominent for psychological services may pose an additional barrier to accessing services. Telephone-based psychological interventions may be an appealing option for those who prefer to receive psychological services in the privacy of their own homes.

Potential Issues and Troubleshooting Tips for Telephone-Based Interventions

There are a number of potential issues to be aware of when delivering telephone-based psychological interventions. One concern raised by both clinicians and patients is the potential impact on rapport and potential for misunderstandings given that many forms of nonverbal communication are lost over the telephone (e.g., smiling, eye contact, body language). Although some patients prefer the anonymity of telephone-based interventions, others find it difficult to establish trust and disclose personal information over the telephone without having already established a relationship with the treatment provider. In such cases, it would be beneficial to first meet in person prior to commencing a telephone-based intervention. If this is not feasible due to physical and practical barriers, other options include using interactive videoconferencing technology that is compliant with privacy regulations or even simply exchanging photos so that the patient has a "face to put to the voice." Clinicians will likely need to spend more time developing rapport prior to engaging in telehealth interventions, pay closer attention to patients' verbal and nonverbal behaviors (e.g., long pauses, change in affect), and be more explicit about their own nonverbal behaviors during the sessions (e.g., having an awareness that patients cannot see their encouraging smiles or nods, informing patients when they are making some notes or scanning homework worksheets so that they understand why the clinician is silent for a moment).

Given that telephone-based interventions occur at a distance, it may be more difficult to explain concepts or skills because both parties do not have a shared focus of attention (e.g., unable to focus on the same handout while the clinician explains a concept or homework exercise), and it may also be more challenging to determine whether patients understand the information being conveyed. For the same reason, it is also more difficult for patients and clinicians to review written homework exercises, such as food records, activity logs, or other worksheets. For these reasons, the sessions may require some additional preparation because clinicians need to send all handouts to patients in advance of each session so that they can both view the same handouts, albeit from different locations. Similarly, patients need to submit their homework for clinicians to review in advance of each session. It is important that clinicians frequently check in with patients to assess their understanding of the information conveyed, for example, by asking them to describe a concept in their own words, to articulate the rationale behind a homework exercise, or to state how a coping skill introduced in the session applies to them personally.

The increased convenience and comfort afforded by telephone-based psychological interventions can also potentially act as a limitation. One of the benefits of face-to-face psychological interventions is that the clinician's office is a sanctuary in a sense, and the regularly scheduled appointments provide protected time to focus on oneself. In contrast, patients may have many more distractions to deal with if they engage in treatment sessions from their own home or office. They may find it more difficult to protect time for treatment sessions if their friends, family, or coworkers spontaneously visit or if other tasks are perceived as more urgent (e.g., feeling stressed about a work deadline and therefore either canceling the treatment session, asking to reschedule it for a later time, or attempting to multitask during the session). In light of these issues, it is important that the clinician set appropriate boundaries regarding their availability and ideally schedule all the sessions at a predictable time so that the patient is aware that this should be treated as protected time for both of them. In addition, it is important to discuss the environment in which patients will be participating in telephone-based interventions to ensure that it is private, safe, and free from unnecessary distractions (e.g., not while driving!). In order for patients to receive the greatest benefit from treatment, they should be encouraged to engage in treatment sessions in a quiet and distraction-free environment with a desk so that they can easily review treatment materials and take notes during the session.

Ethical Considerations in Delivering Telephone-Based Interventions

The delivery of psychological interventions by telephone also raises some unique ethical considerations. In response to these issues, many regulatory bodies have developed ethical guidelines that pertain specifically to the use of telehealth in health care delivery [2,69–72]. When obtaining informed consent before proceeding with telephone-based interventions, it is important to discuss both the benefits (e.g., accessibility, convenience, comfort) and risks (e.g., misunderstandings due to lack of visual cues, potential reduced efficacy compared to face-to-face interventions for certain clinical issues), as well as the security and privacy limitations associated with the particular forms of technology being used in the provision of psychological services (e.g., if the patient will be sending completed homework worksheets to the clinician).

Prior to commencing telephone-based psychological interventions, it is important for the treatment provider to obtain the name and contact information of someone to contact in the case of an emergency. The treatment provider must become familiar with emergency and crisis services in the patient's geographic region. For example, the treatment provider can collaborate with the patient to identify a local healthcare provider to provide backup support if needed, such as the patient's general practitioner, and to determine local emergency telephone numbers including crisis hotlines. The treatment provider should have a plan in place in the event of a physical or psychiatric emergency and discuss emergency procedures with the patient at the start of treatment.

The definition of telehealth and the rules dictating how it is regulated vary widely across jurisdictions. A significant benefit of telephone-based interventions is that geographic barriers are reduced, and patients can theoretically access support from obesity experts who reside in different jurisdictions. Given that there are no universal telehealth regulations, the healthcare provider must become familiar with and honor the local jurisprudence and standards of practice for his or her discipline, as well as the jurisdiction in which the service is being delivered. For example, mandatory reporting requirements and age of consent for treatment may differ across jurisdictions. Healthcare providers must also inform themselves of jurisdictional requirements regarding licensure or certification, which may include being licensed to provide services both in the patient's and the healthcare provider's jurisdictions.

Clinical Vignette Revisited

To recap from the clinical case, Mrs. Edwards has social anxiety and recurrent major depressive episodes with occasional suicidal ideation. Her eating patterns have become chaotic since being off work, and she has been gaining more weight recently. She has historically had difficulty maintaining weight loss and is receptive to a referral to the nearest specialized obesity program, which unfortunately is located 125 kilometers from her home. She cannot financially afford frequent travel to appointments, and she finds it difficult to drive for extended periods.

Mrs. Edwards should be encouraged to attend the initial consultation appointment in person, if feasible, given some of the potential issues with exclusively telephone-based interventions (e.g., impact on rapport, increased risk of miscommunication). If it is not feasible for Mrs. Edwards to attend the first appointment in person, the clinician could consider using telehealth interactive videoconferencing technology for the initial consultation so that they have an opportunity to "virtually" meet each other. With Mrs. Edwards' consent, it would be beneficial to work collaboratively with her local general practitioner for patient monitoring (e.g., weight, blood pressure, blood glucose).

Given Mrs. Edwards' history of recurrent depression and suicidal ideation, it would be particularly important for the clinician to be familiar with emergency and crisis resources in Mrs. Edwards' community and to establish emergency procedures with her prior to commencing treatment. If Mrs. Edwards is amenable to trying a telephone-based intervention after learning about the potential benefits and risks during the informed-consent procedure, the sessions should be scheduled for a regular location and time when she is free of distractions (e.g., at her kitchen table on a regular weekday basis when her children are at school). In light of her current symptoms, a telephone-based CBT intervention (see Chapters 8 and 9) would be a sensible treatment recommendation. As described earlier, some modifications would be recommended to make CBT feasible by telephone, such as the clinician sending treatment handouts and worksheets prior to the sessions and the patient sending homework for the clinician to review during the sessions. Many interactive platforms now exist that can also facilitate review of materials during sessions (e.g., apps for food records and other CBT worksheets that a patient can grant their clinician access to) (see Chapter 15).

Mrs. Edwards' symptoms should be regularly monitored over the course of the treatment to assess the effectiveness of the telephone-based intervention. If her symptoms are not improving, it would be worth revisiting the idea of face-to-face treatment sessions at the specialized obesity clinic given that telephone-based interventions have reduced efficacy for some patients and presenting issues. If her depression symptoms and suicidal ideation are severe or worsen over the course of treatment, increased collaboration with her local general practitioner would be advised, as well as a referral to a local healthcare provider to treat her depression. If symptom monitoring indicates that the treatment is progressing well, the frequency and duration of the sessions could be tapered over time to build Mrs. Edwards' self-efficacy in her ability to maintain changes with less professional support, eventually culminating in self-therapy sessions to prevent relapse.

Summary

This chapter provided an overview of the current state of telephone-based psychological interventions for severe obesity. Telephone-based CBT appears to be a promising protocol-based treatment method with a small but growing evidence base. Health coaching has often been administered via telephone and has resulted in some success related to weight management and health-promoting behaviors. However, evidence for the effectiveness of telecoaching for maintaining weight loss is less clear. Telephone-based motivational interviewing appears to improve lifestyle behaviors such as diet and physical activity, with these changes maintained over time. Several other telehealth interventions relevant to the treatment of severe obesity have been used, including automated interactive voice messages, self-monitoring, and text messaging as a motivational tool. The benefits of telephone-based psychological interventions include accessibility of treatment for those with barriers to treatment access. However, healthcare providers also need to be aware of treatment considerations unique to the delivery of telehealth interventions and familiar with telehealth-related regulations.

Key Points

- Many psychological interventions are being adapted to treat severe obesity using telecommunications.
- Specific promising interventions include telephone-based CBT, health coaching, and motivational interviewing.
- Telephone-based psychological interventions for severe obesity are beneficial in that they increase treatment accessibility and may lessen patients' concerns related to stigma and discrimination.
- Telephone-based psychological interventions also have limitations, including the potential for misunderstanding due to nonverbal communication, difficulties establishing rapport, and competing demands for patients' attention when "attending" therapy from home.
- Regulations and standards related to telehealth interventions vary by location, so it is essential for treatment providers to be familiar with the regulations in the jurisdictions in which treatment is delivered and received.

References

1. US Department of Health and Human Services. Telehealth, 2015. Available at www .hrsa.gov/ruralhealth/telehealth/ (accessed June 17, 2016).

2. Joint Task Force for the Development of Telepsychology Guidelines for Psychologists. Guidelines for the practice of telepsychology. *Am Psych* 2013; **68**: 791–800.

3. T. P. Carmody, C. L. Duncan, J. Huggins, et al. Telephone-delivered cognitive-behavioural therapy for pain management among older military veterans: A randomized trial. *Psychol Serv* 2013; **10**: 265–75.

4. F. W. Ngai, P. W. Wong, K. Y. Leung, et al. The effect of telephone-based cognitive-behavioural therapy on postnatal depression: A randomized controlled trial. *Psychother Psychosom* 2015; **84**: 294–303.

5. J. R. Fann, C. H. Bombardier, S. Vannoy, et al. Telephone and in-person cognitive behavioural therapy for major depression after traumatic brain injury: A randomized controlled trial. *J Neurotrauma* 2015; **32**: 45–57.

6. D. C. Mohr, J. Ho, J. Duffecy, et al. Effect of telephone-administered vs face-to-face cognitive behavioral therapy and depression outcomes among primary care patients: A randomized trial. *JAMA* 2012; **307**: 2278–86.

7. C. Stiles-Shields, M. E. Corden, M. J. Kwasny, et al. Predictors of outcome for telephone and face-to-face administered cognitive behavioral therapy for depression. *Psychol Med* 2015; **45**: 3205–15.

8. K. Ashton, M. Drerup, A. Windover, et al. Brief, four-session group CBT reduces binge eating behaviours among bariatric surgery candidates. *Surg Obes Relat Dis* 2009; **5**: 257–62.

9. J. Beaulac and D. Sandre. Impact of a CBT psychotherapy group on post-operative bariatric patients. *SpringerPlus* 2016; **4**: 764.

10. S. E. Cassin, S. Sockalingam, R. Hawa, et al. Psychometric properties of the Patient Health Questionnaire (PHQ-9) as a depression screening tool for bariatric surgery candidates. *Psychosomatics* 2013; **54**: 352–8.

11. S. E. Cassin, S. Sockalingam, C. Du, et al. A pilot randomized controlled trial of telephone-based cognitive behavioural therapy for preoperative bariatric surgery patients. *Behav Res Ther* 2016; **80**: 17–22.

12. S. Sockalingam, S. E. Cassin, S. Wnuk, et al. A pilot study on telephone cognitive behavioural therapy for patients six-months post-bariatric surgery. *Obes Surg* 2017; **27**: 670–5.

13. I. Muller and L. Yardley. Telephone-delivered cognitive behavioural therapy: A systematic review and meta-analysis. *J Telemed Telecare* 2011; **17**: 177–84.

14. H. Gade, O. Friborg, J. H. Rosenvinge, et al. The impact of a preoperative cognitive behavioural therapy (CBT) on dysfunctional eating behaviours, affective symptoms and body weight 1 year after bariatric surgery: A randomised controlled trial. *Obes Surg* 2015; **25**: 2112–9.

15. R. Boehmer, S. Barakat., S. Ahn, et al. Health coaching interventions for persons with chronic conditions: A systematic review. *Syst Rev* 2016; **5**: 1–7.

16. R. Q. Wolever, L. A. Simons, G. A. Sforzo, et al. A systematic review of the literature on health and wellness coaching: Defining a key behavioural intervention in healthcare. *Glob Adv Health* 2013; **2**: 38–57.

17. A. J. Hutchison and J. D. Breckon. A review of telephone coaching services for people with long-term conditions. *J Telemed Telecare* 2011; **17**: 451–8.

18. J. Sangster, S. Fuber, M. Allman-Farinelli, et al. Effectiveness of a pedometer-based telephone coaching program on weight and physical activity for people referred to a cardiac rehabilitation program: A randomized controlled trial. *J Cardiopulm Rehabil Prev* 2015; **35**: 124–9.

19. L. A. Tucker, A. J. Cook, N. R. Nokes, et al. Telephone-based diet and exercise coaching and a weight-loss supplement result in weight and fat loss in 120 men and women. *Am J Health Promot* 2008; **23**: 121–9.

20. B.W. Saelens, J. F. Sallis, D. R. Wilfley, et al. Behavioural weight control for overweight adolescents initiated in primary care. *Obes Res* 2002; **10**: 22–32.

21. M. Grey, S. S. Jaser, M. G. Holl, et al. A multifaceted school-based intervention to reduce risk for type 2 diabetes in at-risk youth. *Prev Med* 2009; **49**: 122–8.

22. V. Jefferson, S. S. Jaser, E. Lindemann, et al. Coping skills training in a telephone health coaching program for youth at risk for type 2 diabetes. *J Pediatr Health Care* 2011; **25**: 153–161.

23. R. Q. Jeffery, N. E. Sherwood, K. Brelje, et al. Mail and phone interventions or weight loss in a managed-care setting: Weigh-To-Be one year outcomes. *Int J Obes* 2003; **27**: 1584–92.

24. M. A. Kalarchian, M. D. Marcus, A. P. Courcoulas, et al. Optimizing long-term weight control after bariatric surgery: A pilot study. *Surg Obes Relat Dis* 2012; **8**: 710–5.

25. Y. Kim, J. Pike, H. Adams, et al. Telephone intervention promoting weight-related health behaviours. *Prev Med* 2010; **50**: 112–7.

26. B. H. Marcus, M. A. Napolitano, A. C. King, et al. Telephone versus print delivery of an individualized motivationally tailored physical activity intervention: Project STRIDE. *Health Pyschol* 2007; **26**: 401–9.

27. N. E. Sherwood, R. W. Jeffery, N. P. Pronk, et al. Mail and phone interventions for weight loss in a managed-care setting: Weigh-To-Be 2-year outcomes. *Int J Obes* 2006; **30**: 1565–73.

28. V. A. Shrewsbury, B. Nguyen, J. O'Connor, et al. Short-term outcomes of community-based adolescent weight management: The Loozit study. *BMC Pediatr* 2011; **11**: 1–10.

29. J. Opdenacker and F. Boen. Effectiveness of face-to-face versus telephone support in

increasing physical activity and mental health among university employees. *J Phys Act Health* 2008; **5**: 830–43.

30. B. C. Martinson, A. L. Crain, N. E. Sherwood, et al. Maintaining physical activity among older adults: Six-month outcomes of the Keep Active Minnesota randomized controlled trial. *Prev Med* 2008; **46**: 111–9.

31. A. L. Hawkes, T. A. Patrao, A. Green, et al. CanPrevent: A telephone-delivered intervention to reduce multiple behavioural risk factors for colorectal cancer. *BMC Cancer*; **12**: 560–9.

32. W. P. Sacco, J. I. Malone, A. D., Morrison, et al. Effect of a brief, regular telephone intervention by paraprofessionals for type 2 diabetes. *Int J Behav Med* 2009; **32**: 349–59.

33. B. J. O'Hara, P. Phongsavan, K. Venugopal, et al. Effectiveness of Australia's Get Healthy Information and Coaching Service: Translational research with population wide impact. *Prev Med* 2012; **55**: 292–8.

34. W. Anderson-Loftin, S. Barnett, P. Bunn, et al. Soul food light: Culturally competent diabetes education. *Diabetes Educ* 2005; **31**: 555–63.

35. M. F. van Wier, C. Dekkers, I. J. M. Hendrikson, et al. Effectiveness of phone and e-mail lifestyle counseling for long term weight control among overweight employees. *J Occup Environ Med* 2011; **53**: 680–6.

36. B. C. Martinson, N. E. Sherwood, A. L. Crain, et al. Maintaining physical activity among older adults: 24-month outcomes of the Keep Active Minnesota randomized controlled trial. *Prev Med*; **51**: 37–44.

37. S. M. Dennis, M. Harris, J. Lloyd, et al. Do people with existing chronic conditions benefit from telephone coaching? A rapid review. *Aust Health Rev* 2013; **37**: 381–8.

38. D. L. Chambless and T. H. Ollendick. Empirically supported psychological interventions: Controversies and evidence. *Annu Rev Psychol* 2001; **52**: 685–716.

39. M. J. Armstrong, T. A. Mottershead, P. E. Ronksley, et al. Motivational interviewing to improve weight loss in overweight and/or obese patients: A systematic review and meta-analysis of randomized controlled trials. *Obes Rev* 2011; **12**: 709–23.

40. S. R. Rollnick, W. R. Miller, and C. C. Butler. *Motivational Interviewing in Health Care: Helping Patients Change Behavior.* New York, NY: Guilford Press, 2008.

41. A. L. Baker, A. Turner, P. J. Kelly, et al. "Better Health Choices" by telephone: A feasibility trial of improving diet and physical activity in people diagnosed with psychotic disorders. *Psychiatry Res* 2014; **220**: 63–70.

42. M. Clark, S. E. Hampson, L. Avery, et al. Effects of a tailored lifestyle self-management intervention in patients with type 2 diabetes. *Br J Health Psychol* 2004; **9**: 365–79.

43. C. J. Greaves, A. Middlebrooke, L. O'Loughlin, et al. Motivational interviewing for modifying diabetes risk: A randomised controlled trial. *Br J Gen Pract* 2008; **58**: 535–40.

44. G. S. Kolt, G. M. Schofield, N. Kerse, et al. Effect of telephone counseling on physical activity for low-active older people in primary care: A randomized, controlled trial. *J Am Geriatr Soc* 2007; **55**: 986–92.

45. C. A. Befort, N. Nollen, E. F. Ellerbeck, et al. Motivational interviewing fails to improve outcomes of a behavioural weight loss program for obese African American women: A pilot randomized trial. *Int J Behav Med* 2008; **31**: 367–77.

46. K. Resnicow, D. C. Wallace, A. Jackson, et al. Dietary change through African American churches: Baseline results and program description of the Eat for Life Trial. *J Cancer Educ* 2000; **15**: 156–63.

47. H. M. van Keulen, I. Mesters, M. Ausems, et al. Tailored print communication and telephone motivational interviewing are equally successful in improving multiple lifestyle behaviours in a randomized

controlled trial. *Ann Behav Med* 2011; **41**: 104–18.

48. J. A. Bennett, K. S. Lyons, K. Winters-Stone, et al. Motivational interviewing to increase physical activity in long-term cancer survivors: A randomized controlled trial. *Nurs Res* 2007; **56**: 18–27.

49. C. H. Bombardier, D. M. Ehde, L. E. Gibbons, et al. Telephone-based physical activity counseling for major depression in people with multiple sclerosis. *J Consult Clin Psychol* 2013; **81**: 88–99.

50. M. K. Campbell, C. Carr, B. Devellis, et al. A randomized trial of tailoring and motivational interviewing to promote fruit and vegetable consumption for cancer prevention and control. *Ann Behav Med* 2009; **38**: 71–85.

51. E. R. Levensky, A. Forcehimes, W. T. O'Donohue, et al. An evidence-based approach to counseling helps patients follow treatment recommendations. *Am J Nurs* 2007; **107**: 50–8.

52. C. Newnham-Kanas, J. D. Irwin, D. Morrow, et al. The quantitative assessment of motivational interviewing using Co-Active Life Coaching Skills as an intervention for adults struggling with obesity. *Int Coaching Psychol Review* 2011; **6**: 211–28.

53. K. Resnicow, A. Jackson, T. Wang, et al. A motivational interviewing intervention to increase fruit and vegetable intake through Black churches: Results of the Eat for Life trial. *Am J Public Health* 2001; **91**: 1868–93.

54. D. Smith West, J. R. Harvey, R. A. Krukowski, et al. Do individual, online motivational interviewing chat sessions enhance weight loss in a group-based, online weight control program? *Obes* 2016; **24**: 2334–50.

55. J. Woollard, L. Beilin, T. Lord, et al. A controlled trial of nurse counselling on lifestyle change for hypertensives treated in general practice: Preliminary results. *Clin Exp Pharmacol Physiol* 1995; **22**: 466–8.

56. E. Eakin, M. Reeves, S. Lawler, et al. Telephone counseling for physical activity and diet in primary care patients. *Am J Prev Med* 2009; **36**: 142–9.

57. T. A. Wadden, M. L. Butryn, P. S. Hong, et al. Behavioral treatment of obesity in patients encountered in primary care settings: A systematic review. *JAMA* 2014; **312**: 1779–91.

58. E. Eakin, M. Reeves, E. Winkler, et al. Maintenance of physical activity and dietary change following a telephone-delivered intervention. *Health Psychol* 2010; **29**: 566–73.

59. K. H. Webber, D. F. Tate, and L. M. Quintiliani. Motivational interviewing in Internet groups: A pilot study. *J Am Diet Assoc* 2008; **108**: 1029–32.

60. A. L. Hawkes, S. K. Chambers, K. I. Pakenham, et al. Effects of a telephone delivered multiple health behavior change intervention (CanChange) on health and behavioral outcomes in survivors of colorectal cancer: A randomized controlled trial. *J Clin Oncol* 2013; **31**: 2313–21.

61. P. A. Estabrooks and R. L. Smith-Ray. Piloting a behavioral intervention delivered through interactive voice response telephone messages to promote weight loss in a pre-diabetic population. *Patient Educ Couns* 2008; **72**: 34–41.

62. P. Klasnja and W. Pratt. Healthcare in the pocket: Mapping the space of mobile-phone interventions. *J Biomed Inform* 2012; **45**: 184–98.

63. J. Morak, K. Schindler, E. Goezer, et al. A pilot study of mobile phone-based therapy for obese patients. *J Telemed Telecare* 2008; **14**: 147–9.

64. M. I. Fitzgibbon, M. R. Stolley, L. Schiffer, et al. Obesity Reduction Black Intervention Trial (ORBIT): 18-month results. *Obes* 2001; **18**: 2317–25.

65. B. S. Gerber, M. R. Stolley, A. L. Thompson, et al. Mobile phone text messaging to promote healthy behaviors and weigh loss maintenance: A feasibility study. *Health Informatics J* 2009; **15**: 17–25.

66. S. W. Buccholz, J. Wilbur, D. Ingram, et al. Physical activity text messaging interventions in adults: A systematic review. *Worldviews Evid Based Nurs* 2013; **10**: 163–73.

67. M. D. Lara, M. T. Baker, C. J. Larson, et al. Travel distance, age, and sex as factors in follow-up visit compliance in the post-gastric bypass population. *Surg Obes Relat Dis* 2005; 1: 17–21.

68. R. M. Puhl and C. A. Heuer. The stigma of obesity: A review and update. *Obes* 2009; 17: 941–64.

69. Canadian Psychological Association. Draft ethical guidelines for psychologists providing psychological services via electronic media. Ottawa, CA, 2006.

70. H. Daniel and L. Snyder Sulmasy. Policy recommendations to guide the use of telemedicine in primary care settings: An American College of Physicians position paper. *Ann Intern Med* 2015; **163**: 787–9.

71. APA Work Group on Telepsychiatry. Telepsychiatry Toolkit, 2017. Available at https://www.psychiatry.org/psychiatrists/practice/telepsychiatry/telepsychiatry-toolkit-home (accessed October 7, 2017).

72. Standing Committee of European Doctors. CPME Guidelines for Telemedicine, 2002. Available at www.ehtel.eu/publications/ehealth-studies-and-reports/CPME-Guidelines-for-Telemedecine-2002-10-16.pdf/view (accessed October 7, 2017).

Web-Based and Smartphone Application–Based Psychological Interventions in Severe Obesity

Melvyn Zhang, Alvona Loh, and Roger Ho

Case Vignette

Sandra is a 32-year-old woman who has been referred by her psychiatrist to the bariatric wellness program. She has previously been diagnosed with alcohol-use disorder and major depressive disorder. Her psychiatrist noted that Sandra tends to have eating binges whenever her mood is clinically depressed, and she also binges on alcohol at times to cope with her emotions. Her obesity has led to other medical issues, such as hypertension and impaired glucose tolerance. Sandra was keen to undergo an evaluation by the bariatric team to determine if she is a suitable candidate for bariatric surgery.

Sandra was assessed by a multidisciplinary team, and the psychiatrist recommended that she attend a weekly psychosocial intervention program given that psychosocial factors appeared to contribute to her eating binges and alcohol consumption. Hence the team psychiatrist recommended that she attend several sessions with the psychologist prior to them recommending bariatric surgery. Sandra expressed that while she is keen for the surgery, she is not able to return on a weekly basis to engage in the recommended treatment program. In addition to having work commitments, she also lives in the outskirts of the city, and hence it would be very time-consuming for her to travel to see the therapist.

Sandra shared with the team that she was previously recommended some smartphone applications that she uses on a daily basis to rate her mood and self-monitor the amount of alcohol she consumes. She showed the team a list of websites she found and asked them whether they are appropriate. Because her work is highly mobile in nature, she also asked the team to recommend her a smartphone application that she could use to help her in her treatment.

Introduction

Given the rapid advances in technologies that have transformed various aspects of healthcare, this chapter describes how technology can be harnessed as another form of psychosocial intervention in the management of obesity. Internet- and smartphone-based interventions for obesity and weight management will be discussed, and empirical research will be reviewed. The chapter will then discuss the authors' experiences in the conceptualization and implementation of Internet- and smartphone-based obesity interventions. The Case Vignette will be revisited later in the chapter.

Technological Advances and Healthcare Transformation

In the last decade, there have been major advances in technologies, with the introduction of the smartphone as well as wireless wearable devices (e.g., Fitbit). Technology has since become an integral aspect of healthcare as healthcare has shifted from conventional documentations to computerized electronic health records [1]. One of the paradigm changes is the result of the introduction of the smartphone and mobile health (mHealth) [1]. mHealth refers to the utilization of smartphones and their accompanying applications in healthcare delivery [1]. Smartphones and their accompanying applications have been used in the fields of medicine, surgery, and psychiatry. In addition, the introduction of wearable devices has also opened up opportunities for fitness and other personalized data to be collated continuously that could be used for healthcare interventions.

Internet-Based Interventions for Obesity and Weight Management

A recent review was conducted that examined health information on obesity that is available online for pregnant mothers [2]. The objective of the review was largely in determining the quality of the information that is freely available online and to determine whether the Internet is a good medium for disseminating health advice pertaining to weight management to pregnant mothers [2]. The review highlighted that websites that were obesity focused, targeting consumers, and funded by governmental bodies tend to have higher scores on information quality [2]. The review also demonstrated that there is much diversity in the information quality of websites, making it difficult for individuals to determine whether the information made available on a website aligns with evidence-based recommendations [2].

Myriad other studies have reported on the effectiveness of Internet-based interventions for obesity and related conditions. Wagner and colleagues conducted a randomized, controlled trial (RCT) that demonstrated the feasibility and efficacy of an Internet-based cognitive-behavioral therapy (CBT) program for individuals with binge eating disorder (BED) [3]. The Internet-based intervention was developed based on an evidence-based face-to-face and self-help cognitive-behavioral program for BED. The periodic follow-up assessments completed after the intervention indicated that binge eating episodes improved across time among those who received the online intervention. A recent trial demonstrated that Internet-based interventions are not only effective in the longer-term maintenance of weight loss but also cost-effective [4]. In addition, feasibility studies have demonstrated that the Internet is a useful option to reach individuals with obesity residing in rural areas [5]. Meta-analytic studies have shown that Internet-based interventions are effective in reducing weight and waist circumference, which is one of the parameters commonly used in determining whether an individual is obese and at risk for metabolic syndrome [6].

Smartphone Application–Based Interventions for Obesity and Weight Management

With the advances in mHealth technologies, there has been a myriad of healthcare applications on the application store, some of which are created by healthcare professionals, whereas others have been created by developers and commercial companies. Stevens and colleagues reviewed the currently available smartphone applications on three application stores, namely, Apple iTunes, the Blackberry store, and the Google Play store [7]. The objective of the review was to determine the functionalities of the applications related to weight loss surgery and to determine the level of healthcare professionals' involvement in the conceptualization of these applications. The authors identified a total of 38 applications, the vast majority of which were conceptualized by patients and contained either informational content, self-monitoring components (e.g., food logs, step trackers), or patient support forums. Notably, healthcare professional involvement was present in only 43 percent of all the applications reviewed. The authors concluded that the lack of healthcare professional involvement could affect the quality of these applications [7].

Connor and colleagues conducted an even larger review to determine the quality of existing bariatric surgery and obesity applications available on Apple iTunes, the Blackberry store, the Google Play store, as well as the Samsung and Windows application stores [8]. They identified a total of 83 applications, the vast majority of which sought to provide patients with educational information. Discussion forums were also widely available on the applications reviewed. Similar to the review conducted by Stevens and colleagues [7], Connor and colleagues also noted a lack of healthcare professional involvement in the conceptualization of the applications and pointed out the lack of regulations in terms of the governance [8].

In their review, Zhang and colleagues highlighted how smartphones and their accompanying applications have revolutionized and transformed healthcare but also pointed out the issues surrounding the existing applications [9]. One of the core issues pertains to the evidence base of applications. Although some studies have examined functionalities of the applications and included healthcare professional involvement in their design and conceptualization, there remains a paucity of studies that have used objective tools to measure the information quality. Since the introduction of Web 2.0 technologies, there are validated tools that have been used to assess the information quality of websites. Similarly, such tools could potentially be used to assess information quality of smartphone applications. Zhang and colleagues also discussed how healthcare professionals could be more involved in the conceptualization and design of healthcare applications so as to improve the evidence base – a point that will be returned to later in this chapter [9].

Eunjoo and colleagues used an objective rating scale to analyze the information quality of Korean obesity management Smartphone applications [10]. They reviewed a total of 148 smartphone applications that were available on the Korean application stores and applied the Silberg scale in the analysis of the information quality of those applications. The Silberg scale had been used previously to assess the quality of health information available on the Internet, but it had not yet been applied to smartphone applications. The Silberg scale takes into consideration the following aspects in the analysis of the information quality: involvement of healthcare professionals, provision of references, conflicts of interests, and the currency of the information. Of note, only 3 of the 148 applications (i.e., 2 percent of all applications) had a total score of more than 7 points out of a total of 9 points, suggesting that most of the existing applications have poor information quality and a poor evidence base. Given that the study by Eunjoo and colleagues was limited to the analysis of Korean obesity applications [10], Zhang and colleagues conducted a larger review using the Silberg scale to rate the information quality of bariatric applications that could be identified globally in all the application stores [11]. The average Silberg score for the 39 applications reviewed was only 4, suggesting that many existing bariatric applications also have poor information quality and a poor evidence base. Zhang and colleague identified a number of gaps in information quality, including lack of provision of appropriate references, full disclosure of sponsorship, and accurate disclosure regarding whether the application had been modified in the past month [11].

The poor evidence base underlying most of these applications may be accounted for, in part, by the lack of healthcare professional involvement in the conceptualization and design of many applications. Zhang and colleagues recommended that applications on the application stores be subjected to objective tests such as the Silberg scale in order to inform consumers on which applications are more informative and based on clinical evidence [9]. They also recommended that healthcare professionals critically appraise applications prior to making any recommendations and encouraged them to be more involved in the application conceptualization process. Zhang and colleagues have highlighted ways in which healthcare professionals could potentially create simple and informative applications even if they do not have any domain knowledge about application creation [10,11].

Given that most of the applications on the application stores have relatively low information quality and lack healthcare professional involvement in their development, it is important for healthcare professionals to familiarize themselves with the current research evidence and perhaps only recommend smartphone applications that have been evaluated. To date, a few empirical studies have been conducted to evaluate some of the smartphone applications. Mundi and colleagues reasoned that bariatric surgery might not be successful at times for patients due to a paucity of knowledge and lack of motivation to modify certain aspect of their lifestyle [14]. To this end, they conceptualized a smartphone application that could deliver educational materials in the form of a video and use ecological momentary assessment to assist individuals in changing unhealthy behaviors. Their pilot study with 20 patients indicated that the vast majority felt that the application was helpful. Although this pilot study suggests that a well-conceptualized application could potentially be efficacious, a larger-scale RCT is warranted to determine whether the results are replicable, and a longer-term follow-up of these patients after surgery is needed to determine whether the improvements are sustained. Other studies have examined whether the smartphone could be used as an adjunct to behavioral counseling. A study by Allen and colleagues randomized 68 patients with obesity to one of four groups: (1) an intensive counseling intervention, (2) an intensive counseling intervention + smartphone application, (3) a less intensive counseling intervention + smartphone application, and (4) a smartphone application only [15]. The results indicated that patients who received counseling that was augmented with a smartphone application lost the greatest amount of weight, suggesting that appropriately designed smartphone applications can be a beneficial adjunct to treatment.

Essential Features of eHealth and mHealth Obesity Intervention Programs

This section provides an overview of the common domains that Internet- and smartphone-based interventions should include in order to ensure that the intervention is efficacious and the fidelity to the intervention is high. Based on prior research findings, Gilmore and colleagues recommend that the following components ought to be present in any eHealth and mHealth program in order for it to be successful [16].

Behavioral Change Modification Therapy

Behavioral change modification therapy implies the inclusion of a goal-centered therapeutic approach that seeks to help individuals alter their eating patterns and increase their level of physical activity. In addition, these approaches also help to modify their underlying maladaptive thinking patterns that might have contributed to their weight.

Collection of Self-Monitoring Data

Self-monitoring enables individuals to be cognizant of their behaviors, particularly those that affect weight. They could identify behaviors that are productive or counterproductive in maintaining their weight loss. Some commonly available self-monitoring techniques include asking individuals to record their daily dietary intake (food record), record their daily physical activity (activity log), and weigh themselves the same time each week and track their weight over time (weight log). These techniques have all been shown to help maintain weight loss.

Individualized Intervention Program

There have been recommendations for new technologies to include a personalized intervention program. The rationale behind this recommendation is that various guidelines regarding dietary intake and physical activity are too generalized and nonspecific for each individual. Having a more personalized intervention program that takes into consideration a patient's demographic factors, weight, and medical/psychological comorbidities would likely increase patient engagement with the application and assist with weight loss.

Recommendations for Using eHealth and mHealth Interventions to Enhance Patient Care

Internet- and Smartphone-Based Cognitive-Behavioral Intervention

Taking into consideration the current evidence base underlying smartphone applications and the recommendations by Zhang and colleagues [11–13], we collaborated with a team at the Toronto Western Hospital Bariatric Surgery Program to conceptualize and subsequently create an application that integrates the essential features noted earlier and overcomes a number of the limitations noted among previous applications [17]. Based on the aforementioned recommendations, technological interventions for obesity need to integrate behavioral change modification therapies to be successful. Psychosocial factors have been increasingly recognized as a precipitating and perpetuating factor with regard to weight gain. Cognitive-behavioral therapy has been shown to be efficacious for patients with obesity (see Chapters 2, 8, and 9). Patients are equipped with coping skills to help them improve their binge eating, and they learn how to challenge maladaptive thoughts that lead to maladaptive health behaviors. Although CBT is efficacious among patients who complete treatment, attendance and adherence to treatment are suboptimal. This finding may be attributed to issues such as geographic distance from the treatment program and thus difficulty attending weekly sessions. These barriers have been effectively eliminated through the usage of telecommunication technologies, including Internet- and smartphone-based technologies.

The team at Toronto Western Hospital thus conceptualized both an Internet-based and smartphone variant of their CBT program. Making use of low-cost technologies as advocated by Zhang and colleagues [12,13], the online CBT program was built using WordPress as the main content-management server. Zhang and colleagues also suggested that Moodle [18], a free open-sourced online learning platform, could also be used in the creation of an online psychotherapy program. The team modeled the online program of the telephone-based CBT intervention described in Chapter 14 to ensure that the same behavioral change model was included. Some of the core aspects of the CBT program included general principles of CBT, the CBT model of obesity, self-monitoring food intake and weight, identifying alternatives to overeating, identifying and managing triggers for overeating, and challenging counterproductive thoughts. The online module includes interactive features such as worksheets to keep participants engaged.

The smartphone variant of the CBT program included some additional functionalities designed to increase the efficacy of the intervention. For example, the smartphone application prompts patients to record their weight and displays a trend analysis of their weight across a particular period of time. Bariatric surgery patients follow a medication and vitamin regime to help supplement their nutrition, and the medications and vitamins prescribed might differ across patients. The smartphone application enables individuals to take a photo of the pills they are supposed to take and reminds them at fixed times each day. Thus the smartphone application provides a more individualized treatment approach, which has been shown to improve the efficacy of interventions.

Both the Internet-based CBT intervention and the smartphone application have been pilot tested among a small group of bariatric patients who reported that they were receptive toward such a modality of intervention. Some improvements were noted on self-report measures of depression and eating pathology, but the small sample size precluded tests of significant change. This feasibility study indicated that patients are generally receptive to technological interventions.

After-Care Application

The previous reviews of smartphone applications highlighted that the vast majority of obesity-related smartphone applications provide information to patients regarding weight management or allow patients to interact with one another via a support forum. There appears to be a paucity of applications that provide patients with information to self-manage their own conditions after undergoing bariatric surgery. The team at Toronto Western Hospital thus harnessed the potential of the smartphone technologies to provide bariatric surgery patients with information relating to self-management [19]. A Web-based application was conceptualized given that the targeted patient population uses a diverse range of smartphone operating systems.

A questionnaire was administered to participants to collect their feedback after using the application. Patients reported feeling more confident with regard to the self-management of their underlying conditions. They also indicated that they valued the information explaining what is to be expected during their follow-up consultations with each member of the multi-disciplinary team, as well as the information regarding how best to reschedule appointments.

Case Vignette Revisited

In light of the barriers that would make it difficult for Sandra to attend weekly sessions at the bariatric program, she would likely benefit from either an Internet- or smartphone-based obesity intervention. These modalities of intervention would help to make the psychosocial services offered at the bariatric program more accessible to Sandra. If the applications are conceptualized with input from the bariatric psychosocial team, the interventions offered are more likely to align with evidence-based practices versus many of the applications widely available through application stores. There are other benefits of harnessing technology in her treatment. For example, such applications could help her self-monitor behaviors relevant to her treatment, such as dietary intake, physical activity, and alcohol consumption, and this information could also potentially provide the bariatric team with more information about her progress through the treatment program.

Summary

Technology has radically transformed healthcare. Internet- and smartphone-based interventions have an important role to play in the management of severe obesity. Research conducted to date suggests that such interventions are feasible to deliver and acceptable to patients. It is recommended that healthcare professionals are closely involved in the conceptualization and design of technological tools for psychosocial interventions to ensure that the interventions are built in accordance with evidence-based practices.

Key Points

- Technology has transformed healthcare interventions, including that of obesity management.
- The quality of existing health apps for obesity management varies widely; thus it is important that patients and consumers make use of interventions that have undergone rigorous testing and been recommended by institutions.
- There is evidence to support the use of Internet- and smartphone-based cognitive-behavioral interventions for obesity, disordered eating, and related issues.

References

1. M. W. Zhang and R. C. Ho. Enabling psychiatrists to explore the full potential of e-health. *Front Psychiatry* 2015; **6**: 177.

2. B. H. Al Wattar, C. Pidgeon, H. Learner, et al. Online health information on obesity in pregnancy: A systematic review. *Eur J Obstet Gynecol Reprod Biol* 2016; **206**: 147–52.

3. B. Wagner, M. Nagl, R. Dölemeyer, et al. Randomized controlled trial of an Internet-based cognitive-behavioral treatment program for binge-eating disorder. *Behav Ther* 2016; **47**: 500–14.

4. T. M. Leahey, J. L. Fava, A. Seiden, et al. A randomized controlled trial testing an Internet delivered cost-benefit approach to weight loss maintenance. *Prev Med* 2016; **92**: 51–7.

5. T. O'Brien, C. Jenkins, E. Amella, et al. An Internet-assisted weight loss intervention for older overweight and obese rural women: A feasibility study. *Comput Inform Nurs* 2016; **34**: 513–9.

6. D. C. Seo and J. Niu. Evaluation of Internet-based interventions on waist circumference reduction: A meta-analysis. *J Med Internet Res* 2015; **17**: e181.

7. D. J. Stevens, J. A. Jackson, N. Howes, et al. Obesity surgery smartphone apps: A review. *Obes Surg* 2014; **24**: 32–6.

8. K. Connor, R. R. Brady, B. Tulloh, et al. Smartphone applications (apps) for bariatric surgery. *Obes Surg* 2013; **23**: 1669–72.

9. M. W. B. Zhang, S. H. Ho, C. C. S. Cheok, et al. Smartphone apps in mental healthcare: The state of the art and potential

development. *Brit J Psych Advances* 2015; 21: 354–8.

10. E. Jeon, H. A. Park, Y. H. Min, et al. Analysis of the information quality of Korean obesity-management smartphone applications. *Healthc Inform Res* 2014; 20: 23–9.

11. M. W. Zhang, R. C. Ho, R. Hawa, et al. Analysis of the information quality of bariatric surgery smartphone applications using the Silberg scale. *Obes Surg* 2016; 26: 163–8.

12. M. W. Zhang, T. Tsang, E. Cheow, et al. Enabling psychiatrists to be mobile phone app developers: Insights into app development methodologies. *JMIR mHealth uHealth* 2014; 2: e53.

13. M. Zhang, E. Cheow, C. S. H. Ho, et al. Application of low-cost methodologies for mobile phone app development. *JMIR mHealth uHealth* 2014; 2: e55.

14. M. S. Mundi, P. A. Lorentz, K. Grothe, et al. Feasibility of smartphone-based education modules and ecological momentary assessment/intervention in pre-bariatric surgery patients. *Obes Surg* 2015; 25: 1875–81.

15. J. K. Allen, J. Stephens, C. R. Dennison Himmelfarb, et al. Randomized controlled pilot study testing use of smartphone technology for obesity treatment. *J Obes* 2013; 13: 151–97.

16. L. A. Gilmore, A. F. Duhé, E. A. Frost, et al. The technology boom: A new era in obesity management. *J Diabetes Sci Technol* 2014; 8: 596–608.

17. M. W. Zhang, R. C. Ho, S. E. Cassin, et al. Online and smartphone based cognitive behavioral therapy for bariatric surgery patients: Initial pilot study. *Technol Health Care* 2015; 23: 737–44.

18. M. W. Zhang and R. C. Ho. Moodle: The cost effective solution for Internet cognitive behavioral therapy (I-CBT) interventions. *Technol Health Care* 2017; 25: 163–5.

19. M. W. Zhang, R. C. Ho, R. Hawa, et al. Pilot implementation and user preferences of a bariatric after-care application. *Technol Health Care* 2015; 23: 729–36.

Psychosocial Interventions for Other Common Psychiatric Comorbidities in Severe Obesity

Sarah Royal and Danielle MacDonald

Case Vignette

Anne is a 49-year-old woman who lives in the same small town of her childhood. Her family consists of her husband of 24 years and her two adult sons, aged 20 and 22 years. She works full time as an administrative assistant at a local veterinary clinic, a position she has held for the past 10 years. She has a few close friends that she knows from her childhood and socializes with them occasionally on weekends. Anne has a body mass index (BMI) of 51 kg/m^2. Growing up, she was larger than most of her peers, and many of her adult relatives were overweight or obese. Her peers bullied her, typically making hurtful comments about her weight, and she had few friends. These experiences continue to affect her, and she feels very anxious when interacting with others because she fears they will judge or reject her based on her weight, personality, and intelligence. Anne gained a significant amount of weight during both of her pregnancies, and she sustained a knee injury while hiking at age 39 that has limited her mobility. She also has a long-standing eating pattern that often involves skipping breakfast and grazing on small amounts of food throughout the day, followed by a large meal at night with her family. Anne occasionally eats mindlessly in the evening while watching television, choosing potato chips, chocolate, or candy when she is feeling particularly sad or anxious.

Anne has been diagnosed with several obesity-related medical comorbidities, including type 2 diabetes, hypertension, and sleep apnea. She must walk at a slow pace or else she has difficulty breathing. She often feels fatigued and both frustrated and discouraged by the physical complications associated with obesity. Anne continues to have difficulty with mobility due to her knee problems. Her increasing weight has recently required her to rely on a cane to help her move around, which affects her ability to complete tasks at work, such as getting up from her seat to pull charts and assist patients. Working in a veterinary clinic, she used to enjoy interacting with the animals but notices that she is no longer able to bend over to pet and play with them. She finds it difficult to engage in physical activity, including walking and gardening. This affects her mood, and she finds that she no longer enjoys these activities. She spends a lot of time at home and is relatively socially isolated. She drinks alcohol four to five nights per week, usually between three and four drinks per evening but sometimes more if she is feeling especially anxious. Over the past year, she has missed work due to health problems, depressed mood, or having a hangover. This has led to financial difficulties for the family. Her husband and children are worried about her and encouraged her to seek out professional help. She met recently with a psychologist and was diagnosed with major depressive disorder, social anxiety disorder, and alcohol-use disorder.

Introduction

This chapter focuses on psychosocial interventions for common psychiatric comorbidities in individuals with severe obesity. Psychiatric disorders can complicate the clinical picture of a person with severe obesity. While the recommended psychological treatments for each comorbid psychiatric disorder would not necessarily differ from that of a nonobese individual, there are certain aspects of the clinical interventions that require special attention in the context of severe obesity. This chapter begins by reviewing cognitive-behavioral interventions for common comorbid anxiety disorders, in particular, social anxiety disorder and panic disorder, including considerations and treatment adaptations for individuals with severe obesity. Treatments for posttraumatic stress disorder are briefly mentioned, with a particular focus on issues that could arise when working with patients with obesity using a cognitive processing therapy framework. Next, major depressive disorder is covered, including modifications for treating patients with severe obesity using behavioral activation as well as cognitive interventions. Last, treatment for substance misuse is considered, including special considerations for severe obesity and for individuals undergoing bariatric surgery. Although certain eating disorders (e.g., binge eating disorder) are common in individuals with severe obesity, they are addressed in other chapters of this book (see Chapters 6, 9, 10, and 11).

Anxiety Disorders

There is strong empirical evidence for the treatment of the various anxiety disorders using cognitive-behavioral therapy (CBT) as a first-line intervention [1]. Cognitive-behavioral treatments for anxiety disorders are brief, structured treatments that typically focus on psychoeducation, cognitive restructuring, and exposure-based interventions as core components, although the specific nature of these interventions varies by disorder and protocol. For example, CBT for social anxiety disorder involves cognitive restructuring of socially anxious thoughts and engaging in formal graded exposure exercises related to social situations generally as well as specific social fears (e.g., public speaking) [2]. Cognitive-behavioral therapy for panic disorder includes psychoeducation and self-monitoring, cognitive restructuring of misappraisals of bodily sensations, and both in vivo and interoceptive exposures (e.g., intentionally inducing feared bodily sensations) [3]. Key goals of exposure exercises in CBT for anxiety disorders include learning to habituate to anxiety, challenging catastrophic predictions, and learning new, inhibitory responses to the original anxiety-provoking stimulus (e.g., bodily sensations in panic shift from, "I'm having a heart attack!" to "unpleasant but not dangerous") [3]. None of the CBT protocols for anxiety disorders have been specifically modified for patients with severe obesity and subject to empirical evaluation. Nevertheless, there are a number of clinical considerations for treating anxiety disorders in patients with severe obesity based on the integration of related relevant literature.

Weight Stigma and Social Anxiety

For individuals with a diagnosis of social anxiety disorder and those who experience subthreshold social anxiety symptoms, the focus of their anxiety is centered on fear of embarrassing oneself or being subjected to judgment from others [4]. Cognitive-behavioral therapy for social anxiety disorder aims to help patients challenge socially anxious thoughts and practice exposing themselves to social and potentially embarrassing situations to both challenge predictions and learn about realistic outcomes in these situations [2]. For example, a woman with social anxiety who is afraid to voice her opinion in work meetings might have thoughts such as: "Everyone will think my ideas are stupid" and "I'll fumble over my words." She also might avoid meetings altogether, or if she cannot avoid meetings, she might sit in the back of the room and stay quiet instead of contributing. For this individual, CBT for social anxiety would include learning to challenge these anxious thoughts and developing more balanced alternatives (e.g., "It is possible that my colleagues might like my ideas"; "Even if not everyone loves my ideas, some people might be interested"; and "I've spoken in meetings before and haven't fumbled on my words"). For this patient, CBT would also include constructing a hierarchy of feared situations that she could approach in a graded manner (e.g., attending a meeting rather than avoiding, sitting in the front rather than the back of the room, making eye contact with her colleagues, and presenting her opinion in a discussion).

In treating individuals with social anxiety disorder who also have obesity, it is important to consider the role of weight stigma and how this may be relevant to socially anxious thoughts and predictions (see Chapter 3). *Weight stigma* refers to negative perceptions of individuals who are overweight or obese and includes pervasive stereotypes that such individuals are lazy, unmotivated, incompetent, sloppy, and lack self-discipline [5]. Rates of weight stigma are high in the general public; for women in particular, rates of perceived weight stigma are similar to rates of perceived stigma regarding age and race [6]. Furthermore, an abundance of evidence indicates that individuals with obesity are routinely discriminated against and/or stigmatized in a variety of domains, including employment settings (e.g., wage penalties, weight biases in hiring decisions and job evaluations), healthcare (e.g., stereotypes and negative attitudes held by healthcare professionals, perceived biases in treatment), interpersonal relationships (e.g., perceived biases from family and friends), and media (e.g., stigmatization of characters with obesity in TV and film, children's media, and news media) [5]. It is not surprising, then, that perceived and internalized weight stigma has been associated with a variety of adverse mental health outcomes, including depression, anxiety, poor body image, low self-esteem, and disordered eating behaviors among individuals with obesity [5,7].

Weight stigma may also increase vulnerability to *weight-based social identity threat* [8]. A *social identity* refers to deriving part of one's self-concept from one's membership in a particular social group, whether an achieved identity (e.g., firefighter, social worker), an ascribed identity (e.g., black, woman), or a socially devalued identity (e.g., drug user). A social identity threat occurs when membership in a culturally devalued social group threatens aspects of one's identity [9]. Even if individuals do not categorize themselves as being an "overweight," "obese," or "fat" person or view this categorization as central to their self-concept, being obese may nevertheless come to form part of their self-concept if they worry that others will view and stereotype them as such [8]. Therefore, a weight-based social identity threat occurs when individuals are concerned that they will be stereotyped, devalued, rejected, or discriminated against because of their weight [8]. Weight-based social identity threats can be activated not only by experiences of direct or suspected discrimination but also in situations in which discrimination is *anticipated* (e.g., a first date, a job interview) and in response to culturally sanctioned devaluations of obesity (e.g., fat jokes) [8].

Challenging Socially Anxious Thoughts

Although CBT for social anxiety disorder aims to help individuals recognize that their social anxiety – centered on fear of judgment from others – is excessive or unreasonable, individuals who have both obesity and social anxiety face a more complex situation. Although fears of judgment *may be* disproportionate to the situation, there is also abundant empirical evidence showing that individuals with obesity are routinely judged and stigmatized in our society in a manner that is socially normative and even socially sanctioned. The presence of normative and socially sanctioned stigma against individuals with obesity certainly complicates the therapeutic task of challenging anxious cognitions centered on fear of judgment from others. The underlying premise of challenging anxious cognitions in CBT is learning that predictions are often exaggerated and feared outcomes are unlikely to occur. In the previous example of the woman who was afraid to speak up in meetings because of thoughts that her coworkers would think she was incompetent, a typical CBT approach may be to challenge these anxious thoughts, gather objective evidence of her competence, and come up with more realistic appraisals about her coworkers' beliefs about her capabilities. However, if this individual has severe obesity, research evidence indicates that her coworkers may actually judge her as less competent and as a less desirable coworker than her nonobese peers [10]. Cognitive restructuring is designed to make *distorted* thoughts more realistic, and for individuals who have severe obesity, judgment from others may in fact be a realistic outcome in some contexts.

Clinicians should first help the patient determine whether their prediction is in fact accurate – despite the literature, it is possible that some anxious predictions are based on previous experiences of stigma and that those in one's current environment do not actually endorse or communicate these stigmatizing beliefs. For instance, the patient described earlier may have had previous coworkers who treated her as incompetent, which may influence her predictions about her current coworkers. This can be achieved by examining the evidence for the prediction. In instances where there is in fact evidence that anxious predictions about judgment from others may be accurate because of the presence of weight stigma, cognitive restructuring may then be better targeted toward thoughts that make global negative statements about oneself (e.g., "I'm incompetent") compared with thoughts that involve others (e.g., "My coworkers think I'm incompetent"). The former can be targeted using standard cognitive restructuring approaches, such as examining the evidence against the thought (e.g., a list of accomplishments that demonstrate that the person is in fact competent). This may be particularly useful because research indicates that confirming and accepting others' stereotypes of them might be a maladaptive strategy that individuals use to cope with weight stigma [11]. However, it would certainly be remiss for clinicians to ignore the impact of a thought such as "My coworkers think I'm incompetent" on the patient, even if this thought is accurate. To target such thoughts when there is evidence that these thoughts are accurate, clinicians may consider incorporating problem-solving skills and coping strategies to a greater degree, including the self-compassion strategies described in Chapter 11.

Research indicates that individuals with obesity cope with weight stigma in a number of ways [11]. Some of these coping approaches and strategies may be amenable to being adapted and incorporated into CBT. Self-protective strategies, such as learning to attribute the stigma to the prejudices of others or society at large as opposed to one's personal flaws, may buffer one's self-esteem by attributing the stigma to an external source [11]. This strategy nicely complements the cognitive restructuring approach. Additionally, engaging in an activity that helps to bolster self-esteem in the threatened area might help an individual cope with or compensate for the stigma experienced [11]. In the previous example, the woman whose competence is threatened at work might cope by engaging in an activity in which she feels particularly competent. Some individuals may find "size acceptance" social activism literature or groups to be helpful for positive coping [11]. Such groups may help individuals shift their thinking about the meaning of their size and may also double as relatively low-risk situations for CBT social anxiety exposure practices. Finally, considering problem-solving approaches to dealing with weight stigma, such as speaking with a manager or human resources about discriminatory practices in the workplace, might help individuals who have faced weight stigma to address the problem directly.

Social Anxiety Exposures

In constructing social anxiety exposure exercises for individuals with obesity, it is worthwhile for clinicians to consider how weight stigma may affect exposure processes and outcomes. One of the key purposes of exposure exercises in the cognitive-behavioral treatment of anxiety, in addition to learning about anxiety habituation, is to challenge catastrophic predictions and facilitate new learning about realistic outcomes of a given situation. Typically, predictions are examined and challenged prior to entering the exposure situation, under the assumption that most of these predictions are extreme and will not come true. Similar to the discussion of challenging thoughts, the role of weight stigma needs to be considered when constructing exposures because it may affect the accuracy of predictions. For example, a person who avoids taking public transportation because she needs two seats and is worried that others will laugh or stare at her might set exposure goals around taking the subway and challenge these predictions directly. However, for a person with severe obesity, it is possible (and for some individuals perhaps not unlikely) that in fact others will notice that he or she uses two seats and may stare or make stigmatizing comments. Therefore, in this situation, in addition to challenging predictions in advance (e.g., "People might not laugh at me"), the therapist should help the patient come up with coping statements in case these realistic predictions come true (e.g., "It feels uncomfortable to have to use two seats, but it will increase my mobility and quality of life substantially if I can use the subway to get around"; "It really makes me feel bad when people make comments about my weight, but I don't want to let that restrict my lifestyle"; or "Needing two seats doesn't say anything about my worth as a person").

Panic Disorder

Individuals with a diagnosis of panic disorder experience recurrent, unexpected panic attacks and associated symptoms, including persistent concern about having additional panic attacks or about their consequences (e.g., "If this continues, I am going to have a heart attack") and/or significant changes in their behavior related to panic attacks (e.g., avoiding situations in which panic attacks might occur) [4]. Behavioral models of panic disorder posit that the fear accompanying an initial panic attack becomes classically conditioned with the interoceptive cues of the panic attack (e.g., racing heart, hyperventilation). Subsequently, experiencing these interoceptive symptoms elicits anxiety, which potentiates the next panic attack [12]. Therefore, the focus of the fear in panic disorder is the physical symptoms themselves. Cognitive behavioral therapy for panic disorder is centered on formal exposure to bodily sensations and reducing avoidance behaviors. For example, a man with panic disorder had his first panic attack when he got stuck in an elevator. His heart started racing, he began to hyperventilate, and he felt hot and dizzy. These symptoms terrified him because he thought he was not getting enough oxygen and might die.

Subsequently, every time he noticed himself feeling dizzy or hot, he started getting anxious. This escalated his heart rate and respiration, and he started thinking he was not getting enough oxygen to his brain, which would lead to a full panic attack. For this patient, CBT for panic disorder would include formal interoceptive exposures to induced physical symptoms, such as repeated trials of spinning in an office chair to induce dizziness, in order to observe that dizziness is uncomfortable but not dangerous and that although it elicits anxiety, it peaks and passes if he does not escape his anxiety. CBT would also include challenging catastrophic predictions, such as "If I start hyperventilating, I might die" by inducing hyperventilation and assessing actual outcomes, as well as decreasing avoidance or safety behaviors.

Panic Disorder and Medical Comorbidities

In treating individuals with panic disorder who also have severe obesity, it is important to consider the role of actual medical symptoms related to comorbid conditions and how this may be relevant to the interpretation of physical symptoms that accompany panic. Individuals with obesity have an increased risk of a large number of medical comorbidities, including type 2 diabetes mellitus, hypertension, dyslipidemia, cardiovascular disease, thromboembolic disease, various respiratory diseases including obstructive sleep apnea, nonalcoholic fatty liver disease, polycystic ovary syndrome, and a number of cancers [13,14]. Furthermore, the risk of all-cause mortality is significantly elevated compared with the nonobese general population for individuals with class 2 and class 3 obesity (i.e., BMI = 35 to <40 kg/m^2 and BMI $\geq$ 40 kg/m^2, respectively) [15].

Although research studies have not examined the treatment of panic disorder specifically in individuals with obesity, the literature does indicate that rates of certain medical comorbidities are elevated in individuals with panic disorder, such as coronary artery disease (CAD) [16] and chronic obstructive pulmonary disease (COPD) [17]. The relationship between panic and medical symptoms appears to be complex, and these symptoms may have a reciprocal influence on one another [18]. Furthermore, because the symptoms of panic disorder involve catastrophic interpretations of interoceptive symptoms (e.g., "I am having a heart attack"), the treatment of panic disorder is complicated when an individual has both panic disorder and a chronic medical illness in which the symptoms of both problems may present similarly (e.g., chest pain). For example, the symptoms of panic disorder and CAD may be difficult for medical professionals to differentiate, and research indicates that the behavioral presentation is similar between those with comorbid panic disorder and CAD and those with panic disorder but without CAD [16]. As a result, individuals with comorbid panic disorder and medical conditions not only may misinterpret panic symptoms as symptoms of their medical problem, but their interoceptive sensitivity also may result in increasingly selective attention to bodily sensations associated with their medical condition (e.g., thoracic pain) [16]. Although the literature does not address obesity directly, given that obesity increases risk for various medical comorbidities, these clinical challenges may be relevant when treating panic disorder in individuals with obesity and related medical conditions.

There is evidence that CBT is helpful for the treatment of panic disorder in the presence of certain medical comorbidities. In fact, some evidence suggests that CBT for panic disorder may improve medical symptoms or behavioral risk factors associated with some medical illnesses [16,18]. Furthermore, for some conditions such as CAD, data indicates that physical exercise may be a helpful adjunct to CBT in reducing panic symptoms [16].

Accordingly, when treating individuals with panic disorder who are also obese and have obesity-related medical conditions, a collaborative, multidisciplinary approach is warranted in which mental health and medical professionals liaise to provide integrated assessment and treatment. Expert commentary and the National Institute for Health and Care Excellence guidelines both indicate that a medical assessment and clear communication between mental health and medical clinicians is critical for patients with panic disorder in order to rule out medical conditions that may be underlying symptoms and/or to establish and manage medical risk during the treatment of panic disorder [16,19].

Modifying Exposures Due to Physical/Mobility Limitations

In addition to considering medical comorbidities, it is also important to consider how exposure practices may need to be modified for patients who have severe obesity and mobility limitations. For example, many CBT exposures designed to induce interoceptive symptoms involve some type of physical exertion, such as spinning in a chair or a circle to induce dizziness or running on a treadmill to increase heart rate and respiration. For patients who have severe obesity, body size might be prohibitive to engaging in some of the typical exposures. In the earlier example of the man who was stuck in an elevator during his first panic attack, this patient became sensitive to signs of increased respiration and heart rate. Although a typical exposure might involve running to induce these sensations, if this patient had severe obesity, he might be physically unable to run. One alternative is to construct a modified exposure within his mobility limitations (e.g., brisk walking or walking up a flight of stairs if he is able to do so). Another alternative is to induce the symptoms in a different way, such as inducing hyperventilation by breathing through a straw. The specific modifications will depend on the symptoms that the patient is most attuned to, as well as his or her specific mobility limitations. Liaising with medical providers to ensure that exposure modifications are appropriate for the patient given his or her physical abilities and medical condition is also prudent.

Posttraumatic Stress Disorder

A history of trauma is an unfortunate reality for many patients with severe obesity [20,21]. A number of individuals who avoid or do not process their traumatic experiences may develop symptoms of posttraumatic stress disorder (PTSD), which is a disorder comprised of a pattern of symptoms that includes reexperiencing the traumatic event (e.g., nightmares, flashbacks), avoidance of traumatic cues, distorted beliefs and persistent negative emotions, and hyperarousal symptoms [4]. Posttraumatic stress disorder can be a debilitating psychological disorder that is highly disruptive to daily activities and can lead to significant impairment.

There are several empirically supported interventions for PTSD in adults, most notably cognitive processing therapy and prolonged exposure. Either of these treatments could be a good option for a patient with severe obesity who wishes to decrease his or her PTSD symptoms. There are no known adaptations of empirically supported treatments for PTSD in adults with co-occurring severe obesity. This section will focus on cognitive processing therapy because there are several considerations that a clinician will want to reflect on before implementing this particular PTSD intervention.

Cognitive Processing Therapy

Cognitive processing therapy (CPT) relies on research demonstrating that although symptoms similar to PTSD are common immediately after a traumatic experience, many people recover naturally from these symptoms, whereas a minority of individuals remain "stuck" [22,23]. Cognitive processing therapy is a form of cognitive therapy that involves identifying *stuck points*, which are negative beliefs that develop after, or are reinforced by, traumatic experiences that can make it difficult to recover. Stuck points are extreme and rigidly held beliefs such as, "It's my fault that I was assaulted," "I can't trust others," "All men are dangerous," or "If I'm not in control, I will be assaulted again." When a patient learns skills in treatment to address their stuck points, the process can facilitate cognitive change related to how they view their traumatic experiences, as well as the processing of intense trauma-related emotions of shame, guilt, fear, sadness, and anger. Cognitive processing therapy uses Socratic questioning and cognitive worksheets to help patients identify their stuck points, as well as learn skills to challenge their beliefs by examining the evidence and developing alternative perspectives on their traumatic events [22]. For example, a patient who was raped and holds the stuck point, "If I hadn't been drinking, I wouldn't have been raped," would learn to challenge self-blame, examine whether or not the evidence supports a belief that alcohol causes rape, and consider the role of the perpetrator's intentions in causing the traumatic event. As such, the cognitive strategies in CPT are similar to those previously presented earlier in this chapter for the treatment of social anxiety disorder (or CBT more broadly). In CPT, in addition to challenging cognitions about blame, patients also explore beliefs in the areas of safety, trust, power/control, esteem, and/or intimacy that keep the individual "stuck" in PTSD [22]. For individuals with co-occurring PTSD and severe obesity, special considerations around the themes of safety and esteem may be particularly important.

With respect to the safety theme in CPT, individuals with PTSD may hold beliefs about their personal safety (or lack thereof) in the world that significantly affect their day-to-day functioning. For example, a patient with PTSD may endorse beliefs such as, "The world is unsafe" and "I can't protect myself," and may engage in many safety behaviors or significant avoidance in an attempt to increase safety in a way that does not match the objective dangerousness of the situation (e.g., refusing to leave the house after dark). Some individuals who have both obesity and PTSD (particularly related to interpersonal traumas) may endorse beliefs that they are less vulnerable to future trauma at a higher weight (e.g., "Being big protects me from being raped again"). For example, a woman who was sexually abused as a child may have experienced less abuse over time that she erroneously attributed to a co-occurring increase in her weight over time. Alternatively, she may be stigmatized due to her weight and possibly receive less sexual attention from others [24], which could reinforce her belief that her weight protects her from unwanted sexual advances and perpetuate avoidance behaviors (e.g., eating to cope with intrusive memories). When working with this stuck point, the CPT therapist should be sensitive to the relationship between PTSD and the patient's body, while challenging beliefs about weight that may contribute to the maintenance of PTSD. For example, by using Socratic questioning (a foundational strategy in CPT), the therapist can help the patient to critically examine the evidence that having a higher weight prevents rape and consider alternative perspectives besides her size or appearance that might explain why she was victimized (e.g., the perpetrator was interested in children of a particular age or took advantage of a situation).

In CPT, patients also address stuck points related to the esteem theme, which includes views about their own worth and the worth of others. Individuals with obesity may have previously developed rigidly held negative beliefs about themselves and their worth due to weight-stigmatizing experiences. By being rejected by others due to their size, individuals with obesity may internalize these views and associated negative labels (e.g., lazy, worthless, unlovable) leading to a negative self-image. A subsequent traumatic event could serve to reinforce their previous learning and further strengthen their belief in the stuck point. For example, if an individual who already holds a negative belief such as "I am unlovable" is treated coldly by her parents after being raped and is told, "You should have known better than to be alone with him," this may reinforce the belief that she is unlovable. The CPT therapist should be attentive to esteem-related stuck points that may have preceded the trauma and that may have been strengthened or reinforced by the trauma. Furthermore, although patients with PTSD who have severe obesity may have other generalized negative core beliefs about themselves, it is important to ensure that the focus in CPT is on beliefs that developed after and/or were reinforced by the traumatic experience and that appear to be maintaining the PTSD.

Other Trauma-Related Considerations

As noted earlier, for some individuals with obesity and PTSD, there may be a complex connection between their body weight, trauma-related symptoms, and eating behaviors. For example, disordered eating behaviors may function to allow the patient to cope with PTSD symptoms such as intrusive memories or persistent negative emotions [25,26]. If eating behaviors allow the patient to cope with PTSD symptoms, when patients with obesity lose weight or change their eating behaviors, it is possible that the avoided emotions related to trauma could reemerge or intensify and increase their sense of vulnerability. For patients who have recently undergone bariatric surgery, their weight loss occurs at a rapid pace, and they may quickly find themselves in distress. Clinicians working with such patients should be aware of this possibility and be attentive to increasing trauma-related reminders and emotions and help patients adopt more skillful ways of coping.

Depression

Major depressive disorder is a common mental health comorbidity of obesity [27]. Both obesity [15] and depression [28] are associated with significant morbidity and mortality and can independently affect the day-to-day functioning of affected individuals in a negative manner. There is overlap between some depressive symptoms and other experiences of individuals with obesity. For example, when experiencing a major depressive episode, individuals can have physical symptoms such as fatigue, impaired sleep, and appetite changes [4]. These same challenges can also occur separately in individuals with obesity, who may also have sleep apnea that significantly affects their sleep pattern as well as fatigue level or who may engage in irregular or dysregulated eating including, in some cases, binge eating and night eating. Furthermore, the literature indicates a bidirectional relationship between depression and obesity such that obesity increases the risk of depression, and depression increases the risk of obesity [29].

Given that this chapter focuses on psychological interventions for comorbid mental health conditions, this section reviews evidence-based treatment for depression as well as adaptations that may be required for working with individuals with severe obesity. There is an abundance of research that supports the use of CBT in the treatment of major depression in adults [30]. There are no known adapted protocols for treating depression in individuals with severe obesity. Below we highlight several suggestions for adapting components of CBT for depression in severe obesity, including adaptations to be considered when using behavioral activation and cognitive strategies.

Behavioral Activation

Briefly, *behavioral activation* is an intervention that targets the relationships between a person's behavior and his or her environment [31]. It is also a stand-alone treatment for depression that can be combined with cognitive strategies in the administration of CBT. Depression may be maintained when the individual is not receiving positive reinforcement or reward from the environment, such as when an individual with depression stays in bed all day and has little opportunity for pleasurable experiences. As such, engagement in adaptive behaviors may decline, which can lead to worsening mood. In behavioral activation, clinicians educate patients about the connection between their behavioral responses to events and their moods. A core component is tracking their mood throughout the day using self-monitoring and to schedule activities that provide a sense of mastery and/or pleasure. Not only may these activities result in a positive shift in mood, which can be reinforcing, but patients learn to understand the connection between activity and mood. There is evidence that behavioral activation improves symptoms of depression [32].

Following psychoeducation, behavioral activation involves monitoring daily activities and mood using an activity record. This process can help patients to see the connection between what they are doing and how they feel. Subsequently, patients can schedule activities strategically to develop positive contingent relationships between their activities and their mood. A challenge that may arise with individuals with obesity is possible limitations in completing some activities due to their size. For example, they may not physically fit into seating options for some pleasure activities (e.g., a seat at a movie theater, a canoe) if there are no accommodations for larger individuals. Individuals with obesity may also have limited mobility due to their size or potentially related injuries or health conditions or could experience significant fatigue or difficulty breathing with exertion. They may not be able to bend over or move in ways that are easier for people without obesity. As such, some activities such as going for a walk, playing a sport, or exploring a museum may prove difficult.

Clinicians should first assess the patient's abilities and limitations in consultation with his or her family physician and possibly other healthcare professionals, such as physical therapists. When collaboratively reviewing activity records with patients, clinicians should take note of activities that likely contribute to the maintenance of the patient's depressed mood, such as time spent in bed or watching TV. Using problem solving, activities that are within the patient's abilities should be identified and encouraged. If a patient is quite limited mobility-wise, activities could focus on what he or she is able to do within the home, including social contact and other pleasure activities, such as listening to music and painting. Individuals with severe obesity may feel ashamed about their physical limitations; thus therapists should be vigilant in session for behaviors denoting shame when discussing physical limitations, such as avoiding eye contact or a decrease in disclosure of information. By responding in an accepting and nonjudgmental manner, therapists can help to reduce their patients' feelings of shame and increase the likelihood of learning details of their difficult experiences and associated emotions, thoughts, and behaviors. Clinicians should also be alert to maladaptive coping strategies that may be negatively reinforcing (e.g., emotional eating, substance use). An important task is to engage patients in activities that can be helpful to their mood, assist with coping, and not contribute to other problems. In addition to pleasure activities, it is important to schedule in activities or tasks that give a sense of mastery or accomplishment, such as completing errands, scheduling appointments, helping children with homework, or similar tasks. These activities can also be reinforcing and improve mood.

With both pleasure and mastery activities, clinicians work with patients to set small, manageable goals that are realistic and attainable within a particular timeframe. This approach increases the odds that the activity will be rewarding and accounts for limitations the patient may have due to the effects of depressed mood (e.g., difficulty concentrating, fatigue). Patients with severe obesity may feel discouraged or hopeless when they are unable to complete goals to the same degree or in the same amount of time as lower-weight individuals. Clinicians are encouraged to respond with validation and empathy regarding the difficulty of this reality and also engage in cognitive restructuring (see below) to help patients adjust how they are thinking about the situation.

Increasingly, there is research demonstrating the mental health benefits of exercise, in particular regarding improvements in mood [33]. Indeed, the National Institute for Health and Care Excellence guidelines recommend that physical activity be modified when included in treatments for adults with both depression and long-term health problems [34]. As indicated earlier, it is recommended that scheduled activities with a physical activity component increase over time. As always, any exercise program should be reviewed and approved by the patient's treating medical professional to ensure that he or she is exercising in a manner that is safe and within the limits of his or her physical abilities.

Cognitive Strategies

Cognitive-behavioral therapy focuses on the interconnection between thoughts, emotions, and behaviors. As such, a key task in cognitive therapy for depression is identifying and challenging negatively biased cognitions. According to the cognitive model of depression [35], patients with depression have negative views of themselves, others, the world, and/or the future that can distort their interpretations of events that occur in their life. These distorted automatic thoughts, assumptions, or core beliefs can affect how individuals feel and behave in response to events.

In the earlier section on social anxiety in this chapter, we described adaptations to cognitive interventions for patients with severe obesity, such as acknowledging experiences with weight stigma when evaluating their anxious predictions. The suggestions from that section are also relevant when targeting depressed thoughts in CBT. Automatic thoughts, assumptions, and core beliefs in depression often revolve around themes of failure, worthlessness, and being unlovable. Patients with severe obesity may have significant experiences of being judged harshly or shunned by others due to their weight status that could contribute to the development and/or reinforcement of core beliefs such as, "I will be abandoned and rejected by others" or "I'm worthless." Clinicians need to be sensitive to the experiences of rejection and subsequent shame that their patients may experience. They can then skillfully engage their patients in determining whether they are discounting or overlooking any evidence of experiences where they are accepted by others to help develop more adaptive beliefs.

Many individuals with severe obesity have made multiple unsuccessful attempts to lose weight. These experiences may contribute to the maintenance of the core belief "I'm a failure" in some patients with depression. Furthermore, they may receive erroneous messages regarding the controllability of weight from loved ones, as well as healthcare professionals, which can further exacerbate their sense of failure. Clinicians should become educated on relevant literature to help identify any biased beliefs about weight controllability they may hold [36,37]. This can help them to engage their patients in challenging these myths as well.

Substance-Use Disorders

A number of interventions have been used to treat substance-use disorders. Contingency management approaches are behaviorally based interventions that make incentives (e.g., vouchers that can be exchanged for rewards) contingent upon negative toxicology screening results. Cognitive-behavioral therapy approaches for substance use include functional analysis of substance-use behaviors and the use of alternative cognitive and behavioral responses in stressful situations. Other approaches include relapse prevention, which aims to anticipate high-risk situations and plan for skillful coping. Meta-analytic research indicates that contingency management approaches and contingency management approaches combined with CBT may be more effective for substance-use disorders than standard CBT and relapse-prevention approaches [38]. The strongest effects occurred for cannabis- and cocaine-use disorders, though the highest dropouts also occurred for cocaine users, and studies of alcohol-use disorder were not included in this study [38]. Results from another meta-analysis suggest that behavioral couples therapy, which uses standard CBT approaches and also includes increasing the coping skills of the partner, has superior efficacy over individual interventions for treating adults with alcohol- and other substance-use disorders [39]. Despite the popularity of motivational interviewing approaches, which aim to increase readiness for change, research indicates that motivational interviewing has moderate efficacy compared with no treatment or weak control conditions in the treatment of alcohol- and other substance-use disorders but no advantage over other active treatments or strong comparison groups [40,41]. Nevertheless, motivational approaches appear to be helpful for engaging patients with substance-use disorders [41], which may be an important first step to change. Finally, despite the popularity of 12-step approaches such as Alcoholics Anonymous, the efficacy of such interventions is difficult to evaluate empirically given that anonymity is embedded as a key element of such programs.

Commonalities between Overeating and Substance-Use Disorders

In treating patients with substance-use disorders and comorbid obesity, one important consideration is the ways in which problematic substance-use and eating behaviors may interact or overlap. Although obesity does not appear to increase the risk of substance-use disorders, and in fact, some evidence suggests that individuals with obesity are overall at lowered risk, some subsets of individuals with obesity may nevertheless be at risk for problematic patterns of substance use [42]. Some research indicates that there may be shared neurobiological, environmental, cognitive-affective, and behavioral processes between problematic patterns of eating and substance use that may be relevant for those with both substance-use disorders and obesity.

In recent years there has been an explosion of interest in *food addiction* as a construct. The concept of food addiction has been likened to substance-use disorders following observations that for some individuals, eating behaviors and associated problems resemble substance-use behaviors and their consequences in those with substance-use disorders [43]. The validity of this construct continues to be investigated, but there is emerging evidence to suggest a number of conceptual similarities between the proposed construct of food addiction and substance-use disorders. For example, a recent review of the literature noted a number of similarities between food addiction and substance-use disorders, including appetites for both food and substances are cued by environmental stimuli; evidence of "appetizer effects" and "priming effects" indicate that a small "first taste" of both food and drugs precipitates increased desire for each, respectively; there is evidence of the abstinence violation effects in both the eating and substance-use literature; the existence of cravings as a motivator for both eating and drug-use behaviors; the occurrence of bingeing behaviors for both food and substances; and reward and wanting as key motivators of both eating and substance-use behaviors [44]. There is also some evidence of neurobiological similarities in individuals with eating and substance-related behaviors [43,45,46], although the implications of such similarities remain under investigation.

Given that there may be common neurocircuitry associated with problematic patterns of both eating- and substance-related behaviors [45], some researchers have postulated that food and drugs may therefore compete for reward sites in the brain [47]. For example, there is some evidence of an inverse relationship between BMI and both alcohol and marijuana consumption for individuals with obesity, which may suggest that food-related reward actually protects from substance-related reward (although it is noted that the data on which this interpretation is based are correlational, and therefore such conclusions should be interpreted cautiously) [48,49]. Nevertheless, it is important to note that the validity of the food addiction construct continues to be investigated.

Bariatric Surgery and Alcohol Use

There is some evidence that individuals without alcohol problems who undergo bariatric surgery are at increased risk of prospectively developing subsequent alcohol problems after surgery. For example, a rigorous multisite study followed participants undergoing bariatric surgery and matched controls prospectively for 20 years [50]. At baseline, all participants had low-risk alcohol use and did not have alcohol-use problems. In the 20-year follow-up period, individuals who underwent bariatric surgery were at significantly increased risk of engaging in alcohol use that was classified as medium risk or greater and were at significantly increased risk of self-reported alcohol problems and alcohol-abuse diagnoses compared with matched control patients. When various surgical procedures were compared, gastric bypass surgery conferred the greatest risk compared with other types of surgical procedures [50]. Although the mechanism for this finding is unknown, there is evidence that gastric bypass surgery alters alcohol metabolism such that peak alcohol levels are higher and alcohol elimination times are longer [51].

Treatment Considerations

Given these data, there are some considerations for the psychological treatment of substance-use disorders in individuals with obesity. First, given the research on eating- and substance-related behaviors and the dopaminergic system, clinicians should be attentive to the functional role of eating and substance-use behaviors, particularly functional similarity or overlap between these behaviors. More specifically, if eating and substance use serve a similar function (e.g., emotion regulation, self-soothing), one clinical concern is that as the substance use improves, eating behaviors may worsen. This may be of particular concern for individuals who engage in binge eating or emotional eating. In order to assess whether this is the case, clinicians can undertake a functional assessment of both problematic eating and substance-use behaviors to determine the primary antecedents cuing the behaviors and reinforcing consequences of the behaviors. For example, if a woman with an alcohol-use disorder drinks to relieve stress after work, she may find that as her alcohol use decreases, she begins to overeat after work instead as an alternative way to cope with stress and soothe herself. A detailed functional analysis would likely reveal that both eating and alcohol use are cued by work-related stress and that comfort, relaxation, and stress reduction are reinforcing consequences of both behaviors. When behaviors are functionally similar, clinicians should point out this observation to patients and help patients make explicit plans for skillful coping so as not to rely on another functionally similar problem behavior. The patient described earlier may make plans for adaptive stress reduction after work, such as taking a hot shower, having a cup of tea, and engaging in a pleasant activity. She may also make an eating plan for after work so that she is not relying on making food-related decisions during times of high stress. Clinicians might also consider assigning self-monitoring of eating behaviors and/or checking in regularly about the status of eating behaviors in the context of substance-use treatment to determine whether any problematic patterns have emerged as a substitute for substance use.

Another point of consideration in the treatment of substance use with patients with obesity is that withdrawal from certain classes of substances – namely, stimulants (e.g., cocaine, amphetamines) and tobacco – may increase appetite [4]. Clinicians should provide information about these symptoms and assist patients in planning for how they will handle increased appetite as they withdraw from substances. Furthermore, liaising with a medical team for medical monitoring and appropriate medical care during substance withdrawal is important, particularly given that many individuals with obesity face increased medical risks. Relatedly, patients with obesity who have undergone bariatric surgery, particularly gastric bypass surgery, should be provided with information and education around increased risks associated with alcohol use after surgery. Liaison and multidisciplinary collaboration with the patient's medical team are indicated in such situations as well.

Clinical Vignette Revisited

Anne has symptoms meeting criteria for major depressive disorder, social anxiety disorder, and alcohol-use disorder. Prior to starting any psychological intervention, she underwent a medical evaluation by her family physician to determine any physical limitations and considerations that might inform psychological treatment planning. When treating her depression using a CBT framework, Anne's therapist engages her in behavioral activation by monitoring her activities and mood and strategically planning both pleasure and mastery activities to help improve her mood. Anne previously enjoyed walking and gardening. Her therapist helps her to determine how to incorporate these activities safely given her physical limitations, including difficulty walking and inability to bend over. They decide that she would walk in her backyard for a length of time she can tolerate while subsequently increasing the intensity, duration, and frequency of this activity. Anne identified that a benefit of walking was observing nature, which gave her a sense of pleasure. She and her therapist also decide to include time in her week to drive out to a beautiful area of town and spend some time in nature. With respect to gardening, they set a goal to create a small garden box that can be kept on a table in the sunlight so that she is able to easily tend to the plants. Anne and her therapist also set goals to increase the time she spends with her family and her childhood friends, which they noted usually leads to a positive shift in her mood. They also plan for coping at work, where she is unable to bend over and play with many of the animals. Anne notices that she is still easily able to pet the larger dogs and includes more of this activity into her workday.

When challenging both depressed and socially anxious thoughts, Anne's therapist should remain cognizant of her past history of being bullied and judged based on her weight. Anne also notes that presently strangers often stare at her when she is walking on the street and sometimes make hurtful comments about her size and tell her to lose weight. Her therapist acknowledges that her automatic thoughts such as, "People don't like me because of my weight," may not be entirely inaccurate in that there are in fact some people who judge her based on her weight. The therapist's role is to acknowledge and incorporate these experiences while also helping Anne to challenge the extreme nature of some of her thoughts and beliefs. Anne learns to consider, and also starts to track, experiences where she is not judged and in fact receives positive feedback from others and also develop ways to cope with discrimination. This is especially important when evaluating the outcome of exposures when treating her social anxiety using a CBT framework.

Anne also wishes to address her alcohol use in treatment and sets a goal of abstinence. Her therapist works with her on this goal using contingency management and CBT. While completing this task, Anne and her therapist monitor her eating patterns because, after engaging in behavioral analysis, they discover that alcohol use and eating both serve to regulate her emotions and allow her to cope with stress. They also work on developing skills to self-soothe in a more effective manner.

Summary

In summary, this chapter focused on adapting mainly cognitive-behavioral interventions when treating individuals with severe obesity who also have mental health comorbidities. When engaging patients in behavioral interventions, clinicians need to be aware of physical limitations that might prevent them from completing some activities. Clinicians also need to be creative in determining pleasure and mastery activities and designing exposures that are safe as well as effective in shifting mood or approaching anxiety-provoking stimuli, respectively. Furthermore, challenging beliefs is a critical component of CBT, and clinicians need to educate themselves about the influence of weight-based stigmatizing experiences on the development and maintenance of maladaptive beliefs that underlie various mental health conditions. Finally, problem solving and adaptive coping should take a central role because these issues arise in treatments for depression, anxiety disorders, posttraumatic stress disorder, and substance-use disorder in individuals with severe obesity.

Key Points

- Clinicians should have their patients with severe obesity undergo a medical evaluation to determine any risks or physical limitations of engaging in psychological treatment.
- When challenging cognitions in CBT, clinicians who are treating individuals with severe obesity should be sensitive to any experiences with weight-based prejudice and discrimination.
- When engaging individuals with severe obesity in behavioral interventions, such as behavioral activation or exposures, clinicians should ensure that they make adaptations that address any physical limitations.

References

1. A. C. Butler, J. E. Chapman, E. M. Forman, et al. The empirical status of cognitive-behavioural therapy: A review of meta-analyses. *Clin Psychol Rev* 2006; **26**: 17–31.

2. C. L. Turk, R. G. Heimberg, and L. Magee. Social anxiety disorder. In D. H. Barlow, ed., *Clinical Handbook of Psychological Disorders: A Step-by-Step Treatment Manual* (4th edn). New York, NY: Guilford Press, 2008: 123–63.

3. M. G. Craske and D. H. Barlow. Panic disorder and agoraphobia. In D. H. Barlow, ed., *Clinical Handbook of Psychological Disorders: A Step-by-Step Treatment Manual* (4th edn). New York, NY: Guilford Press, 2008: 1–64.

4. American Psychiatric Association. *Diagnostic and Statistical Manual of Mental Disorders* (5th edn). Arlington, VA: American Psychiatric Association, 2013.

5. R. M. Puhl and C. A. Heuer. The stigma of obesity: A review and update. *Obesity* 2009; **17b**: 941–64.

6. R. M. Puhl, T. Andreyeva, and K. D. Brownell. Perceptions of weight discrimination: Prevalence and comparison to race and gender discrimination in America. *Int J Obes* 2008; **32**: 992–1000.

7. S. Papadopoulos and L. Brennan. Correlates of weight stigma in adults with overweight and obesity: A systematic literature review. *Obesity* 2015; **23**: 1743–60.

8. J. M. Hunger, B. Major, A. Blodorn, et al. Weighed down by stigma: How weight-based social identity threat contributes to weight gain and poor health. *Soc Pers Psychol Compass* 2015; **9**: 255–68.

9. B. Major and L. T. O'Brien. The social psychology of stigma. *Annu Rev Psychol* 2005; **56**: 393–421.

10. M. V. Roehling. Weight-based discrimination in employment: Psychological and legal aspects. *Personnel Psychol* 1999; **52**: 969–1016.

11. R. Puhl and K. D. Brownell. Ways of coping with obesity stigma: Review and conceptual analysis. *Eat Behav* 2003; **4**: 53–78.

12. M. E. Bouton, S. Mineka, and D. H. Barlow. A modern learning theory perspective on the etiology of panic disorder. *Psychol Rev* 2001; **108**: 4–32.

13. D. D. Hensrud and S. Klein. Extreme obesity: A new medical crisis in the United States. *Mayo Clin Proc* 2006; **81**: S5–10.

14. V. J. Lawrence and P. G. Kopelman. Medical consequences of obesity. *Clin Dermatol* 2004; **22**: 296–302.

15. K. M. Flegal, B. K. Kit, H. Orpana, et al. Association of all-cause mortality with overweight and obesity using standard body mass index categories: A systemic review and meta-analysis. *JAMA* 2013; **309**: 71–82.

16. A. Sardinha, C. G. S. Araujo, G. L. F. Soares-Filho, et al. Anxiety, panic disorder and coronary artery disease: Issues concerning physical exercise and cognitive behavioral therapy. *Expert Rev Cardiovasc Ther* 2011; **9**: 165–75.

17. N. Livermore, L. Sharpe, and D. McKenzie. Prevention of panic attacks and panic disorder in COPD. *Eur Respir J* 2010; **35**: 557–63.

18. N. B. Schmidt and M. J. Telch. Nonpsychiatric medical comorbidity,

health perceptions, and treatment outcome in patients with panic disorder. *Health Psychol* 1997; **16**: 114–22.

19. National Institute for Health and Care Excellence (NICE). *Panic Disorder Overview*, 2017. Available at http://path ways.nice.org.uk/pathways/panic-disorder #content=view-index&path=view%3A/pat hways/panic-disorder/panic-disorder-overview.xml (accessed April 26, 2017).

20. C. M. Grilo, R. M. Masheb, M. Brody, et al. Childhood maltreatment in extremely obese male and female bariatric surgery candidates. *Obes Res* 2005, **13**: 123–30.

21. T. B. Gustafson and D. B. Sarwer. Childhood sexual abuse and obesity. *Obes Rev* 2004; **5**: 129–35.

22. P. A. Resick, C. M. Monson, and K. M. Chard. *Cognitive Processing Therapy for PTSD: A Comprehensive Manual.* New York, NY: Guilford Press, 2016.

23. P. A. Resick and M. K. Schnicke. Cognitive processing therapy for sexual assault victims. *J Consult Clin Psych* 1992; **60**: 748–56.

24. E. Y. Chen and M. Brown. Obesity stigma in sexual relationships. *Obes Res* 2005; **13**: 1393–7.

25. L. S. Talbot, S. Maguen, E. S. Epel, et al. Posttraumatic stress disorder is associated with emotional eating. *J Trauma Stress* 2013; **26**: 521–5.

26. K. Trottier and D. E. MacDonald. Update on psychological trauma, other severe adverse experiences and eating disorders: State of the research and future research directions. *Curr Psychiatry Rep* 2017; **19**: 45.

27. S. L. McElroy, R. Kotwal, S. Malhotia, et al. Are mood disorders and obesity related? A review for the mental health professional. *J Clin Psychiatry* 2004; **65**: 634–51.

28. L. Culpepper. Understanding the burden of depression. *J Clin Psychiatry* 2011; **72**: e19.

29. F. S. Luppino, L. M. de Wit, P. F. Bouvy, et al. Overweight, obesity, and depression: A systematic review and meta-analysis of longitudinal studies. *Arch Gen Psychiatry* 2010; **67**: 220–9.

30. P. Cuijpers, M. Berking, G. Andersson, et al. A meta-analysis of cognitive-behavioural therapy for adult depression, alone and in comparison with other treatments. *Can J Psychiatry* 2013; **58**: 376–85.

31. C. R. Martell, M. E. Addis, and N. S. Jacobson. *Depression in Context: Strategies for Guided Action.* New York, NY: W.W. Norton, 2001.

32. I. Soucy Chartier and M. D. Provencher. Behavioural activation for depression: Efficacy, effectiveness and dissemination. *J Affect Disorders* 2013; **145**: 292–9.

33. G. Stathopoulou, M. B. Powers, A. C. Berry, et al. Exercise interventions for mental health: A quantitative and qualitative review. *Clin Psychol Sci Prac* 2006; **13**: 179–93.

34. National Institute for Health and Care Excellence (NICE). Depression in adults with a chronic physical health problem: Recognition and management, 2017. Available at www.nice.org.uk/guidance/cg91 (accessed November 6, 2017).

35. A. T. Beck. *Cognitive Therapy and the Emotional Disorders.* New York, NY: Meridian, 1976.

36. F. L. Greenway. Physiological adaptations to weight loss and factors favouring weight regain. *Int J Obes* 2015; **39**: 1188–96.

37. P. Sumithran and J. Proietto. The defense of body weight: A physiological basis for weight regain after weight loss. *Clin Sci* 2013; **124**: 231–41.

38. L. Dutra, G. Stathopoulou, S. L. Basden, et al. A meta-analytic review of psychosocial interventions for substance use disorders. *Am J Psychiatry* 2008; **165**: 179–87.

39. M. B. Powers, E. Vedel, and P. M. G. Emmelkamp. Behavioral couples therapy (BCT) for alcohol and drug use disorders: A meta-analysis. *Clin Psychol Rev* 2008; **28**: 952–62.

40. B. L. Burke, H. Arkowitz, and M. Menchola. The efficacy of motivational interviewing: A meta-analysis of controlled clinical trials. *J Consult Clin Psychol* 2003; **71**: 843–61.

41. B. W. Lundahl, C. Kunz, C. Brownell, et al. A meta-analysis of motivational interviewing: Twenty-five years of empirical studies. *Res Soc Work Pract* 2010; **20**: 137–60.

42. R. A. Sansone and L. A. Sansone. Obesity and substance misuse: Is there a relationship? *Innov Clin Neurosci* 2013; **10**: 30–5.

43. J. Hebebrand, O. Albayrak, R. Adan, et al. "Eating addiction," rather than "food addiction," better captures addictive-like eating behavior. *Neurosci Biobehav Rev* 2014; **47**: 295–306.

44. P. J. Rogers. Food and drug addictions: Similarities and differences. *Pharmacol Biochem Behav* 2017; **153**: 182–90.

45. N. D. Volkow and R. A. Wise. How can drug addiction help us understand obesity? *Nat Neurosci* 2005; **8**: 555–60.

46. G-J. Wang, N. D. Volkow, P. K. Thanos, et al. Similarity between obesity and drug addiction as assessed by neurofunctional imaging: A concept review. *J Addict Dis* 2004; **23**: 39–53.

47. M. W. Warren and M. S. Gold. The relationship between obesity and drug use. *Am J Psychiatry* 2007; **164**: 1268.

48. K. D. Kleiner, M. S. Gold, K. Frost-Pineda, et al. Body mass index and alcohol use. *J Addict Dis* 2004; **23**: 105–18.

49. M. Warren, K. Frost-Pineda, and M. Gold. Body mass index and marijuana use. *J Addict Dis* 2005; **24**: 95–100.

50. P-A. Svensson, A. Anveden, S. Romeo, et al. Alcohol consumption and alcohol problems after bariatric surgery in the Swedish Obese Subjects Study. *Obesity* 2013; **21**: 2444–51.

51. G. A. Woodard, J. Downey, T. Hernandez-Boussard, et al. Impaired alcohol metabolism after gastric bypass surgery: A case-crossover trial. *J Am Coll Surg* 2011; **212**: 209–14.

Chapter 17

Integrated Models of Obesity Care

Sanjeev Sockalingam and Raed Hawa

Case Vignette

Laura is a 42-year-old woman who has been struggling with her weight since her first pregnancy when she was 32. She had a difficult pregnancy, and she had preeclampsia. Postpartum, she experienced mood symptoms that required pharmacologic intervention. She was put on sertraline 150 mg, which helped her to feel better. She attempted to discontinue sertraline, but her mood symptoms returned.

She has a full-time job as a high school teacher. Her husband is a business executive and travels a lot. She describes her life as "on the go" but overall "happy." She finds pleasure helping people. She is the "go to" person for friends who have problems or need help. Her mother has been sick lately, and she is being investigated for possible dementia. Laura is her only support.

Despite keeping a happy face, Laura struggles with her body image. She has attempted several weight loss programs with little success because she finds that the demands of the program are "too much." She avoids looking at herself in the mirror and has been avoiding intimate contact with her husband, claiming that she is feeling tired. She feels "ugly" at times and has doubts about her husband's love for her.

She reports that she has a weakness for chips and cookies. She enjoys the crunchiness of the food. She usually misses breakfast and has a "healthy" lunch. She eats a large meal at supper but does not feel full. She indulges in more chips and cookies after supper, and at times she wakes up at night to eat her favorite snacks. She has been feeling more down recently as a result of her increased weight.

At her last appointment with her primary care physician, she was told that her blood pressure is high and her lipid profile is abnormal. She became very concerned because she has a family history of heart disease. She asked her physician if there is anything that can be done to help her with her weight and to prevent weight-related complications.

Introduction

Previous chapters in this book have outlined the role of psychological treatments to support severe obesity management. Models of care where psychosocial care is integrated as a core component of treatment are needed to support their delivery. In this chapter, we review the role of integrated care models to provide psychological care to patients with severe obesity. Following a review of the general evidence base for integrated care, this chapter provides a summary of obesity-specific integrated care models and outlines an approach for integrating psychological treatments for severe obesity care within these interprofessional contexts.

Integrated Models of Care

Integrated care has often been used interchangeably with the term *collaborative care*, and there is confusion between these terms. Katon and colleagues originally defined collaborative care as a specific type of integrated care model using the chronic care model with the goal of improving access to mental health treatment within primary care settings [1,2]. Moreover, three levels of collaboration and integration have been described in the literature, specifically coordinated services, collocated services, and integrated services [3]. *Coordinated* services consist of communication of patient care needs between mental health and primary care providers when needed, but care is delivered in separate settings. *Collocated* services consist of mental health and primary care providers working in a shared space, which increases the likelihood of communication, education, and overall patient care as a result of proximity. At this level, there are no formal, structured communication and coordination processes. Last, *integrated* services consist of a team approach with one joint treatment plan. The latter is the goal of established evidence-based models of integrated care and would support a team-based approach to severe obesity care.

With the evolution of the integrated collaborative care model, there have been several attempts to define the core components of this model. A joint report by the American Psychiatric Association and the Academy of Psychosomatic Medicine identified four essential elements of integrated collaborative care [4]. These four elements include the following:

1. **Team Driven.** Care is coordinated by a multidisciplinary group of healthcare delivery professionals, who are empowered to work at the top of their professional training.
2. **Population Focused.** The team is responsible for the provision of care and health outcomes of a defined population of patients.
3. **Measurement Guided.** The team uses systematic, disease-specific, patient-reported outcome measures to drive clinical decisions on care.
4. **Evidence Based.** The team applies evidence-based treatments to individual clinical contexts to improve patient outcomes.

It is through these elements that collaborative care has achieved its improved clinical outcomes and resulted in high levels of satisfaction among providers and patients.

Several collaborative care models have been reported in the literature. One of the most well known models is the Improving Mood-Promoting Access to Collaborative Treatment (IMPACT) model for depression [5–7]. IMPACT is based on a model where a depression care manager provides evidence-based interventions and systematic monitoring. The care manager connects the primary care physician and psychiatrist, and the latter consults with the care manager on patients with ongoing mental health issues not responding to initial treatment provided by the care manager. The model has been adopted widely in the management of a range of diseases, such as diabetes and cancer [5,6].

Additional integrated care models developed to address issues related to geographic isolation have been studied. These models may use telephone, videoconferencing, and telemedicine modalities to bridge the gap between academic and more rural settings. An example is the Project Extension of Community Health Outcomes (ECHO), which originated in New Mexico. This integrated care model uses videoconferencing technology to link specialist teams, often consisting of a medical specialist, behavioral health specialist, and other healthcare professionals (e.g., pharmacist, social worker), with primary care clinicians practicing in local communities [8]. Project ECHO uses weekly clinics where multiple primary care clinicians attend virtually to discuss cases with specialist teams and with one another. The case discussions are supplemented with focused teaching related to evidence-based practice and treatment algorithms and guidelines. The ECHO model uses measurement-based care, team collaboration, and evidence-based treatment approaches with a defined patient population to improve outcomes. Given its focus on chronic and complex diseases, Project ECHO is a promising model for building primary care capacity for managing obesity, including psychosocial aspects of obesity care.

Evidence for Integrated Collaborative Care

As mentioned earlier, collaborative mental health care has been studied across a range of diseases, such as diabetes [2], cardiovascular disease [9], cancer [10], and chronic pain [11]. In a seminal study by Katon and colleagues, integrated care for depression in the context of multiple physical health conditions was studied in 14 primary care clinics in a single-blind randomized, controlled trial (RCT) [9]. The study demonstrated greater 12-month improvement in glycated hemoglobin (for diabetes) levels, cholesterol, systolic blood pressure, and depression scores and also showed greater patient satisfaction with care. In an integrated collaborative care treatment RCT for depression care in patients with cancer, those receiving collaborative care experienced less depression, anxiety, pain, and fatigue than those receiving usual care [10]. Moreover, a large systematic review of 79 RCTs involving 24,308 participants showed significant improvements in depression and anxiety long term with collaborative care [12]. Therefore, there is clear evidence for the effectiveness of this model for comorbid health conditions, namely, physical and mental health conditions, suggesting that there may be a potential role for collaborative care in the management of severe obesity.

As mentioned earlier, Project ECHO uses components of integrated care and has shown to be effective in improving patient outcomes. A seminal prospective cohort study on hepatitis C showed comparable treatment outcomes for patients managed in ECHO rural primary care sites and patients managed by specialists in an academic health center [13]. Following this seminal ECHO study, there have been additional studies demonstrating improved patient outcomes in diabetes and dementia [14]. Data from a mental health and addictions ECHO has also shown improvements in building primary care clinicians' knowledge and self-efficacy [15]. Although trials on Project ECHO in obesity are lacking, anecdotal reports of ECHO for obesity care suggest that the ECHO model may be another vehicle for integrated care delivery in severe obesity.

Implementation of Integrated Care Programs

Although integrated care models are supported by a large evidence base, their implementation has been a challenge, and there is literature identifying key barriers in implementation. Kathol and colleagues used key informant interviews with 11 nationally recognized sites delivering integrated physical and mental health care [16]. Analysis of these interviews identified several barriers to integrated care implementation. First, the culture of organizations was identified as a key barrier. Some clinical programs did not see mental health as part of total health and did not feel that mental health professionals were a necessary part of the team to support medical clinicians in delivering mental healthcare to patients. Second, the lack of understanding of clinicians' roles in cross-disciplinary process was another barrier. A third barrier was the changes to mental health specialists' work habits (e.g., moving from 50-minute time slots to the responsiveness necessary for primary clinician support, such as case review rounds and indirect consultations). Fourth, a lack of management practices supporting the development of relationships between mental health providers, physical health providers, and care managers was an additional barrier to implementing integrated care. Recognition of these barriers early in the planning and reassessing these factors during the implementation phase of integrated care programs are critical to mitigating potential roadblocks to integrated care.

Several factors have been identified as being critical to the success of integrated care programs [16]. First, it is important to foster collaborative relationships between program leads and staff participating in the physical and mental healthcare. Second, team members should be educated about the value of integrated care and receive training in the provision of integrated services, especially for complex patients. This should focus on training in physical healthcare for mental health professionals and mental healthcare for physical health professionals. Third, it is critical to have longitudinal champions for both the physical and mental healthcare within these models. They are important to cultivating the culture of integrated care and to perpetuate collaborative relationships between care providers. Fourth, collocation of services can support these collaborative relationships and increase interprofessional communication. Lastly, consolidated health records where documentation, measurement, and communication of both physical and mental needs are a core component of integrated care models to further support integration across professions. These ingredients are core features of successful and sustainable integrated care models and should be considered when developing integrated care programs for severe obesity care.

Integrated Care Models in Severe Obesity

Although integrated collaborative care has an established evidence base, the use of collaborative care in severe obesity treatment has been limited despite its potential. Guidelines for obesity management advocate for a multidisciplinary approach to obesity care, which aligns with the team-based approach to integrated care [17]. Moreover, the focus on both mental and physical health and the team-based approach to care resonate with severe obesity care given the high rates of psychiatric comorbidity and multiple factors precipitating and perpetuating obesity.

As discussed previously, patients with severe obesity have high rates of psychiatric illness (see Chapter 1). Integrated care models go beyond collocation and can be used to further integrate behavioral health assessments and treatments within bariatric medicine and bariatric surgery programs. Further, systematic screening and measurement can facilitate a stepped-care approach, where psychological treatments discussed in this book can be used early in the care of patients with severe obesity. For example, patients after bariatric surgery may be screened by nurses or dietitians within the program and identify early signs of loss of control over eating and emotional eating. Recognition of these symptoms may prompt referral to a mental health clinician through an activated care pathway, which may begin with a support group (see Chapter 13) or a clinician-guided Internet-based cognitive-behavioral therapy (CBT) intervention (see Chapter 15). Failure to respond to this first intervention may progress to a second level of intervention based on patient preference and access, which may include telephone-based CBT (see Chapter 14) or mindfulness-based eating awareness therapy (MB-EAT; see Chapter 10). Through an integrated care model, these pathways of care can be applied in a systematic manner, and timely access to mental health treatment can be implemented in this measurement-based care approach. Using this model, patients would receive the recommended multidisciplinary approach but also address issues with access and timely interventions to prevent weight regain after treatment for severe obesity.

Evidence for Integrated Care Models in Severe Obesity

Currently, there is a paucity of evidence for the efficacy of integrated care in treating obesity. The Partnership Overweight Netherlands (PON) initiative is a collaborative network of multiple healthcare professionals across the healthcare system aimed at delivering an integrated health standard to manage and prevent obesity [18]. PON uses a stepped-care approach based on clinical practice guidelines to match treatment intensity with patients' weight-related health risk. In a pilot cross-over study focused on childhood obesity management, primary care providers supported by obesity specialists via telehealth showed benefit compared with patents managed by primary care providers only [19]. The group treated first with the integrated care approach reduced their body mass index (BMI) to a greater extent than the group receiving primary care management only. Moreover, the integrated care group experienced a significant reduction in BMI from baseline compared with the comparison group; however, there was no significant difference in BMI at six months between both groups. In another study using a less formal integrated care approach consisting of preceptor-ships and virtual communities, primary care physicians' and nurses' self-efficacy in managing obesity within their local settings improved significantly [20]. These studies demonstrate the emerging evidence for integrated care in severe obesity management but also highlight the need for further research in this area.

Based on integrated care data suggesting improvements in chronic disease adherence, the use of integrated care in obesity has promise in supporting patient engagement and adherence to obesity treatment. Given that studies have shown poor adherence rates to bariatric surgery care [21,22], there is a role for using integrated care approaches to enhance patient engagement and adherence to obesity treatments to support long-term weight loss and health benefits. The use of telephone-based peer support within an integrated care setting has not been shown to be effective in improving metabolic indices in a target patient population with type 2 diabetes mellitus [23]. While the components of integrated care align with the potential care needs in severe obesity, further research is needed to explore the impact of integrated care on obesity outcomes and to examine the effectiveness of specific methods of integrated care delivery.

Case Vignette Revisited

Laura's primary care physician refers her to a specialized weight loss and wellness clinic that follows an interdisciplinary care model. This model is based on self-management that is facilitated by a multidisciplinary team of healthcare professionals that consists of a primary care physician, a nurse practitioner, a dietician, a social worker, and a psychologist. A care manager coordinates the treatment that is described in her individual healthcare plan, and Laura is a partner in the treatment plan. An intensive lifestyle treatment is proposed that incorporates dietary support, physical activity, and behavioral therapy. The aim of the treatment (the clinic refers to the treatment as "the patient's journey") is to achieve a sustainable improvement in lifestyle that not only leads to a healthier weight but also prevents a relapse in the long run. Laura's journey should ideally include the following components:

- A thorough medical chart review should be performed using a standardized evaluation, verifying medical history, surgical history, medications, and BMI for the 18 months before and after the baseline evaluation.
- Given Laura's mood symptoms, her mood and anxiety should be assessed at baseline (using self-report inventories) to guide treatment and response as needed. Sertraline should be reassessed to determine whether it is still helping her mood, contributing to her weight, or needs to be changed.
- A thorough dietary assessment should be conducted to determine whether Laura is having symptoms suggestive of binge eating or night eating. A review of her diet, daily intake, and triggers for her overeating is important as well.
- Metabolic markers should be assessed over time, including HbA1c (marker for dysglycemia), lipoproteins ApoB (marker of atherogenic low-density lipoprotein), and ApoA1 (marker of protective high-density lipoprotein). Consideration should be given to use diet to control Laura's abnormal lipid profile, including the use of lipid-reducing medications.
- Given that objective measurements of exercise capacity in patients are usually better than self-reports, the six-minute walk test (6MWT) could be used [24,25]. A 6MWT measures the distance an individual can walk in six minutes. It is a simple index that estimates Laura's functional capacity and can be used to predict morbidity and mortality.
- A weight loss readiness tool (WLRT) based on Prochaska and DiClemente's Stages of Change model could be used to evaluate Laura's readiness regarding weight management, nutrition, and physical activity.
- Given that Laura has identified body image issues as distressing to her mental health, a valid questionnaire such as the Multidimensional Body-Self Relations Questionnaire (MBSRQ) can be used to assess body image dissatisfaction [26].

Close follow-up and coordination of services are essential for the proper management of Laura's comorbidities. Psychoeducation and encouragement with special attention to barriers and enablers are important to help Laura sustain any lifestyle changes that she achieves.

Summary

Obesity is a complex chronic condition requiring a team-based approach to care. The interplay of physical and mental health comorbidity further reinforces the value of an integrated care approach to obesity management that involves an interprofessional team. Evidence has clearly demonstrated the effectiveness of integrated collaborative care models for psychological symptoms across a range of medical patient populations. While further research is needed to evaluate the effectiveness of collaborative mental healthcare in obesity treatment settings, there are merits to using team-driven measurement- and evidence-based approaches in a systematic way in obesity care. Given the range of psychological interventions discussed previously in this book, integrated collaborative care approaches offer a necessary vehicle for delivering these psychological treatments and assessing response in an organized and efficient manner. Models such as Project ECHO offer an additional capacity-building and collaborative approach to obesity care. Given the high rates of psychiatric comorbidity in obesity, it is paramount that future research focuses on the efficacy, implementation factors, and cost-effectiveness of collaborative mental healthcare models in obesity.

Key Points

- Integrated care is a cost-effective evidence-based model of care demonstrating improvements in mental health and physical outcomes.
- Given the multimorbidity and complexity of obesity care, integrated care models should be considered as an evidence-based model to bridge the gap of physical and psychosocial care for patients with obesity.
- While models of integrated care specific to obesity are still emerging, integrated care models may support team-based approaches, care coordination, treatment access, and patient adherence to recommendations in obesity care.
- Further research should focus on evaluating multicomponent integrated care models in obesity, specifically identifying their impact on patient quality of life and health outcomes.

References

1. W. Katon, J. Russo, E. H. Lin, et al. Cost-effectiveness of a multicondition collaborative care intervention: A randomized controlled trial. *Arch Gen Psychiatry* 2012; **69**: 506–14.

2. W. Katon, J. Unutzer, M. Y. Fan, et al. Cost-effectiveness and net benefit of enhanced treatment of depression for older adults with diabetes and depression. *Diabetes Care* 2006; **29**: 265–70.

3. A. Blount. Integrated primary care meets health reform. *Fam Syst Health* 2010; **28**: 77.

4. E. R. Vanderlip, J. Rundell, M. Avery, et al. *Dissemination of Integrated Care within Adult Primary Care Settings: The Collaborative Care Model*. Washington, DC: American Psychiatric Association and Academy of Psychosomatic Medicine, 2016. Available at www.psychiatry.org/psychia trists/practice/professional-interests/integra ted-care/get-trained/about-collaborative-care (accessed October 10, 2017).

5. J. Unutzer, H. Harbin, M. Schoenbaum, et al. *The Collaborative Care Model: An Approach for Integrating Physical and Mental Health Care in Medicaid Health Homes* (Health Home Information Resource Center Brief). Washington, DC: Centers for Medicare and Medcaid Services, 2013. Available at www.chcs.org/resource/the-collaborative-care-model-an-approach-for-integrating-physical-and-mental-health-care-in-medicaid-health-homes/ (accessed October 10, 2017).

6. J. Unutzer, W. Katon, J. W. Williams Jr., et al. Improving primary care for depression in late life: The design of a multicenter randomized trial. *Med Care* 2001; **39**: 785–99.

7. J. Unutzer and M. Park. Strategies to improve the management of depression in primary care. *Prim Care* 2012; **39**: 415–31.

8. S. Arora, S. Kalishman, D. Dion, et al. Partnering urban academic medical centers and rural primary care clinicians to provide complex chronic disease care. *Health Aff (Millwood)* 2011; **30**: 1176–84.

9. W. J. Katon, E. H. Lin, M. Von Korff, et al. Collaborative care for patients with depression and chronic illnesses. *N Engl J Med* 2010; **363**: 2611–20.

10. M. Sharpe, J. Walker, C. Holm Hansen, et al. Integrated collaborative care for comorbid major depression in patients with cancer (SMaRT Oncology-2): A multicentre randomised controlled effectiveness trial. *Lancet* 2014; **384**: 1099–108.

11. S. K. Dobscha, K. Corson, N. A. Perrin, et al. Collaborative care for chronic pain in primary care: A cluster randomized trial. *JAMA* 2009; **301**: 1242–52.

12. J. Archer, P. Bower, S. Gilbody, et al. Collaborative care for depression and anxiety problems. *Cochrane Database Syst Rev* 2012; **10**: CD006525.

13. S. Arora, K. Thornton, G. Murata, et al. Outcomes of treatment for hepatitis C virus infection by primary care

providers. *N Engl J Med* 2011; **364**: 2199–207.

14. C. Zhou, A. Crawford, E. Serhal, et al. The impact of Project ECHO on participant and patient outcomes: A systematic review. *Acad Med* 2016; **91**: 1439–61.

15. S. Sockalingam, A. Arena, E. Serhal, et al. Building provincial mental health capacity in primary care: An evaluation of a Project ECHO mental health program. *Acad Psychiatry* 2017 (in press).

16. R. G. Kathol, M. Butler, D. D. McAlpine, et al. Barriers to physical and mental condition integrated service delivery. *Psychosom Med* 2010; **72**: 511–8.

17. D. C. Lau, J. D. Douketis, K. M. Morrison, et al. 2006 Canadian clinical practice guidelines on the management and prevention of obesity in adults and children (summary). *CMAJ* 2007; **176**: S1–13.

18. J. C. Seidell, J. Halberstadt, H. Noordam, et al. An integrated health care standard for the management and prevention of obesity in the Netherlands. *Fam Pract* 2012; **29** (Suppl. 1): i153–6.

19. A. Fleischman, S. E. Hourigan, N. H. Lyon, et al. Creating an integrated care model for childhood obesity: A randomized pilot study utilizing telehealth in a community primary care setting. *Clin Obes* 2016; **6**: 380–8.

20. J. P. Baillargeon, D. St-Cyr-Tribble, M. Xhignesse, et al. Impact of an integrated obesity management system on patient's care: Research protocol. *BMC Obes* 2014; **1**: 19.

21. S. Larjani, I. Spivak, M. Hao Guo, et al. Preoperative predictors of adherence to multidisciplinary follow-up care postbariatric surgery. *Surg Obes Relat Dis* 2016; **12**: 350–6.

22. S. Sockalingam, S. Cassin, R. Hawa, et al. Predictors of post-bariatric surgery appointment attendance: The role of relationship style. *Obes Surg* 2013; **23**: 2026–32.

23. J. C. Chan, Y. Sui, B. Oldenburg, et al. Effects of telephone-based peer support in patients with type 2 diabetes mellitus receiving integrated care: A randomized clinical trial. *JAMA Intern Med* 2014; **174**: 972–81.

24. R. J. Butland, J. Pang, E. R. Gross, et al. Two-, six-, and 12-minute walking tests in respiratory disease. *Br Med J (Clin Res Ed)* 1982; **284**: 1607–8.

25. S. Solway, D. Brooks, Y. Lacasse, et al. A qualitative systematic overview of the measurement properties of functional walk tests used in the cardiorespiratory domain. *Chest* 2001; **119**: 256–70.

26. T. F. Cash and T. Pruzinsky. *Body images: Development, Deviance, and Change.* New York, NY: Guildford Press, 1990.

Chapter 18

An Integrated Psychological Approach to Obesity Care

Stephanie E. Cassin, Raed Hawa, and Sanjeev Sockalingam

Case Vignette

Karl is a 57-year-old married man with three adult children. He lives in an apartment in a large city with his wife and daughter (age 26). His eldest son (age 30) resides in the same city with his wife and their two children (ages one and three). His youngest son (age 22) attends university across the country. He has been working as a taxi driver for the past 10 years.

Karl has a history of major depressive disorder and alcohol-use disorder. He experienced his first major depressive episode at the age of 18, shortly after starting university. He also began drinking pretty heavily around the same time. Initially, his drinking was limited to social occasions with friends from his dorm and his varsity football team, but it began interfering with his academic and athletic performance. He felt like a disappointment for not succeeding in the two areas he typically excelled in and began isolating himself and drinking more heavily to numb his feelings. He was kicked off the football team due to poor performance and attendance at practices, became increasingly depressed, and withdrew from university at the end of his first year.

Karl met his first wife at the age of 20, and they married a few months later. His alcohol use caused a lot of friction in their relationship, and she threatened to divorce him if he did not seek help for his addiction. He briefly attended a self-help support group with her continued "nagging," but she informed him that it was "too little too late" and ended the relationship. He reported that he first experienced suicidal ideation at this time and had a plan in mind, but he did not make an actual attempt. He continued attending the support group, found a sponsor to turn to for additional support, and was able to significantly cut back on his drinking.

Karl met his current wife at the age of 24, and he describes their 33-year marriage as having "some ups and downs but generally happy." His drinking has been well controlled throughout their marriage, but his weight has increased substantially. He had previously had an athletic build from playing competitive sports, but after he stopped playing football, he continued eating at least the same amount of food but did not engage in any consistent physical activity – and this pattern has continued throughout his adulthood. In addition, he began turning to food for the same reasons he had previously turned to alcohol – to numb negative emotions, cope with boredom, and reward himself. He has eating binges approximately twice per week and is growing increasingly concerned about his weight, physical health, and mental health.

Karl attended an appointment with his family physician. On examination, he weighed 415 pounds at a height of 6 feet, 1 inch (body mass index [BMI] = 55 kg/m^2). In the context of his progressive weight gain, Karl had developed type 2 diabetes mellitus, hypertension, and obstructive sleep apnea. He was taking oral hypoglycemics to manage his diabetes, but his blood sugar levels were not well controlled. He was also taking medication for his blood pressure (ramipril), and he was intermittently adherent with his continuous positive airway pressure (CPAP) machine for his sleep apnea.

Karl sought treatment recommendations from his physician, who informed him that bariatric surgery is the most effective treatment for long-term weight loss and improvement of obesity-related comorbidities for an individual of his weight. Karl felt that surgery was too drastic a measure, and he wanted to try something less invasive. His physician informed him that a number of psychosocial interventions may also be helpful in improving his eating habits and other health behaviors and referred him for a psychosocial consultation at a program that offers both surgical and nonsurgical treatments for obesity.

Introduction

This book has discussed psychosocial issues common among individuals with severe obesity (see Chapter 1), provided a rationale for incorporating psychosocial interventions as a component of integrated care models (see Chapters 2 and 17), and described a variety of psychosocial interventions that are relevant to obesity care using illustrative case vignettes and clinical dialogues (see Chapters 5 to 18). Severe obesity is a complex and chronic disease that warrants an integrated and long-term approach to care, which may necessitate numerous medical and psychosocial interventions in sequence or combination for sustained improvement over time. In this final chapter, we use a Case Vignette to illustrate an integrated psychological approach to obesity care. This approach requires that a thorough psychosocial assessment be conducted in order to develop a personalized case conceptualization and identify problem areas that warrant psychosocial intervention. Consistent with evidence-based practice, psychosocial interventions are then recommended that take into consideration the best available scientific evidence, expert opinion, and clinical expertise and the patient's characteristics, values, and preferences [1].

An Integrated Psychological Approach to Obesity Care

A number of psychosocial interventions appear promising in the treatment of severe obesity and associated comorbidities, including motivational interviewing (MI; see Chapters 5 to 7), cognitive-behavioral therapy (CBT; see Chapters 8 and 9), mindfulness-based interventions (see Chapter 10), compassion-focused interventions (see Chapter 11), family-based interventions (see Chapter 12), and support group interventions (see Chapter 13). This is by no means an exhaustive list of all psychosocial interventions that have been used in the treatment of severe obesity. The chapters in this book describe interventions that currently have the greatest evidence base supporting their use in individuals with severe obesity, as well as interventions that have not yet been empirically tested specifically in individuals with severe obesity but hold promise given their effectiveness and/or efficacy for related issues, such as weight loss, treatment adherence, disordered eating (e.g., binge eating, emotional eating), health behaviors (e.g., physical activity, dietary changes), body image disturbance, and psychological comorbidity (e.g., mood disorders, anxiety disorders, substance-use disorders).

One recurring theme in this book is that even the psychosocial interventions currently considered most effective in the treatment of severe obesity result in modest weight loss in the short term (typically 5 to 10 percent total weight loss), and the weight loss is very difficult to maintain over time (see Chapter 2). In fact, the benefit of these psychosocial interventions may be their ability to maintain current weight in the context of a history of progressive weight gain over years, which may not align with patients' expectations. It is important that patients be made aware of realistic weight loss outcomes at the outset of treatment and be encouraged to set treatment goals that extend beyond weight loss, such as improved eating habits (e.g., increased fruit, vegetable, fiber, and water consumption; decreased binge eating and emotional eating), physical activity, physical health (e.g., reduced blood pressure, cholesterol, blood sugar; medication reduction or discontinuation), psychological functioning (e.g., improved mood and anxiety), and quality of life.

In light of the large number of biological, psychological, and social factors contributing to the onset and maintenance of obesity, it is perhaps not surprising that a time-limited psychosocial intervention would result in only modest and short-term weight loss. The recognition of obesity as a complex and chronic disease calls for a care approach similar to those used to manage other chronic diseases such as cardiovascular disease, diabetes, and hypertension – specifically, a multifaceted and integrated approach that includes regular ongoing contact with a multidisciplinary team over the long term within a system that patients can easily navigate [2].

The empirical literature examining psychosocial interventions specifically for individuals with severe obesity is still in its infancy. Many of the interventions described in this book have been empirically tested using pre-post designs with no control group (i.e., did patients improve following the psychosocial intervention?) or by comparing the psychosocial intervention with a control group (i.e., did individuals in the psychosocial intervention group improve more than individuals in a control group – such as compared with standard care?). A smaller number of studies have examined the efficacy of a combined psychosocial treatment approach (e.g., does the addition of motivational interviewing to behavioral weight loss treatment improve outcomes?) or a combined psychosocial-medical treatment approach (e.g., does the addition of cognitive behavioral therapy improve bariatric surgery outcomes?). Given the modest weight loss outcomes that have been reported in studies examining specific time-limited psychosocial interventions, a more comprehensive treatment approach is likely warranted, particularly in cases in which significant obesity-related comorbidities are also present.

Guidelines for managing chronic diseases typically include a framework for developing and executing a multifaceted and integrated treatment plan [2]. Ideally, such a framework would include algorithms or decision trees to guide the sequence of care – for example, providing recommendations for coordinating the patient's care or plotting the sequence of interventions. Although the psychosocial interventions described in this book appear to be beneficial in the management of severe obesity, currently no clinical guidelines exist to determine which type(s) of psychosocial interventions should be offered to particular patients, how those interventions should be integrated or sequenced, how long each intervention should continue, and when each intervention should be offered in the course of obesity care (e.g., if a patient chooses to undergo bariatric surgery, should psychosocial interventions be offered before and/or after surgery?). Given the lack of published scientific research examining optimal care pathways that integrate psychosocial and medical/surgical interventions in the management of obesity, these clinical decisions are typically made on the basis of expert consensus, clinical expertise, and team discussion, while considering the patient's characteristics and preferences and the resources and expertise available within a particular program.

Application of an Integrated Psychological Approach to Obesity Care

A thorough psychosocial assessment should be conducted to develop a personalized case conceptualization that identifies target issues warranting intervention. Returning to the Case Vignette, Karl has severe obesity (BMI = 55 kg/m^2), and a number of factors are likely contributing to his increasing weight trajectory, including a sedentary lifestyle, overeating, and binge eating. He uses food to numb negative emotions, cope with boredom, and reward himself. He has a history of major depressive disorder and alcohol-use disorder, both of which have been well controlled for some time now; however, he is growing more concerned about his mental health. He also has a number of obesity-related medical comorbidities, including type 2 diabetes, high blood pressure, and sleep apnea, which could benefit from interventions aimed at improving treatment adherence. Psychosocial interventions with an evidence base supporting their effectiveness for improving those particular issues should be recommended (see Table 18.1).

Table 18.1 Applications of Psychosocial Interventions in the Management of Severe Obesity

Psychosocial intervention	Potential applications
Motivational interviewing	• Raising the topic of a patient's weight if it is posing a medical concern • Providing personalized feedback regarding a patient's weight or obesity-related comorbidities • Providing psychoeducation regarding weight regulation or obesity-related comorbidities in a way that minimizes the risk of eliciting shame or defensiveness • Preparing patients for medical or surgical treatments for obesity • Resolving ambivalence about changing certain behaviors (e.g., increasing physical activity, improving eating behaviors) • Enhancing self-efficacy for change • Increasing adherence with treatment plans (including medical treatments) • Treating psychological comorbidities (e.g., substance-related disorders)
Cognitive-behavioral therapy	• Setting health-related goals • Improving eating behaviors (e.g., normalizing eating patterns, reducing binge eating and emotional eating) • Improving physical activity and self-care behaviors • Improving body image • Challenging distorted (self-sabotaging) thoughts implicated in the maintenance of obesity • Developing coping strategies to improve health-related behaviors and reduce vulnerability to disordered eating • Maintaining behavioral and cognitive changes over time (relapse prevention) • Treating psychological comorbidities (e.g., depression, anxiety, substance-related disorders)

Table 18.1 (cont.)

Psychosocial intervention	Potential applications
Mindfulness-based interventions	• Identifying hunger and satiety • Reducing emotional eating and binge eating • Reducing pain • Reducing stress • Reducing depressive relapse
Compassion-focused interventions	• Reducing self-criticism and shame • Improving self-acceptance • Improving body image • Improving disordered eating (e.g., binge eating) • Coping with thoughts that are not necessarily "distorted" • Reducing weight bias internalization
Family-focused interventions	• Involving the patient's family or support network in the treatment process • Providing psychoeducation about weight regulation and the treatment of obesity • Reducing stigma regarding obesity • Identifying family member behaviors that could sabotage the patient's treatment • Identifying health behaviors that family members can engage in together • Identifying support that family members can provide to the patient • Identifying familial stressors and enhancing problem-solving and coping skills • Enhancing family cohesion, communication, and conflict management
Support group interventions	• Providing a sense of community for patients and their families • Providing informational, practical, and emotional support • Learning from, and being inspired by, others with lived experience who are coping successfully • Increasing accountability for making and maintaining health-related improvements
Telephone-based interventions	• Increasing treatment accessibility • Using a stepped-care treatment approach (i.e., telephone sessions as a lower-intensity intervention) • Supplementing face-to-face interventions with telephone contact (e.g., periodic "booster" sessions by telephone following a face-to-face intervention)
Smartphone applications and Internet-based interventions	• Increasing treatment accessibility • Using a stepped-care treatment approach (i.e., smartphone and Internet-based interventions as a lower-intensity intervention) • Self-monitoring health-related variables (e.g., food intake, physical activity, weight, mood) and tracking them over time • Supplementing face-to-face interventions with smartphone applications or Internet-based resources (e.g., self-monitoring apps, treatment worksheets) • Maintaining health-related changes over time (relapse prevention)

In light of Karl's current BMI, bariatric surgery would be considered the most efficacious treatment option for significant and sustained weight loss and improvement of obesity-related comorbidities [3]. However, this treatment option is not aligned with Karl's current treatment preferences. He considers surgery too invasive and prefers to try a medically supervised psychosocial intervention instead. Cognitive-behavioral therapy is an evidence-based treatment recommendation for improving health behaviors, such as eating behaviors and physical activity (see Chapters 2 and 8), and for various forms of disordered eating, including binge eating (see Chapters 2 and 9). Of note, CBT is also an evidence-based treatment recommendation for both major depressive disorder and alcohol-use disorder (see Chapter 18) should these issues resurface for Karl.

Case Vignette Revisited

Karl completed 24 sessions of CBT with a psychologist at the obesity program. His primary treatment goals were to "lose weight" and "feel better." The psychologist had a candid discussion with him about realistic weight loss outcomes following CBT and collaboratively set SMART goals with Karl that extended beyond weight loss (see Chapter 8). Following this discussion, his broad treatment goals were to reduce binge eating, eat smaller portions of meals at regular time intervals throughout the day, and increase physical activity. In light of Karl's treatment goals, the psychologist used the CBT strategies described in Chapters 8 and 9. The psychologist also referred Karl to a dietician within the program early in his treatment to develop a personalized meal plan. In addition, he attended a few sessions with a physical therapist periodically throughout treatment that recommended suitable exercises and developed an exercise plan of increasing duration and intensity. The psychologist monitored his progress with the meal plan and exercise plan each week while reviewing his food and activity records in session and collaboratively set new specific goals with him each week.

By all accounts, Karl had a successful psychosocial treatment outcome. He significantly reduced his eating binges from twice per week to one per month on average. He reduced his portion sizes and increased his intake of fruit, vegetables, fiber, and water. He increased his physical activity, primarily through daily walks and some strength training exercises. His daily blood glucose control improved with these changes in nutrition and activity and resulted in an overall improvement in his hemoglobin A1C. Moreover, he was able to use his CPAP machine more consistently after he received education on the impact of untreated sleep apnea on his fatigue, mood, and overall health. As a result of these changes, he reported that he was sleeping better and had more energy throughout the day. He lost 9 percent of his total body weight, reducing his weight from 415 to 378 pounds and his BMI from 55 to 50 kg/m^2.

Karl was able to take credit for the changes he made to his eating and activity level, but he reported feeling disappointed that he did not lose more weight. He felt optimistic initially because the weight came off quickly, but as it began to plateau around 380 pounds, he felt that he would be unable to lose much more weight through diet and exercise alone (or at least not in a way that he could maintain as a long-term lifestyle change). He was also hoping that his lifestyle changes were going to have a greater impact on his diabetes management and physical fitness, but he was not able to discontinue any medications and, although he was able to walk more, his weight made it difficult to engage in more vigorous exercise, keep up with his busy grandchildren, and travel by plane to visit his son.

Karl and his psychologist revisited the idea of bariatric surgery. At a BMI of 50 kg/m^2, Karl would be a candidate for surgery. The psychologist informed Karl that bariatric surgery typically results in 20 to 30 percent total body weight loss (60 to 70 percent excess weight loss) long term [3,4] and significant improvement in obesity-related comorbidities, including type 2 diabetes [5]. The psychologist recommended that Karl attend an information session about bariatric surgery at the obesity program to gather more information. Following that session, Karl decided that he wanted to be evaluated for bariatric surgery.

As part of the multidisciplinary psychosocial evaluation for bariatric surgery, Karl met with a nurse, dietician, social worker, and psychologist. The psychologist completed a psychodiagnostic assessment, which indicated that Karl previously met criteria for major depressive disorder and alcohol-use disorder, both of which were currently well controlled, and binge eating disorder, which is currently characterized by low-frequency binges.

Karl and his wife both attended the assessment with the social worker, and they were asked to share their feelings about, and expectations for, surgery. Karl and his wife both expressed some ambivalence about the surgery. Karl shared his perception that bariatric surgery is a "vanity surgery." He knew of two women, but no men, who underwent bariatric surgery and was worried how others might respond to him having the procedure. However, he felt that the potential benefits of the surgery outweighed the risks. Karl's wife mentioned his recent weight loss and shared her belief that "if he just tries harder, he can lose more weight on his own." She also admitted to feeling very worried about surgical complications ("death!") while also acknowledging the health risks associated with his current weight.

Karl had some blood drawn as part of the nursing assessment, and the results indicated that he had a small amount of alcohol in his system. When this was brought to his attention, he admitted that he was not entirely forthcoming during his psychodiagnostic assessment because he felt that it would jeopardize his opportunity for bariatric surgery. He disclosed that he had, in fact, been abstinent from alcohol for many years but that he had recently started drinking again when he had the urge to binge eat. He assured the nurse that he was not drinking excessively and that he would be able to stop completely if approved for the surgery.

Case Conceptualization Revisited

Case conceptualizations should be revisited throughout obesity care and revised accordingly in light of new information and changing circumstances. Returning to the Case Vignette, Karl's treatment preference has changed since the time his physician referred him for obesity treatment such that he is now interested in pursuing bariatric surgery. The list of identified target issues warranting intervention has also shifted over time. Karl and his wife both express some ambivalence regarding bariatric surgery. Although both of them acknowledge the potential health risk associated with obesity, Karl perceives bariatric surgery to be a "vanity surgery," and his wife worries about surgical complications and holds some stigmatizing beliefs regarding his obesity, specifically concerning the controllability of weight. Karl's binge eating and overall quantity and quality of food consumption have improved significantly; however, there is evidence that Karl has been consuming alcohol again, and it may be serving the same functions as food had previously (i.e., to numb negative emotions, cope with boredom, and reward himself). Alcohol consumption should be prioritized as a treatment target because problematic substance use is a contraindication to bariatric surgery.

Case Vignette Revisited

Karl's psychologist used motivational interviewing to explore his alcohol use, including the perceived short- and long-term benefits and costs of consuming alcohol. She asked about his understanding of the impact of alcohol use on bariatric surgery, as well as potential issues that could arise postoperatively as a result of alcohol use and, with his permission, provided some additional information and clarified some of his misconceptions. Karl did not feel that his current alcohol use was problematic, but he understood that it could affect his eligibility for surgery at the current time and/or pose issues if his alcohol use continued or escalated postoperatively.

The psychologist recommended that they revisit CBT, this time focusing on coping skills to manage his alcohol use. The psychologist explained that given the similar functions that alcohol and food appear to serve in Karl's life and the shared mechanisms underlying them, many of the CBT skills he used to effectively improve his eating behaviors and reduce his eating binges (see Chapters 8 and 9) could be applied to alcohol use as well. For example, in reviewing the cognitive-behavioral conceptualization of binge eating, Karl noticed that alcohol consumption is similar to binge eating in that they both function to increase pleasure and reduce distress in the short term but then further increase negative emotions as well as vulnerability for eating binges or alcohol consumption. He began recording alcoholic beverages on the CBT self-monitoring record (see Figure 8.2) that he had already been using to monitor his food consumption and physical activity in order to increase awareness of his alcohol use and its relation to his thoughts and emotions. The psychologist explained that the activities that Karl had been engaging in to reduce his vulnerability to binge eating and to ride out urges to binge eat could also be used when he has the urge to drink alcohol. In addition, CBT thought records (see Figure 8.3) could be used to challenge negative thoughts or assumptions that increase vulnerability to drinking, and problem-solving skills could be used to identify triggers for alcohol consumption and develop effective ways of coping with them. A brief CBT intervention focused on applying the coping skills he previously learned to his alcohol use was effective in eliminating his alcohol consumption. He reported that bariatric surgery was a motivating factor for making this lifestyle change.

The psychologist scheduled an appointment with both Karl and his wife to provide some psychoeducation on the various contributors to weight and weight regulation, as well as information on the magnitude of weight loss that can be expected from various psychosocial and surgical interventions. The purpose of the psychoeducation was to challenge some common misconceptions about the controllability of weight that were also held by Karl's wife, including the expectation that Karl should be able to lose his excess weight if he simply tried harder. The psychologist also provided some general information about typical improvements following bariatric surgery, as well as potential complications that Karl's wife was concerned about but encouraged the two of them to write down all their questions so that they could remember to ask the bariatric surgeon during the surgical consultation appointment. In addition, the psychologist encouraged Karl and his wife to attend the bariatric surgery support group offered through the obesity program so that they could learn more about what to expect from bariatric surgery from patients at various stages of the process. Karl was also pleased to see other men at the bariatric surgery support group given that he did not personally know of any men who had undergone the surgery. Karl ultimately decided that he did want to receive bariatric surgery, and the interdisciplinary obesity team felt that he was currently a good candidate for the procedure.

Karl did not experience significant complications as a result of bariatric surgery, and he had a good outcome over the first postoperative year. He reduced his BMI from 50 to 37 kg/m^2 and experienced resolution of his type 2 diabetes and reduction in the CPAP pressure that was needed to control his apnea. Although his mood was quite stable prior to surgery, he reported significant improvements in the first few months following surgery and noted that his eating binges had completely stopped because he could no longer consume large portions at one sitting. However, he also noted that he had started grazing on food more recently and had the same feeling of loss of control over eating despite not being physically able to consume much food at one sitting. He acknowledged feeling disappointed lately because he had not lost quite as much weight as he had hoped and was not optimistic that he would be able to meet the weight loss goal he set for himself. In addition, he reported feeling ashamed about his body due to the excess skin that developed as he lost weight, which he attributed both to the appearance of the excess skin and the anger he felt toward himself for "allowing" himself to become obese in the first place. Despite these critical thoughts concerning his weight and body image, he was still able to take credit for the changes he had made, including stopping drinking, improving his food choices, and regularly engaging in physical activity even when he was not feeling particularly motivated.

Case Conceptualization Revisited

Healthcare professionals need to remain vigilant to a number of issues that may arise following bariatric surgery and that may have an adverse impact on long-term medical and psychological outcomes. Returning to the Case Vignette, Karl had a positive outcome in the first postoperative year – he lost a significant amount of weight, his physical health improved, his eating binges stopped, and his mood improved. These are all typical outcomes in the first year following bariatric surgery [6]. Although Karl's eating binges stopped because he was physically unable to consume large amounts of food within one sitting postoperatively, he started to engage in other forms of disordered eating (i.e., grazing and loss-of-control eating) that have been shown to predict suboptimal weight loss as well as weight regain postoperatively [7,8]. His appraisal that he should have lost more weight and that he would be unable to meet his weight loss goal lead to feelings of frustration and pessimism. In addition, although the majority of bariatric surgery patients develop excess skin postoperatively, Karl's appraisal that he "allowed" himself to become obese likely heightened his self-criticism and shame. In light of evidence that deterioration of mood and mental quality of life is common among bariatric surgery patients after the first year [9] and that weight bias internalization, self-criticism, and shame have a negative impact on health behaviors, including physical activity and eating behaviors (see Chapters 3 and 11), these factors should be closely monitored. This recommendation is particularly fitting in Karl's case given his past history of major depressive disorder because postoperative depression has been shown to predict poorer surgical outcomes [10].

Case Vignette Revisited

Karl's psychologist referred him to a mindfulness-based eating awareness training (MB-EAT) group (see Chapter 10) facilitated by another psychologist and dietitian within the obesity program. In addition to reducing his subjective sense of loss of control over eating and his grazing between meals, he found the group helpful because he realized that other patients were experiencing similar issues with their eating postoperatively. He also continued to attend the bariatric surgery support group because he found it to be a supportive environment and informative resource, and it also helped to keep him accountable for sticking with the goals he set for himself.

Following the MB-EAT group, Karl met with his psychologist for another brief CBT intervention. They reviewed the CBT skills that Karl learned during his previous sessions and discussed how he could apply those skills to cope with his current concerns. For example, they identified and challenged some of the negative automatic thoughts leading to feelings of disappointment and pessimism, including "I should have lost more weight" and "I'll never be able to reach my weight loss goal." Karl realized that some cognitive distortions may be present in these thoughts, such as *should* statements, fortune-telling error, all-or-nothing thinking, and discounting the positive. The psychologist reviewed typical weight loss outcomes following bariatric surgery to challenge Karl's belief that he should have lost more weight and helped him to generate alternate thoughts: "Although I was personally hoping to lose more weight by now, my current weight loss is on track, and I'm continuing to exercise regularly." In addition, she encouraged him to consider improvements beyond the number on the scale, particularly those affecting his quality of life. Karl acknowledged that his physical health had improved and that he was able to discontinue some of his medications. His physical fitness had also improved, and he had more energy to play with his grandchildren. He was also able to fit into an airplane seat and, as a result, was able to visit his youngest son at university and go on vacation with his wife.

The CBT intervention also integrated self-compassion strategies with the aim of improving Karl's self-criticism and shame (see Chapter 11). The psychologist provided some psychoeducation on the adverse impact of self-criticism and shame on health behaviors and illustrated the feedback cycle using a CBT model. For example, when looking in the mirror, Karl reported that he frequently thought, "My body looks disgusting, and it's my own fault," which lead to feeling ashamed and, in turn, increased vulnerability to maladaptive behaviors such as grazing, inactivity, and social isolation. By helping Karl to be mindful of these emotions when they arise (e.g., "This is really hard right now"; "It's difficult to feel so critical of myself") and to recognize that they are common experiences (e.g., "Many people are dissatisfied with their bodies"; "Many people find it difficult to control their eating"; "Many people struggle with their weight"), the psychologist was able to encourage Karl to treat himself with self-compassion rather than self-criticism (e.g., "Let me be kind to myself and give myself the compassion I need"). When struggling to treat himself with compassion, Karl found it helpful to imagine what he might say to his daughter if she was having similar thoughts and feelings or to imagine what his daughter might say to him. He had made a few close connections in the bariatric surgery support group, and he also tried to imagine the advice he might give to one of those people if they were having similar thoughts and feelings.

Karl and his psychologist focused on relapse-prevention strategies for the final few sessions, which were tapered in frequency (see Chapter 8). They revisited Karl's original treatment goals and reviewed the progress he made throughout his time in the obesity program. They discussed his triggers for maladaptive behaviors, such as grazing, binge eating, and alcohol consumption, and anticipated future events that could increase vulnerability to these behaviors. They reviewed the CBT and compassion-focused strategies they had worked on together, as well as the mindfulness exercises Karl learned at the MB-EAT group. They also discussed the social supports available to Karl, including his wife and children, the interprofessional team at the obesity program, the bariatric surgery support group as a whole and the specific group members he connected with, and his family physician. Karl set some specific and realistic goals that he was planning to continue working on following treatment. The psychologist suggested that a smartphone application might be helpful in maintaining the progress he made throughout his treatment and to prevent relapse (see Chapter 15). She recommended a CBT application that he could use to monitor his food intake, physical activity, weight, and alcohol use and that also included interactive worksheets similar to the ones he completed during treatment (e.g., CBT thought records and problem-solving worksheets). Karl reported that he had already downloaded a smartphone application with a variety of guided mindfulness exercises, and it had been helpful in encouraging him to practice mindfulness regularly. In light of evidence that regular, ongoing contact is needed to effectively manage chronic diseases and that healthcare providers often need to initiate the contact [2], the psychologist scheduled a brief follow-up telephone call with Karl one month later.

Summary

Severe obesity is a chronic disease that warrants an integrated and long-term treatment approach. Given the complexity of obesity, a comprehensive approach to obesity care may necessitate numerous medical and psychosocial interventions in sequence or combination for sustained improvement over time. A number of psychosocial interventions appear promising in the treatment of severe obesity and associated comorbidities, including motivational interviewing, cognitive-behavioral therapy, mindfulness-based interventions, compassion-focused interventions, family-based interventions, and support group interventions. A personalized case conceptualization should be developed to identify problem areas that warrant intervention and to develop evidence-based treatment plans that take into consideration the best available scientific evidence, expert opinion, and clinical expertise and the patient's characteristics, values, and preferences [1].

Key Points

- Obesity is a complex chronic disease that requires an integrated and long-term treatment approach.
- Psychosocial interventions are increasingly being recognized as an important component of obesity management.
- A number of psychosocial interventions appear promising in the treatment of severe obesity and associated comorbidities, including motivational interviewing, cognitive-behavioral therapy, mindfulness-based interventions, compassion-focused interventions, family-based interventions, and support group interventions.
- Little empirical research to date has examined optimal approaches for sequencing or integrating treatment approaches in obesity care.
- A thorough psychosocial assessment should be conducted to develop a personalized case conceptualization and identify target problems that warrant intervention, and psychosocial interventions with an evidence base supporting their effectiveness for improving those problems should be recommended.

References

1. D. Sackett, S. Strauss, W. Richardson, et al. *Evidence-Based Medicine: How to Practice and Teach EBM* (2nd edn). Edinburgh: Churchill Livingstone, 2000.

2. Ministry of Health and Long Term Care. Preventing and managing chronic disease: Ontario's framework, 2007. Available at www.health.gov.on.ca/en/pro/programs/cdpm/pdf/framework_full.pdf (accessed November 2, 2017).

3. J. Picot, J. Jones, J. L. Colquitt, et al. The clinical effectiveness and cost-effectiveness of bariatric (weight loss) surgery for obesity: A systematic review and economic evaluation. *Health Technol Assess* 2009; **13**: 1–190.

4. H. Buchwald, J. N. Buchwald, and T. W. McGlennon. Systematic review and meta-analysis of medium-term outcomes after banded Roux-en-Y gastric bypass. *Obes Surg* 2014; **24**: 1536–51.

5. P. R. Schauer, D. L. Bhatt, J. P. Kirwan, et al. Bariatric surgery versus intensive medical therapy for diabetes-3-year outcomes. *N Engl J Med* 2014; **370**: 2002–13.

6. J. L. Colquitt, K. Pickett, E. Loveman, et al. Surgery for weight loss in adults. *Cochrane Database Syst Rev* 2014; **8**: CD003641.

7. M. J. Devlin, W. C. King, M. A. Kalarchian, et al. Eating pathology and experience and weight loss in a prospective study of bariatric surgery patients: 3-year follow-up. *Int J Eat Disord* 2016; **49**: 1058–67.

8. J. E. Mitchell, N. J. Christian, D. R. Flum, et al. Postoperative behavioral variables and weight change 3 years after bariatric surgery. *JAMA Surg* 2016; **151**: 752–7.

9. S. Sockalingam, R. Hawa, S. Wnuk, et al. Psychosocial predictors of quality of life and weight loss two years after bariatric surgery: Results from the Toronto Bari-PSYCH study. *Gen Hosp Psychiatry* 2017; **47**: 7–13.

10. C. S. Sheets, C. M. Peat, K. C. Berg, et al. Post-operative psychosocial predictors of outcome in bariatric surgery. *Obes Surg* 2015; **25**: 330–45.

Index